THE
LEFT-HANDER SYNDROME

THE
LEFT-HANDER
SYNDROME

The Causes and Consequences
of Left-Handedness

Stanley Coren

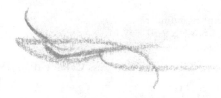

THE FREE PRESS
A Division of Macmillan, Inc.
NEW YORK

Maxwell Macmillan Canada
TORONTO

Maxwell Macmillan International
NEW YORK   OXFORD   SINGAPORE   SYDNEY

The Free Press
A Division of Macmillan, Inc.
866 Third Avenue, New York, N.Y. 10022

Maxwell Macmillan Canada, Inc.
1200 Eglinton Avenue East
Suite 200
Don Mills, Ontario M3C 3N1

Macmillan, Inc. is part of the Maxwell Communication Group of Companies

Printed in the United States of America

printing number
3 4 5 6 7 8 9 10

Library of Congress Cataloging-in-Publication Data

Coren, Stanley.
   The left-hander syndrome: the causes and consequences of left-handedness / Stanley Coren.
      p. cm.
   Includes bibliographical references and index.
   ISBN 0–02–906682–4
   1. Left- and right-handedness. I. Title.
QP385.5.C68 1992
152.3'35—dc20   91–26505
                                           CIP

This book is dedicated to my co-investigators:

Diane Halpern, Clare Porac, and Alan Searleman.

Without their research contribution and their insight,
much of the knowledge and theory
that is presented in this book would not exist.

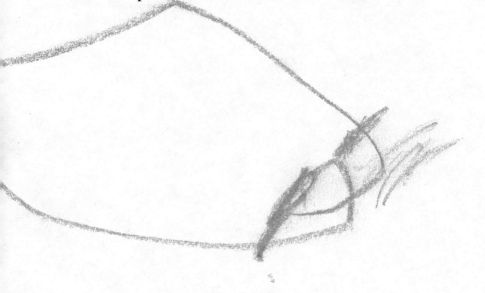

Contents

Preface

At various times in history, left-handedness has been regarded as many things: a nasty habit, a social inconvenience, or a mark of the devil. It has also been taken as a sign of neurosis, rebellion, creativity, artistic ability, musical ability, psychopathology, mental retardation, criminality, homosexuality, genius, sports proficiency, or empathy. Our long fascination with handedness is shown by its mention in the Bible; references to it appear in some Egyptian tomb writings.

The problem of handedness has caught the attention of many thinkers and scientists including Charles Darwin, Benjamin Franklin, William James, and Thomas Carlyle. Over the past twenty years or so, researchers have shown that left-handedness is more than a minor difference. Increasingly we are coming to understand that left-handedness has social, educational, and psychological implications and affects many aspects of health, well-being, and even life span.

This book focuses on all that distinguishes right- and left-handers. It demonstrates that handedness is only one part of sidedness, which also includes footedness, eyedness, and earedness, and shows readers how to measure their own sidedness. The book answers some common questions such as: Where does handedness come from? Is it coded in the genes? Does it stem from social pressure? Might it indicate some damage or injury? Is it related to the organization of the brain, and how?

Further, the book examines the differences between left- and right-handers in terms of intelligence, personality, creativity, and a number of other domains.

Left-handers may be one of the last unorganized minorities in our society, with no collective power and no real sense of common identity. Yet they are a minority that is often discriminated against by social, educational, and religious institutions. Social customs and even our language set the left-hander apart as "different" and probably "bad."

This book in some sense records a journey of exploration begun when a scientist came across a surprising set of research findings. The resulting program of investigation, which extended over more than ten years, led that scientist to the shocking conclusion that left-handers probably die younger than right-handers. He also found that most risks to which left-handers are especially vulnerable have to do with the way in which the right-handed majority treats the unseen left-handed minority. This scientist here offers ways in which the left-hander can be made both safer and more comfortable in a right-handed world.

Acknowledgments

I would like to thank many people who helped me directly and indirectly in the preparation of this book. People in my laboratory at the University of British Columbia over these many years—including David, Wong, Wayne Wong, Marion Buday, Susan Dixon, Kevin Donelly, Geof Donelly, Miriam Blum, Richard Cropp, Jeannie Garber, Susan Louie, Murray Armstrong, Tania Jackson, Kathy Cooper, Colin Ensworth, Jean Porac, Keven Wright, Dereck Atha, Lynda Berger, Sung Il Park, Geof Grover, and far too many others to list—have aided in various aspects of my research. Colleagues Darrin Lehman and Peter Suedfeld made useful comments, both formal and informal, on parts of this manuscript. Mike McKinnell did some of the figures for chapters 13 and 15. My lovely wife Joan read through the entire manuscript for continuity and even had the psychological stamina to stay married to me throughout the writing process. I must, of course, also thank the Natural Sciences and Engineering Research Council of Canada and the Medical Research Council of Canada, who have funded my research over the past two decades. Finally, my gratitude goes to my invaluable co-investigators over the years: Diane Halpern, Clare Porac, and Alan Searleman, to whom this book is dedicated.

S. C.
Vancouver, Canada

1

Beliefs and Stereotypes About Handedness

A neglected minority group constitutes about 10 percent of the present human population. Like many other minority groups it has been subject to prejudice, humiliation, and discrimination—not on the basis of race, religion, age, or national origin, but simply on the basis of the hand that its members use for such everyday acts as brushing teeth or cutting food. This group consists of left-handers. Right-handers might feel that words such as "discrimination" used with reference to left-handers are a bit overdone or melodramatic. I (a right-hander) certainly would have felt that way when I began researching the psychology and neuropsychology of handedness some twenty years ago. But through that research it became clear to me that most of us do have a set of often-unacknowledged attitudes toward left-handers that express themselves in condescension and even scorn.

Language and the Left

For proof of negative attitudes toward left-handers we need go no further than our own language. The very word *left* in English comes from the Anglo-Saxon word *lyft*, which means "weak" or "broken." No less an authority than the venerable Oxford English Dictionary[1] defines *left-handed* as meaning "crippled," "defective," "awkward," "clumsy," "inapt," "characterized by underhanded dealings," "ambiguous," "doubtful," "questionable," "ill-omened," "inauspicious," and "illegitimate."

Common phrases in the English language demonstrate a negative view of left-handedness. For instance, a *left-handed complement* is actually an insult. A son from the *left side of the bed* is illegitimate. A *left-handed marriage* is no marriage at all, but an unconsecrated or adulterous sexual liaison, as in the phrase, "a *left-handed honeymoon* with someone else's husband." Thus, a *left-handed wife* is really a mistress. A *left-handed diagnosis* is wrong, and *left-handed wisdom* is a collection of errors. To be about *left-handed business* is to be engaged in something unlawful or unsavory. Sailors speak of ships that are left-handed, meaning that they are unlucky or "wrong" in some way. Someone talking about your sex life who calls you left-handed has labelled you a homosexual; *bent to the left* carries the same meaning.

Not one positive phrase is to be found in the language surrounding "left" or "left-handed." *Right* and *Right-handed* seldom seem to connote anything more than favoring the right hand for various activities. A *right-handed wife* simply describes a married woman who favors the use of her right hand. In those few instances where there is any emotional content, *right* carries a positive connotation. Thus to be someone's *right-hand man* means to be important and useful to that person.

One must not suppose that speakers of the English language have a unique dislike of left-handers. The tendency appears to be universal. For example, in French the word for left is *gauche*, which also conveys the meanings "crooked," "ugly," "clumsy," "uncouth," and "bashful." The word *gauche* has been taken over directly in English with its negative connotations intact. A person who acts inappropriately in a social situation is said to be "gauche."

The German word for left-handed is *linkisch*, which also gets the dictionary definition of "awkward, clumsy, and maladroit." The left-hander does no better in Spanish, where the word for left-handed is *zurdo*. It is used in phrases such as *no ser zurdo*, which means "to be very clever," but literally translates as "not to be left-handed." A similar picture appears in Italian where a left-hander is *mancino*, which is derived from crooked or maimed (*mancus*) and is also used to mean "deceitful" or dishonest." The bad press of the left-hander in Italy, however, is a historical carry-over from the Latin, in which the word for left is *sinister*, closely related to the noun *sinistrum*, meaning evil.

Eastern European languages continue the tradition of denigrating left-handers. In Russian, to be called a left-hander (*levja*) is a term of insult. One variant of this term is used to refer to a black-marketeer, while from the same root comes the phrase *na levo*, meaning "sneaky." The word for left in Polish is quite similar (*lewo*); it also conveys the idea of "illegal," and is often used to refer to a sneaky or underhanded "trick." Similarly, in Romany (the language of the Gypsies) we find *bongo*, also the term used to describe a crooked card game, a fixed horse race, or a wicked and dishonest person.

If a word meaning continues to endure, that fact suggests that the idea or usage has been generally accepted by the speakers of the language as correct and useful. Thus our language says that we feel that the left-handers are not a very nice group of people and that they are definitely "wrong" in many ways. What is the origin of these negative attitudes?

I doubt that handedness really entered my consciousness to any degree when I was a child. I knew that left and right were different, because I remembered my father telling a story about the problem of remembering which was which. My father's story had to do with a difficulty encountered in teaching military recruits to march. When one sergeant tried to move raw recruits along in step, shouting the usual "Left, right, left, right," so many didn't know which foot was which that only chaos resulted. The usual tactics of shouting "I said left! Not that left foot, your other left foot!" or loud swearing didn't work with this particular group of soldiers. Exasperated, the sergeant resorted to a *mnemonic* or memory device. He tied a piece of hay to the left foot of each man and resumed the march, shouting, "Hayfoot, right, hayfoot, right," until the group finally mastered close-order drill and the concepts of left and right.

As a child I could distinguish left from right and knew that my right hand did most of the work, such as writing, putting food into my mouth, brushing my teeth, and holding tools. My left hand was merely the "other" one. It helped out, but didn't seem to bear its full share of the burden.

Perhaps the first left-hander that I remember was my cousin Steve. Steve was a few years younger than me. Since his parents lived less than a city block from our house and the families frequently visited, I knew him pretty well, or at least I thought I did. One night, at one of those large family dinners where everybody squeezes together around a table to eat, I found my cousin Steve seated next to me on my right side. Dinner started with bowls of hot soup. As we began to eat, because of the close quarters, disaster struck. Somehow my right arm, heading mouthward with a spoon full of soup, snagged on Steve's left arm, which was similarly engaged. My startled hand dropped and jerked a bit in surprise, but Steve's left hand caught the edge of his bowl, dumping hot chicken soup into his lap and splashing some over onto me.

His sister Eleanor immediately barked, "Stephen, you are so clumsy. You are always doing things like that!"

Merely amazed, I asked, "Why did you do that? Why didn't you use your *regular* hand?"

Two things were happening at that moment in my life. First, I was learning that some people had a different "regular" hand, and it wasn't their right hand. Second, I was being exposed to my first bit of negative propaganda about left-handers as my Aunt Sylvia buzzed around trying to clean Steve up, while muttering, "Stephen, you really have to be more careful. You certainly are the sloppiest child I've ever seen."

From across the table my Aunt Frieda advised, "You really ought to teach him to eat with his right hand. He is intelligent enough to do that, isn't he?"

The conversation continued for a while, as the family discussed whether Steve was simply an uncoordinated and awkward child, whether he was using his left-handedness as a means of "getting attention," or whether he was simply being stubborn and intractable by not using his right hand. None of it was very complimentary. For a ten-year-old who had just discovered that left-handedness existed, this was all fascinating (though I'm sure that Steve didn't think so). What I didn't know is that I was receiving my first systematic indoctrination from society suggesting that left-handers are different and somehow "wrong," perhaps inferior, and may require correction.

Today, from the perspective of a psychologist, I would say that I was beginning to form a stereotype about left-handers. Stereotypes are impressions of whole groups of individuals.[2] In a stereotype we mentally assign common characteristics to all members of a particular group. Examples of stereotypes are: "the British are reserved and formal," "Italians are emotional," "librarians are serious," "accountants are dull," "doctors are wealthy," "blacks are athletic," "Jews are materialistic," "teenagers are tactless," "women are more sensitive than men," and "used-car salesmen can't be trusted as far as you can throw them."

Stereotypes are based on a number of grouping principles. Notice in my examples that some group impressions were based upon nationality and others upon occupation, race, religion, sex, and age. Visible physical or behavioral characteristics play an important role in forming stereotypes. Thus we might form the stereotype that "redheads are hot-tempered" and "large muscular men are dumb 'jocks' and certainly not interested in poetry or intellectual pursuits." Handedness, of course, involves visible behaviors that mark an individual as a member of the "left" or "right" group.

An important prerequisite for stereotype formation is recognition of the characteristics that distinguish one group from another, a process called social categorization. Up to the night of that dinner with my cousin Steve, for instance, I had been unaware that the characteristic of handedness defined a particular group. Now, amid the sploshes of chicken soup, I had become aware of the differences associated with handedness. This stereotype was subsequently to be shaped in a negative way, on its way toward becoming a *prejudice.*

Another important prerequisite for stereotype formation is development of a notion of "us" versus "them." Psychologists refer to "us" as the *ingroup,* to which we belong, and "them" as the *outgroup.* For me, of course, the ingroup was right-handers, while the outgroup was left-handers. The very act of making this distinction starts to change the way that we think of the outgroup. A classic study illustrates this psychological process.

In the summer of 1954 a small group of boys arrived in Robbers Cave State Park in Oklahoma. All were eleven years old, white, healthy, well adjusted, and from middle-class family backgrounds. For about a week, the boys played together in a densely wooded 200-acre area of the park, hiking, swimming, boating, and camping out, in other words, engaging in the normal activities of summer camp. Within a short time, the boys gave themselves a group name and began to mark that name on their T-shirts and caps. They had formed an ingroup identity.

What the boys didn't know is that they were actually part of an elaborate study conducted by the social psychologist Muzafer Sherif and his associates,[3] one in which their parents had agreed to let them participate. What the boys also didn't know is that they were not the only group in the park. Two groups had been brought to the park, one calling itself the "Rattlers" and the other, the "Eagles." When the two groups were brought together in sports competitions, virtually overnight they turned into hostile antagonists. For instance, when they were asked their opinions about their own group they described their ingroup as being "brave," "tough," and "friendly." They described the other group (the outgroup) as "sneaky," "stinkers," and "smart alecks." In other words, the boys had formed a positive stereotype about their ingroup and a negative stereotype (a prejudice) about the outgroup.

This study is a microcosm of what goes on in real life. We develop stereotypes indicating that the group we belong to is "good" and that people who do not belong to that group are "bad." What is particularly interesting from a psychological point of view is that group membership does not have to be based on anything important or involving. As long as you feel that you are part of a group, you begin to form such ingroup-versus-outgroup stereotypes.

I witnessed one example of how even apparently petty and inconsequential factors can serve to define a group and may result in an unfavorable stereotype of people who are not part of it. A few years ago I attended the Pacific National Exhibition, which is much like a county fair, with animals on display, games, exhibitions and so forth. It is held each year in Vancouver, Canada. One of the events, this particular year, was pig racing. The way this piece of trivial entertainment worked is that four pigs were let out of a large holding shed into four chutes. Which pig squiggled into which chute was purely random. A sort of colored collar or cape in red, yellow, green, or blue was then fitted onto each pig to identify it. The spectators in the stands were seated in four sections, containing colored benches that were also red, yellow, green, or blue. The announcer then encouraged the crowd to "root for your pig," that is, for the pig whose cape was the same color as the benches in a section. In other words, for the duration of this competition, the people sitting on the yellow benches were supposed to be a group, and the people on the red, green, and blue benches were different groups. There were several races in each set, each lasting about a minute or two as the pigs ran around a narrow track to reach the finish·line, where they got a bit of food.

Even though most of the people seated in the stands did not know each other, it became clear after only one or two races that an ingroup-versus-outgroup mentality had formed, based solely upon the colored bleachers people found themselves on. Evidence that a group stereotype was forming appeared almost immediately after the first race, from the shouted comments of the spectators. First there was praise for their own ingroup: Shouts like, "All of the smart people picked the red group!" or "All of the winners belong to us greens!" began to be heard. These suggested that "us" (the ingroup) are good. However, soon there were indications of a negative stereotype of the outgroups. Some teenagers in the "blue group" began to jeer a group of senior citizens who had clustered together in the "red group," with comments like, "Your pigs are as old and as slow as you are!" One noisy group of individuals in the "yellow group" jeered at some overweight people in the "green group," saying, "There are more pigs on the green benches than on the track!" Quite clearly, then, the other side of the equation was being filled out, indicating that "them" (the outgroup) are bad. These insults were coming from a population of Canadians who normally pride themselves on their politeness and tolerance and who live in a city that annually sponsors one of the largest peace and pro-environment parades in North America. The psychologically important finding is that this hostility toward complete strangers was a consequence of the formation of an ingroup versus outgroup relationship.

Such processes of social categorization and group identity are responsible for the set of negative impressions that cluster around left-handers. For right-handers, the left-hander appears "different" and therefore not part of the ingroup. When the natural tendency to praise "us" and downgrade "them" begins to assert itself, the fact that left-handers are relatively sparsely distributed through the population makes it rather easy for the right-hander to feel that he or she is part of a large ingroup with similar behavior patterns. The other side of the coin is that the left-hander often considers himself or herself to be socially isolated, not part of a group that they can turn to for support.

Numbers alone might be enough to support a negative stereotype of left-handers, but other factors also play a role. First is the effect of labelling on our stereotypes of left-handers. We often learn our stereotypes and prejudices from our parents, friends, and society in general. Such learning is supported or initiated by labels. If I hear the phrase "Arab terrorists" frequently enough, after a while any mention of "Arab" makes me think "terrorist," with all the negative connotations of the label.

Even a label that has a basis in fact may also have an emotional effect. Simply labelling individuals negatively often results in the development of strong prejudices.[2] If news reports label the current party in power as "corrupt and uncaring," whether the label is based in fact or not, its repetition will cast a negative emotional cloud over anyone associated with that party. If you hear a product referred to as "cheap and chintzy," you are not apt to buy it. In the dinner table episode, my cousin Steve was instantly labelled "clumsy" by Cousin Eleanor, "sloppy" by Aunt Sylvia, and "dumb" by Aunt Frieda. As my arm had tangled with Steve's arm, these labels could have been applied as accurately to me. However, I was a member of the ingroup of right-handers at the table, while as a left-hander Steve was a member of the outgroup. The outgroup is always seen as wrong in confrontations with the ingroup. I was supplied by my ingroup relatives with labels that could also be applied to other members of that outgroup. In other words, I was starting to learn a stereotype about left-handers.

Stereotypes are strengthened and maintained through simple repetition. My newly learned prejudice toward left-handers was bound to be strengthened and reinforced in normal conversations when I heard phrases like "a left-handed compliment" used in their usual negative sense.

Another important factor in the development of the negative stereotype is similarity. A popular dictum states that "opposites attract." However, research over the past hundred years has shown it to be more likely that "birds of a feather flock together." For example, we tend to be attracted to people who behave as we do or even look like us. People who are most similar to one another tend to form more lasting friendships and relationships.[4] Some evidence suggests that we try to avoid individuals dissimilar to us in behavior or attitudes.[5] Such a preference for similarity and dislike of difference might make the majority of right-handers uncomfortable with people who differ from them by using their left hands for everyday activities.

A third factor is the effect of familiarity. Psychological research contradicts the proverb "familiarity breeds contempt." Familiarity breeds comfort, positive feelings, and attraction. Simply being exposed to something, such as a face or a behavior, makes us like it better.[6] We prefer the music we hear on the radio, the faces we frequently encounter in the news, and the foods we are regularly exposed to. These effects can be extremely subtle. For example, in one psychological study the investigators photographed college women and prepared prints showing both the original face and its mirror image. These prints were then shown to the women and their friends. Their friends and lovers thought that the correctly printed pictures were more flattering. The women themselves had a strong preference for the mirror-image prints of their faces, because they were more familiar with their own faces as they appeared in a mirror.[7] Similarly, almost-subliminal influences make us feel less comfortable with left-handers' actions simply because they are less familiar to us. Right-handed actions appear more natural and preferable. Possibly, those who live with a left-hander are less negatively affected by left-sided behaviors.

Handism

The average right-hander may be astonished by the assertion that left-handers are stereotyped and deny any feelings of superiority or disdain. We have to scratch the surface of the right-hander's mind a bit to dig up these feelings. Consider the following incomplete snippet from a conversation:

"How did it go?"

"He acted like a complete_____."

By filling in the blank we can indicate whether things went well or badly. If we fill in the blank with "idiot" or "oaf," clearly things did not go well. If we fill in the blank with "genius" or "hero," then things did go well.

But what happens if we fill in the blank with "left-hander"? I once tried this experiment with a group of university students, whom I asked to interpret the second speaker's intended meaning. Ninety-one percent of the group described the second sentence as indicating that the subject was "clumsy," "socially inept," "dumb," "out of place," "rude," or any of a number of equally negative descriptions. The remaining 9 percent (possibly the left-handers in the group) were noncommittal in their responses, offering comments like "need more information to answer" or "it doesn't make much sense." Of 104 responses, not one was positive, which suggests a strong negative stereotype about left-handers.

Other psychological research confirms this stereotype. For instance, G. William Domhoff[8] asked a group of children from the first through the ninth grade, "Does the word 'left' remind you of good or bad?" Even among the first graders, the majority felt that left was bad, and the size of that majority increased with age. The older the children were, the more strongly they held the negative stereotype, with sixth graders (about 12 years of age) already showing as strong a negative bias as adults. Thus, by puberty we have already entrenched our negative (outgroup) prejudices toward the left in general and left-handers in particular.

Why do these negative prejudices and stereotypes about left-handers persist in our language and in the minds of right-handers? One reason has to do with what psychologists call the *Just World Phenomenon*. It goes something like this. People tend to feel that the world is, with a few bumps here and there, pretty much a fair place, where people generally get what they deserve and deserve what they get. This notion of a just world results from our training as children that good is rewarded and evil is punished. A natural conclusion can be drawn from that kind of reasoning: Those who are rewarded must be good, and those who suffer (even from our own discrimination and prejudice) must deserve their fate. A bizarre example comes from a German civilian who was shown the concentration camp at Bergen-Belsen at the close of World War II.

He remarked, "What terrible criminals these prisoners must have been to receive such treatment." In other words, because bad things had happened to the prisoners, they must be bad people. The same type of thinking helps the right-handed majority to preserve its negative view of left-handers. Since left-handers have been *labelled* as being "bumbling," "wrong" or even "evil" by the very language that we use, they must *be* bumbling, wrong and evil people.

Up to now we have been talking about how the negative feelings, stereotypes, and prejudices toward left-handers develop, what they are, and why they persist. Unfortunately these prejudices have implications, not only for attitudes, but also for actions. Ultimately they can cause friction and disharmony between the left- and right-handed segments of society.

The term *discrimination* is used to describe behaviors directed against individuals who belong to a certain group of people simply because of their membership in that group. Discrimination often occurs when group identities are strong and an emotional or stressful situation arises. For example, in the Robbers Cave Park experiment described earlier, the negative feelings that the "Rattlers" and the "Eagles" had for each other eventually exploded into discriminatory action and violence. Group flags were burned, cabins were ransacked, and a food fight exploded in the mess hall and turned into a veritable riot.

Discrimination usually is most harmful when social institutions such as governments, schools, religions, and professional organizations support or reinforce it. These entities tend to introduce specific policies, practices, customs, or procedures that may be formalized into laws. The effect is to limit the behaviors or opportunities of members of the "marked" group. Discrimination may take many forms: racism and sexism are two familiar ones. What I am suggesting now is that what we can call *handism* is another. Right-handers, clearly believing that their handedness pattern is associated with superior abilities, form the majority group in a pattern of behaviors, prejudices, and discriminatory practices. Beliefs and behaviors distinguishing right-handed from left-handed actions have become formalized into the everyday practices and even the religions of most societies.

The Unlucky Left

It is a simple step from the notion that left-handers are a different and inferior minority group to the idea that left-handers, and anything to the left, will be unlucky as well. For example, John Gay, writing in the eighteenth century, included the following bit of verse in one of his fables:

> That raven on your left-hand oak
> (Curse his ill-betiding croak)
> Bodes me no good.

A large number of similar sayings and signs associate the right side with good luck and the left side with bad luck. For example (to stay with the subject of birds on either side), the Irish have several similar superstitions. If you are on a journey and see three magpies on your left, it is bad luck; but two on your right is good luck. Even better, if you hear a cuckoo on your right, you will have a full year of good luck.

Twitches, itches, and buzzes also indicate either good or bad luck depending upon which side they are on. Let's consider a short catalog of some of these superstitions.

• If your right palm itches, you will receive money; if your left itches, you will lose money. This superstition, quite widespread, can be found in Scotland, in Morocco, among the Gypsies, and in North America. An interesting variation ties things back directly to the action of the hands. A Middle Eastern belief holds that if your beard itches and you scratch it with your right hand you will receive something, but if you scratch it with your left hand you will not get anything.

• If your right eyelid twitches it means that some absent member of your family will return or that some other pleasant event will occur. The Greek poet Theocritus, who lived about 270 B.C., wrote, "My right eye itches now, and shall I see my love?"[9] A twitch from your left eyelid, however, may foretell a death in the family or some other unpleasant occurrence, according to widespread customs in North Africa.

• Ears work just as well, as long as we keep left and right in mind. In the Caribbean and in various places on the British Isles they say that if your right ear rings or buzzes you are going to hear some good news, a friend is calling your name, or a kind word is being said about you. If your left ear rings it means bad news is coming, an enemy is using your name, or someone is backbiting or slandering you.

• In Roman times a sneeze to the right meant good fortune, but a sneeze to the left predicted bad luck.

We can add to these omens. For instance, itching of the sole of the right foot means a successful journey, whereas itching of the left big toe means misfortune. The same story is told in many forms for eyebrows, cheeks, sides of the nose, sides of the head, shoulders, and even for the buttocks. Simply put, something that happens on the right means good fortune, something that happens on the left means misfortune. *Left-handed luck* is bad luck.

An interesting variation on the theme is the interpretation of moles, those harmless dark skin blemishes. Ashwell Stoddart[10] in 1805 and John Brand[11] in 1842 collected several centuries of traditions associated with these body marks. Maps have been made of the human body to show the precise location of moles and their interpretation. All of these maps convey the common theme that the right side is fortunate and the left unfortunate. For instance, a mole on the left side of the chest is a clear sign of a wicked person, while a mole on the right side of the chest indicates a very talented individual.

Although this bit of bodily fortune-telling may seem a harmless game, it became a matter of life and death during the days of witch hunters. A standard procedure in trial of an accused witch was the public examination of her naked body. Among the many possible "proofs" of witchcraft was a blemish or mole on the left side, which was always interpreted as a mark of the Devil. The left, as we shall see, "belongs to the Devil."

The Devil and the Left

One common superstition holds that it is unlucky to spill salt. When you do, however, you are supposed to throw a pinch of salt over your left (not your right) shoulder to offset the bad luck. Few people who practice this harmless ritual know the reason for this action: Tradition has it that you lessen your bad fortune by throwing the salt in the face of the devil or evil spirit that is lurking at your left side.

The notions that tie the left side to evil and devils are quite old. The word *Satan*, which is the most common name given to the Devil, has no connection with the left in its derivation. In Hebrew the word simply means "adversary" or "opponent." Any angel in God's court could fill the office of Satan, functioning much like a prosecutor in a trial. The Talmud, which is a vast collection of the oral law of the Jews, along with elaborations, explanations and commentaries from rabbis and scholars, explains that there was a chief adversary, or a Chief of Satans. He is the one who ultimately became the Prince of Demons. His name, *Samael*, is clearly associated with the Hebrew word for left side, *se'mol*. Apparently, according to heavenly protocol, the angel Michael is on God's right and

Samael is on the left. After Samael was thrown out of heaven, he was replaced by Gabriel, who doesn't seem to carry the taint of the left (except, perhaps, in his ordained job as the one who will announce the end of the world).

The notion that the right side was blessed and left side cursed finds its way into a number of practices. Dr. Samuel Johnson, famous as a poet, and critic and as the author of the first complete English dictionary, published in 1755, wrote, "To enter the house with the skir or left foot foremost brings down evil on the inmates." This distinction is based upon much earlier traditions among the Romans. When entering a friend's home, guests were careful to do so with the right foot forward. When entertaining, they would post a slave next to the door to be sure that every guest entered with the right foot first. From this foot-watching slave comes the first use of the term *footman*.

This attribution of evil to the left and good to the right appears in various forms throughout the world. An interesting version comes from Polynesia. Among the Maori of New Zealand helpful, fortunate, strengthening, and life-giving influences enter through the right side of the body, while death and misery find their way to the center of our being through the left side.

Weak and potentially at risk, the left side has to be protected. Amulets in the form of copper bracelets, silver arm bands, and various rings worn on the left side have served this purpose. From this tradition we have developed the custom of wearing a ring on the fourth finger of the left hand. Circling the weakest finger on the weakest hand, it is intended to protect us from temptations and to keep other bad things away from us.

If the left side is evil, then it would seem to follow that evil things should be done with the left hand. It is only a short step further to the presumption that an evil person must be left-handed and that the Prince of Evil, the Chief of Satans, the Devil himself, must be left-handed. Anthropologists have found many examples of the evil of the left and left-handers. For instance, among the Eskimos every left-handed person is viewed as a potential sorcerer.[12] In Morocco left-handers are considered to be *s'ga*, a word that can be interpreted as indicating either a devil or a cursed person.[13]

The idea that the Devil is sinister, in hand use as well as in his other behaviors, has been institutionalized in many ways. Most artistic representations of the Devil show him to be left-handed. For example, Figure 1.1 displays two Tarot cards in the classic design. Taken from the version published by Claude Burdel in 1751,[14] they represent variations of the

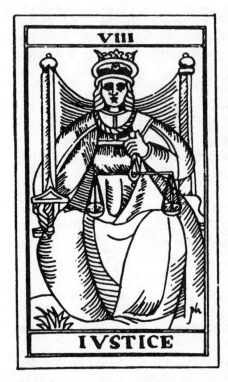 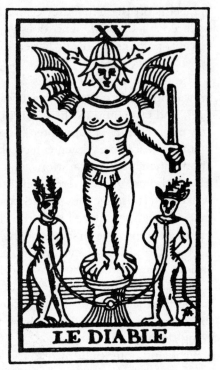

FIGURE 1.1: In the classic tarot Justice is right-handed and the Devil is left-handed, as can be seen from the hands that they use to hold their sword *(from the Burdel tarot classic cards, 1751).*

most familiar designs still in circulation. Notice that Justice, who is good, holds her sword in her right hand. The Devil, being evil, holds his sword in his left hand.

The left had became quite important in witchcraft and many aspects of demonology, where it served as the expression of evil. It was the left hand that was used to harm or curse another person.[15] To effect a curse, witches were instructed to silently touch the recipient with the left hand. Through it the curse, already prepared through ritual and incantation, would be directly conveyed to the victim.

The left hand also played an important role in the rituals of the *Black Mass* or *Witches' Sabbath*. Margaret A. Murray researched these practices and described the Black Mass as it supposedly occurred around 1609.[16] In the typical witch gathering, the leader of the ceremony was the Queen of the Sabbath. As the witches gathered they hailed the queen, holding the left hand high and then lowering it, with the fingers pointing downward, in salute. The left hand was also used in making offerings to the witch queen and in passing wine from one witch to another. If the sabbath was successful, Satan himself appeared. The Devil then gave the gathering of witches a benediction, always with the left hand, as opposed to the right-handed blessing of the Christian church. Often, each individual was reconsecrated to the Devil. Usually this ceremony involved some form of baptism or anointing, which Satan performed with his left hand. Such a ceremony is shown in the drawing in figure 1.2, taken from a manuscript published in 1626. Finally, the Devil applied his talons to each of the participants. Talon marks were considered by witches to be marks of honor. These marks were made on the left arm or the fingers of the left hand, on the left eyelid, the left shoulder, the left thigh, or the left side of the chest. Such marks, blemishes, or moles, particularly on the left side, were often all the evidence that witch hunters needed to condemn an individual to torture, inquisition, and even death. Another potential sign of sorcery or witchcraft was evidence of left-handedness itself.

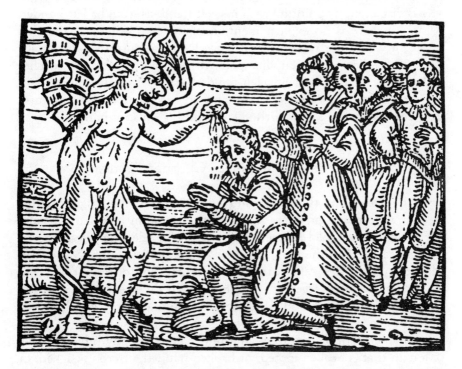

FIGURE 1.2: The Devil baptises his followers using his left hand (*From Guazzo, Compendium Maleficarum, 1626).*

It is interesting to speculate about a celebrated case in which a woman was burned as a witch. The French National Archives in Paris contain an official copy of the trial of Joan of Arc. According to this transcript, Joan told the panel who sat in judgment of her, "I was 13 when I had a voice from God for my help and guidance. . . . I heard this voice to my right. . . ." Surely the voice from the right must be from God, just as that voice from the left would be from the devil.

This same trial record, however, contains a hint that there may have been diabolical forces at work and evil hidden within the "Warrior Maiden." In the margin of one page is a sketch that is believed to be a portrait of Joan done from life. In it she is wearing a skirt (not the man's armor that we have come to picture her in) and is holding her unsheathed sword in her left hand. This sinister observation is also corroborated by another source. A miniature painting of Joan in a fifteenth-century manuscript of Enguerrand de Montrelet now resides in the British Museum. This painting is so nearly contemporary with Joan of Arc that it is believed to be a truthful portrait painted from memory by one who had actually seen her. She is shown identifying the Dauphin, who is disguised, by pointing with her left hand, as would a left-hander. Although there is no explicit mention of her handedness in the trial record, it would not be surprising, since Joan was burnt for witchcraft, if she had followed the familiar pattern generally ascribed to witches and their ways by displaying left-handedness. Certainly, being a left-hander would have counted against her in the opinion of her inquisitors, who doubtless knew of the Devil and his sinistral hand use.

Handedness and the Judeo-Christian Tradition

Both the Jewish and the Christian traditions are strongly right-handed in their nature and practices. For instance, Judaism holds to the rules laid down in the Old Testament in Leviticus for selecting priests to perform sacraments in the Holy Temple.[17] Maimonides (Rabbi Moses ben Maimon, 1135–1204 A.D.) wrote the interpretation of these rules, and his version has been accepted in rabbinical law. In essence, Jewish priest had to be free of any bodily defects. Maimonides listed one hundred blemishes that a priest must not have. A priest must not be "a blind man, or a lame, or he that hath anything maimed, or anything too long, or a man that is broken-footed, or broken-handed, or crook-backed, or a dwarf. . . ." Included in this list of blemishes is left-handedness.[18]

This negative feeling toward left-handedness is consistent with other

Jewish beliefs. We mentioned that the Hebrew word *se'mol* means left when we spoke about Samael, who became Satan. The same word plays a part in the *Zohar*, the Jewish book of mysticism, which sets out various interpretations for certain passages from the Old Testament. The name of the serpent who lured Eve into sin in the Garden of Eden was *Sammael*, another derivative of the Hebrew word for left. We are even told that this serpent Sammael represents "the personification of evil, the other, or left side."[19]

Among the clergy of both the Jewish and the Christian religions benedictions and blessings are always given with the right hand. Thus in Judaic tradition the blessing of the firstborn son is given by placing the right hand of the father upon his child's head. Thus Moses used the blood of a sacrificial ram to consecrate Aaron and his sons as priests, applying it to the tip of the right ear, the thumb of the right hand, and the big toe of the right foot of each of them.[20]

The Jewish traditions consistently express the notion not only that the right side was good but also that the left was bad. The angel Michael, seated at God's right, is usually depicted as more supportive of Israel than is Gabriel, who is far left as a replacement for Samael. (Sameal was at the far left as the antagonist to Israel before he was completely driven from Heaven to become Christianity's Satan). From this heavenly seating protocol, eventually some generalizations were made; Jews came to believe that the *yezer-tob* (the angel whose influence is toward the good) is always found on the right side, while the *yezer-ha-ra* (the angel whose influence is toward wickedness) is on the left side of every person. Based upon these assumptions, Orthodox Jews have developed certain traditions associated with the *tephillin*, or phylacteries, a word derived from the Greek word meaning an amulet or safeguard. *Tephillin* are two small leather boxes that contain parchment strips inscribed in Hebrew with passages from the Old Testament. These boxes are attached to the body in a prescribed manner with leather straps, on the forehead and on the left arm. The one on the forehead serves as a reminder to keep the sacred laws, and the one on the left arm serves as a barrier between the wearer and the evil influences of *yezer-ha-ra*, the angel on the left.

Christianity is even more strongly oriented toward the right than is Judaism. For instance, at communion, one of the holiest activities for Catholics, Anglicans, Episcopalians, and some other denominations, the priests present the wafer with the right hand; it is supposed to be taken by the communicant with the right hand uppermost, supported by the left, and then brought to the mouth. Similarly, the chalice is held in the priest's right hand and must be grasped by the worshipper with the right hand first, holding the left hand lower as a support.

Christianity carries on the Jewish tradition that all benedictions must be made with the right hand, as the hand of the priest symbolizes the "strong right hand of God." Many paintings of Christ giving a blessing or benediction to an individual or a group illustrate this tradition. I examined reproductions of sixty-three such paintings, each by a different artist, produced over a period of 1500 years, which all had one thing in common: Jesus is shown bestowing the blessing with his right hand raised. Of course, you probably could have guessed this outcome in advance, since we have mentioned that giving a benediction with the left hand was the province of the Devil, or part of the Black Mass or Witches' Sabbath ceremonies. It would be unthinkable to have the Pope giving an Easter blessing with his left hand.

The preference for the right hand is also apparent in the act of confirmation that confers full church membership upon an individual, as well as strengthening and affirming that individual's faith. In the Roman Catholic, Eastern Orthodox, Lutheran, and Anglican churches this ceremony involves an anointing with a mixture of oil and balm. These actions are performed by a bishop, who uses the right hand. There is provision for large congregations, however, where the candidates may be presented in pairs and the bishop may use both hands in the ritual. In England there are some superstitions about this practice. I have heard reports that there is often a bit of scramble during such confirmations, caused by parents who attempt to make sure that their child is confirmed with the bishop's right hand. Many believe that a child confirmed with the left hand will always be unlucky.

Most of the other Christian rituals are similarly right-handed. The personal ritual of shaping the sign of the cross is always performed with the right hand, even if the person is left-handed. Similarly, a child is always baptized by the right hand of the priest. In Scotland there is even a saying used to describe a particularly unlucky person, which goes "He must have been baptized by a left-handed priest".

The Bible is particularly strong in its damnation of the left. Much more attention is paid to the right than to the left in the Scriptures. If we omit references to turning one way or another, we find that the right hand is mentioned eighty times while the left hand or side is referred to only twenty-one times. Typically, the Bible uses the right to represent good and honor and the left to represent bad and dishonor. The right hand is the symbol of honor and strength in passages such as, "The voice of rejoicing and salvation is in the tabernacles of the righteous: the right hand of the Lord doeth valiantly. The right hand of the lord is exalted; the right hand of the Lord doeth valiantly."[21] Compare this description to the uses of the left hand recounted in the Bible, where it is used almost exclusively to represent dishonor, damnation, and inferior choices. For instance, God tells Jonah about the wickedness of the city of Nineveh by telling him that the city contains people who are so sinful that they "cannot discern between their right hand and their left hand."[22] This phrase implies that the people of Nineveh cannot differentiate between good (right) and bad (left).

One particular passage has been often used to show the evils of the left. The Roman Catholic principal of a Catholic elementary school quoted me this passage which he used as scriptural justification for the practice of forcing left-handed children to write with their right hands. The passage, with its ominous prejudice against the left, is part of the Last Judgment, according to Matthew:

> When the Son of Man shall come in his glory, and all the holy
> angels with him, then shall he sit upon the throne of his glory:
> And before Him shall be gathered all nations; and He shall separate
> them one from another, as the shepherd divideth his sheep from
> the goats: And He shall set the sheep on His right hand, and the
> goats on the left. Then shall the King say unto them on his right
> hand, Come ye blessed of my Fathers, inherit the Kingdom prepared
> for you from the foundation of the world. . . . [there follows a catalog
> of the kindnesses to be bestowed upon the sheep on the right hand
> before the King deals with the poor goats on the left.] Then shall
> he say also unto them on the left hand, "Depart from me, ye cursed,
> into everlasting fire, prepared for the devil and his angels. . . ."
> [After a catalog of the sins of the goats, Matthew closes by saying]
> And these shall go away into everlasting punishment: but the righ-
> teous into life eternal.[23]

From such writings it was simple for Christians to deduce that all things left, including the use of the left hand and left-handers in general, must be evil and ultimately must be damned to serve the most evil of all left-handers, the Devil. Remember that, of the two thieves crucified on either side of Christ, it was the one on his right that reached heaven, after all!

Other Religions and Customs

Although the Judeo-Christian sects are familiar to most North American readers, handism in the form of bias against left-handers exists in virtually all of the major religions to much the same extent. Let us briefly consider some cases.

In early Egyptian religion, the god *Set* became the equivalent of Satan. He is identified with evil and destruction and is called "The Left Eye of the Sun." Of course Horus, the god of life, is called the "Right Eye of the Sun." Similarly, the Egyptians believed that the "air of life" enters the right ear and the "air of death" enters through the left ear.

During the Greek classical era, Plato described the harmonies that govern the universe, noting that the left side was reserved for the infernal gods and lower attributes while the right was reserved for high honors and the gods of Olympus and the city.[24]

In Buddhism, when the Buddha expounds upon the path to Nirvana (the state of enlightenment and salvation), he describes a road that divides into two paths. The left-hand road, the wrong way of life, is to be avoided, while the right-hand road is to be followed because it is the eightfold path to enlightenment.

In Central America, the ancient Mayan and Aztec ritual that served the same blessing, protection, or benediction functions as the sign of the cross in Christian worship involved touching the middle finger of the right hand (of course) to soil and then to the lips.

A ritual in Islam involves washing before prayer and before touching the sacred text, the *Koran*. Among fundamentalist Moslems, the washing is done three times. First the right hand and arm are washed, up to the elbow, and then the left hand and forearm. While washing the right hand the worshipper says, "O my God, on the day of judgment place the book of my actions in my right hand and examine my account with favor." When he washes the left hand he says, "Place not at the resurrection the book of my action on my left hand."[25] Here again the right hand is salvation and the left hand damnation.

Contemporary Islamic countries are an interesting example of how handism, as expressed in religious traditions, can also influence more secular activities. In most Islamic countries people are forbidden to eat with their left hand, which is considered "unclean" because it is used for cleaning the body after defecation. Since toilet paper is a relatively recent invention, distinguishing the unclean hand from the hand used for eating would seem to be sensible hygienic practice. Nonetheless, custom does show the influence of handism. Why not simply declare the nonpreferred hand to be the unclean hand? If such were the case, left-handers could eat with the left hand and perform the toilet act with the right, while right-handers could reverse the process. The answer is, of course, that the left hand has been associated with evil by the right-handed majority, and that association has been entrenched in religious doctrine. Therefore, dextral behavior is forced upon the left-hander to such an extent that "public display of use of the left-hand" is against the law in some Islamic countries, including Saudi Arabia.

I recently encountered a particularly striking example of how the secular and religious aspects of Islam interact when it comes to handedness. A political scientist who knew about my work on handedness told me a story about the Ayatollah Khomeini, who served as the rallying point in the revolution that toppled the Shah of Iran. During his exile in France, the Ayatollah wrote a large number of propaganda pamphlets and proclamations. In one of these, he claimed to have proof that the Shah was cursed by Allah. His proof was that the Shah's firstborn son was left-handed!

This list of examples of bias against the left and left-handers is far from complete. However, it should serve to illustrate how left-handers are discriminated against, not only by the language and attitudes of society, but also in overt and explicit ways by custom, superstition, and religion. While we might be uncomfortable about the nature of this handism, the very fact that it exists prods one to ask whether there are any *real* differences between left- and right-handers which could justify such discrimination. Is there any way that left-handers are psychologically, physically, or genetically distinct from their right-handed counterparts? To answer these questions we must learn about the nature of handedness and also about a concept that I will call *sidedness*.

2

The Lopsided Animal

Throughout the ages, human beings have wondered about the properties of mind or behavior that set them apart from other species. Religions and philosophies have always suggested that humankind is, in some ways, quite different and unique, with extraordinary capacities. The alternative to this "special status" idea is the view that animals and people are similar in their abilities, behavior patterns, and predispositions. Belief in a fundamental continuity between human beings and other animals leads to the conclusion that we differ only in the degree to which we display certain characteristics. Human beings, in this view, have the same mental and behavioral patterns as other animals but are a bit smarter and a bit more skillful. Resolution of this debate is of vital importance to psychological theorizing, since it determines whether we can construct general theories that apply to all species or whether we must reserve some part of our psychological theories to apply to humans only.

The question of whether human beings are distinctly different from other animals is not neutral but is charged with all sorts of moral, religious, and social implications. Many inconsistencies are found in the relationships of human beings with animals. We use and exploit other animals for our own needs, and thus seem to have a vested interest in believing that we are fundamentally different and, of course, superior to them. Conversely, there has always been a strong human tendency to assume that animals have humanlike characteristics: emotions, consciousness, and even a world view just like our own. Consequently an objective and unemotional consideration of the question is difficult.

Perhaps the viewpoint that best characterizes modern biological thought on this issue was expressed by the father of evolutionary theory, Charles Darwin. He wrote in *The Descent of Man* that "the difference in mind between man and the higher animals, great as it is, certainly is one of degree and not of kind"[1] He probably would have been pleased with recent findings in biochemistry that suggest that, at the molecular and genetic levels, human beings and chimpanzees are at least 98 percent identical. The degree of similarity is so great that it has been proposed that crossbreeding to make a hybrid species might be possible.[2] Presumably, moral and ethical considerations would forbid such a genetic experiment, but the finding does illustrate how similar human beings are to other primates.

On the other hand, the idea that humankind and animals differ in a fundamental way was suggested by the French scientist and philosopher René Descartes. Writing in the early 1600s, he suggested that one factor that fundamentally separated human beings from animals was language, with all of its apparent flexibility and variety. Other researchers have considered different distinctions. For example, paleontologist Stephen Jay Gould suggests that the characteristic distinguishing human beings from lower animals is consciousness, which he calls "our one great evolutionary invention."[3] Some anthropologists have suggested that the unique aspect of human behavior is our ability to use tools.

Unfortunately for theorists who believe that human beings are unique, the scientific data have not been kind. As to the issue of language in nonhumans, Beatrix and Allen Gardner point out that many failures in training animals to use language might be due to the fact that the trainers were expecting the animals to use a spoken language. As most primates lack the control of tongue, lips, palate, and vocal cords that humans have, they may not be able to actually speak even if they can use language. Reasoning along these lines, the Gardners began to teach a chimpanzee *Ameslan*, the *American sign language* used by the deaf. Ameslan employs hand signals, which chimpanzees can easily learn, rather than spoken words. Starting with the chimpanzee Washoe, the Gardners have shown that primates other than humans can learn an extensive vocabulary (over 150 signs), can form simple sentences, can use grammar, can put together novel ideas, and possess many of the other abilities comprising a level of language use similar to that of a young child.[4] David Premack has gone one step further. By using plastic symbols for words, he was able to teach the chimpanzee Sarah to read and write![5] Although not all psychologists agree that the language learned by chimpanzees has all of the complex qualities of adult human language, most would agree that these "linguistic animals" make it likely that language is not uniquely human after all.

Much the same fate seems to have met the other "special" aspects of behavior that distinguish human beings from the other primates. The anthropologist Jane Goodall has been able to show that animals use tools. She has observed chimpanzees breaking off a branch, trimming away the side shoots, and then using the prepared stick as a tool to poke around inside a termite nest in order to gather insects to eat.[6] This and similar behaviors certainly qualify as primitive toolmaking and tool use.

Next, consider the issue of consciousness. Although some researchers and theorists doubt the existence of consciousness in animals other than human beings they often define consciousness in a way that is unfair to lower species. Such definitions may require language ability to express internal feelings, which is impossible for nonverbal animals. However, when we concede that animals (except for trained apes) cannot express themselves linguistically, ample evidence remains that animals have the same sort of conscious awareness that humans have.[7] Furthermore, if we examine the language output of chimpanzees such as Washoe and Sarah, it provides that they have a consciousness of past, present, and future, much as humans do, suggesting a conscious awareness similar to our own.

If animals have the behavioral abilities associated with language, consciousness, and tool use, does any other unique set of behaviors distinguish human beings from subhuman species? The answer seems to be a qualified "Yes" and has to do with the issue of handedness.

Handedness in Animals

Before we consider whether or not animals are handed (or pawed, as the case may be), it is important to note that handedness, considered from the viewpoint of survival of the species, might appear to be a deficit rather than an advantage.

Handedness is a form of asymmetry in which one side is proficient and the other is less so. In the case of most actions, the ability to respond symmetrically seems more useful than any advantages to be derived from asymmetry. Suppose that you set out to design an animal that can move efficiently through the world. It would make sense to design the beast so that its limbs were of the same size and strength and to place them in symmetrical pairs. Otherwise, the animal would not naturally move in a straight line but would tend to veer to one side. To survive, the animal needs to be able to react with equal speed and coordination in either direction. Certainly predators and other dangers can come from either side, and food or prey are equally likely to appear on the right or the left. Symmetry seems to be beneficial and perhaps vital to survival. An animal who is skillful and swift in dealing with situations arising to one side but awkward and slow when situations arise to the other side is disadvantaged relative to more symmetrical competitors. Despite the apparent logic of this argument, asymmetry of paw or hand use is quite common in the animal world.

Suppose that one wants to measure the handedness (or more accurately pawedness) of some animal such as your family cat. Remember that usually the dominant hand is defined as the hand that is regularly used in tasks that require only one hand. Thus, the cat must be placed in a situation where it can use only one paw but can choose which paw to use. In the laboratory we use a fairly simple task that measures pawedness in cats. We provide a tube wide enough that the animal can get one paw into it comfortably, but not wide enough to hold both paws simultaneously. We then (with great attention-getting fanfare) place a cat treat in the tube and walk away. The cat, after a sniff or two and maybe one or two attempts to shove its head into the opening, will eventually put one paw into the tube and pull out the bit of food. For the majority of cats, the paw used will always be the same one. If the cat uses the same paw in 90 percent of the test trials, we declare that to be the dominant paw. Thus, we have determined whether the cat is left- or right-pawed.

With a few additional scientific safeguards, this procedure has been used to measure the pawedness of cats, rats, and mice.[8] We find that for slightly more than half the animals (54 percent) a dominant paw is consistently used much as we use a dominant hand. There is, however, a major difference between human beings and these other mammals in their handedness patterns. Although approximately 90 percent of all humans are right-handed, cats, rats, and mice that show handedness seem to be equally split between right- and left-pawedness.

Rats and cats, considerably lower on the evolutionary scale that human beings, might not be the appropriate test subjects. The closer a species is to humankind on the evolutionary scale, the more likely it is to display characteristic human behaviors, such as handedness. Accordingly, we might find more convincing evidence for handedness in primates such as the monkey or chimpanzee.

Extensive controversy has been aroused on the subject of handedness in primates. For example, Peter MacNeilage, Michael Studdert-Kennedy, and Bjorn Lindblom assembled all of the known scientific studies of monkey handedness. Twenty-five eminent researchers who reviewed their summary of the data concluded that very little evidence supported the idea that handedness in monkeys is much like handedness in humans.[9] Of many reasons for this conclusion, two are most telling. The first reason is that, as with the cats, rats, and mice, only about half of the monkeys showed consistent handedness, while about nine out of ten human beings do.

The second reason has to do with the pattern of the handedness that we find in monkeys that seem to have a dominant hand: only about 50 percent are right-handed. In contrast, the vast majority of human beings are right-handed. This observation has been verified so many times that we can claim right-handedness to be the predisposition of our species. No scientifically verified report of any culture or country, no matter how isolated, has found left-handers to be in the majority. For instance, Clare Porac and a group of researchers from the University of Victoria reviewed every published study of handedness in the scientific literature over the past thirty years.[10] They looked at sixty-four published reports, covering 156,810 measured individuals. The sample included a variety of racial groups (Caucasian, Negro, Asian, Indian, etc.) and covered geographic locations ranging from North, South, and Central America through Europe, China, Africa, Australia, and the South Pacific. Although the various groups display some minor differences in the specific percentages, every racial and geographic group measured was found to be predominantly right-handed. If we examine only studies of 500 or more adult individuals (to insure reliability in the statistical sense), we find that the percentage of right-handed individuals varies from a high of 96.9 percent to a low of 84.6 percent. Over the whole set of studies we find an average of 91.1 percent right-handedness. This pattern is certainly distinct from the roughly 50 percent right-handedness characterizing the half of the monkey population that shows handedness.

So, perhaps there are some distinguishing behavioral characteristics which set humans apart from the rest of the animal world. Not only have human beings developed a dominant hand, but also they exhibit a species-wide preference for the right hand as the dominant one. In no other species are these two characteristics, consistent handedness and right-sidedness, both present.

While considering asymmetrical handedness as evidence that man is unique among animals, I am reminded of another interpretation of this set of behaviors. The ancient Greek philosophers viewed any departure from symmetry as an example of man's ungodly imperfection. A tale told by Aristophanes declares that man had actually been created round, like a ball. This spherical being had his moon face pointed toward heaven. On the other end was his large spherical bottom, firmly held down by gravity, like one of those inflatable toy clowns that you knock over, only to have it bounce cheerily back upright again. For these completely symmetrical beings there was no front or back, nor left or right. However, as human beings are wont to do, they brought about their own downfall. They eventually became so arrogant and haughty that Zeus grew angry with them. To punish them, he split them into halves and tossed these to the god Apollo, who turned the new-made faces and genitals of each of these "raw" hemispheres forward. This was so that they might better attend to their god's warning, "If they continue impenitent, I shall split them once more and they will hop along on one leg."[11] According to this story, our asymmetry is a sign of our imperfection, not a sign of our special status among the other animals of our world.

If the Greeks were correct, we are truly imperfect beings. The preference for the right side is a particularly human characteristic not limited to hand use. Human asymmetrical behavior patterns involve the foot, eye, and ear as well. In each case humankind shows the same rightward bias that it shows for handedness. What we are speaking about comprises a general set of symmetrical behaviors that encompass the notion of *sidedness*. As you will see, it is sidedness that is really a species-wide human characteristic.

Sidedness

It is important to remember that the general plan of the human body is symmetrical. This means that if we drew an imaginary line vertically so that it passed through the nose and navel, the left and right sides would be very similar, except they would be mirror images of each other. When we look at the left and right sides of the body they seem to offer a balanced and harmonious appearance. Yet when we examine them closely, we find that this apparent symmetry of the human form is actually an illusion. The human form seems symmetrical only because of our habit of looking at general similarities, not paying attention to the many structural differences that make the body asymmetrical.

Portrait artists are very aware of the asymmetries in every human face.

Perhaps the mouth may have a slight downward turn on one side and not the other. One cheek might have a dimple or indentation that the other does not. The eyes and the ears also exhibit differences. One eye is frequently somewhat larger than the other or is positioned slightly lower. Research has shown that in most people the right ear is placed lower on the head than the left ear. There are also small but detectable differences in the size and shape of the ears. For these reasons, portrait artists argue that a truly symmetrical face would be unnatural and unlikely and, what is worse for artist, uninteresting.

Other structural differences exist between the right and left sides of the body, many of which involve the internal placement of organs. For instance, the liver is on the right side of the body, and the spleen is on the left. Returning to external features, we often find differences in limb length or hand and foot size in many structurally normal adults. The most common finding is that the dominant hand is somewhat larger than the other hand, and the arm attached to the dominant hand is somewhat longer. There is even evidence that the right testicle in most men is generally larger and placed somewhat higher than the left testicle, while the left breast of most women is larger and lower than the right.

Although structural differences are visible to careful inspection, the right hand, foot, eye and ear, even if different in detail from their left-sided counterparts, are designed along the same lines and carry out the same functions. Observation of your two hands, for example, reveals no structural differences that predict the complex set of different behaviors that show up as handedness. Considering only the structure of the two hands cannot determine that one hand can competently draw, write, or manipulate small objects while the other is clumsy and awkward at these tasks. If one hand were shaped like a pair of tongs and the other like a hammer, we would expect a difference in function, as one would be designed to grasp things and the other to hit things. Such hands would be called *morphologically* different (differing in shape and structure); the difference in morphology predicts a difference in function. The puzzle in human beings is that the two hands are morphologically similar and functionally very different.

Handedness includes some of the most easily observed functional differences between the right and left sides. Whenever people write, throw a ball, or use a toothbrush, they are performing an activity that is best done with one hand and not two. To observe which hand the person prefers for such activities is to observe that person's handedness. There are many such one-handed tasks, which differ somewhat in the amount of strength needed, the amount of dexterity involved, and the size and particular set of muscles involved. In observing drawing, sewing, picking up small objects, dropping coins into slots, or unscrewing lids from jars, we find that, for most people, the hand that performs all or most of these tasks tends to be the same one. It is a really rare to find a person who can write and perform all of these activities equally well with both hands. Such a person would be called *ambidextrous*, where *ambi* is Latin for "both" and *dexter* is Latin for "right" as in right-handed. Thus an ambidextrous person is deemed equivalent to a person with two right hands for all tasks.

Footedness

Although handedness is the primary problem that we are concerned with, it is important to note that we are actually *sided*, since we also have other biases toward the right or left. After handedness, the most obvious functional asymmetry is in the use of our feet. Just as we have a preferred or dominant hand, we have a preferred or dominant foot. Footedness shows itself in many situations. For example, most people use a particular foot to kick a ball, to step on a bug, to stamp out a match, or to pick up a small object with their toes. Most use the same foot for all of these tasks and, as in the case of handedness, we are biased toward favoring our right side. In a study that tested 5,147 people for sidedness,[12] we found that 88 percent of the people were right-handed and 81 percent were right-footed. This means that although humans have a right-sided bias for their foot use, the tendency is not quite as strong as it is for handedness. It is also the case that a right-hander exhibits a strong tendency to be right-footed as well. Of our group, 84 percent had their dominant hand and dominant foot on the same side.

Eyedness

Virtually everybody knows about handedness, and many know about or suspect the existence of footedness, but most people are completely unaware of some other forms of sidedness. These little-known forms have to do with our paired sense organs, our eyes and our ears. Just as we have a preferred hand or foot for tasks in which only one limb can be used, we also have a preferred eye and ear for tasks in which only one sense organ can be used.

Eyedness shows itself in typically one-eyed tasks such as viewing with a telescope, looking into a microscope, sighting down a rifle, or other tasks that require aligning a near and a far target. A task that measures eyedness was described by Giam Baptista del Porta in 1593. To perform a simple version of this task, first pick as a target a spot on a distant wall. Keeping both eyes open, quickly move your arm up and point a finger at the target. Hold your hand where it stopped at the end of the pointing movement. Try not to move it, while you close first one eye and then the other. You will notice that, when you close one eye, the finger seems to be aimed reasonably well at the target. When you close the other eye, the finger appears to point well off to one side. The eye that is open when your finger is most accurately pointing at the target is your *dominant eye*. Because most people are right-eyed, most find that the target and finger seem to be in alignment when viewed with the right eye; when viewed with the left eye, the alignment seems quite poor.

The mechanism of this phenomenon is simple: During the brief time that elapsed while you aimed your finger, your nondominant eye was, for all intents and purposes, shut off. The effect was the same as if you had deliberately closed one eye before aiming your finger. In fact, a mental switch shuts one eye off when you align a near object with a distant one. The information reaching your nondominant eye is just not processed by the brain in that situation. If the brain used information from both eyes, the resultant double images would make pointing impossible. You can see these double images by holding your finger out again to point at the distant target. Fix your eyes on the distant target, but pay attention to your fingertip. You will see one target but two fingertips. Now fix your eyes on your fingertip but pay attention to the distant target, and you will see one fingertip but two targets. You now see the problem presented to the brain. How can you point at one target with two apparently separated fingertips? Alternatively, how can you point at two apparent targets with one fingertip? Of course, simply closing one eye eliminates the double images leaving one target and one fingertip in view, making the act of pointing unambiguous. Having a dominant eye solves the problem of double images without requiring the eyelid to close. Rather, the eye not used in the aiming task is simply "turned off" for a moment.[13]

Like handedness, eyedness is mostly a right-sided matter in human beings. Our survey showed that 71 percent of the population is right-eyed. Also, 74 percent of human beings have their dominant hand and their dominant eye on the same side, a weaker relationship than that found between handedness and footedness.[12]

Eyedness has some other interesting characteristics. Although it might seem likely that the dominant eye would always be the "better" eye, this is far from true. Eyedness seems to be present from quite early in life, and it has been reliably measured in infants at the age of 44 weeks.[14] Once eyedness is established, even moderate losses in the visual ability of the dominant eye won't shift it, and a visually poorer eye often will remain the dominant eye. Quite large decreases in the visual acuity of the preferred eye are needed before eyedness will shift to the other eye.[15]

Some evidence suggests that, in visually normal observers, information received by the dominant eye is processed faster than information to the nondominant eye.[16] Furthermore, there is some evidence that colors appear to be a bit richer to the dominant eye.[17] Judgments of direction are also affected by eyedness. When asked to locate a position in space that they think is "straight ahead" of them, people tend to pick a position shifted toward the side of their dominant eye.[18] The visual system seems to interpret "straight ahead" to mean "straight ahead of your dominant eye."

Earedness

Of all the aspects of sidedness, *earedness* has been the least well studied. Earedness is tested by a set of tasks in which people must select which ear they will use when only one ear can be used. The testing thus resembles that for handedness, footedness, and eyedness. Such tasks might be used to determine which ear is pressed against a clock to hear it ticking, or against a door to hear a sound from the next room or is chosen to wear a single earphone from a portable radio. From such a set of ear-preference measures, we found that 59 percent of the more than five thousand people that we tested were right-eared. Notice that this percentage is much smaller than the percentage of people who are right-handed, right-footed, and right-eyed. The association between earedness and handedness is also considerably weaker than for the other aspects of sidedness. Only 63 percent of the population have their dominant hand and their dominant ear on the same side.[12] Earedness is similar to eyedness in that the most sensitive ear is not always dominant.

Sex and Sidedness

Up to now we have pooled all human beings in the population together to estimate how sidedness is distributed. When we do so, we find a systematic relationship that is almost too neat to be true. We can summarize the basic pattern of human sidedness with the approximations that:

- 9 out of 10 people are right-handed.
- 8 out of 10 people are right-footed.
- 7 out of 10 people are right-eyed.
- 6 out of 10 people are right-eared.

These approximations are reasonable if we consider the adult population and lump men and women together.

However, differences turn up in the pattern of sidedness shown by men and women. Overall, women tend to be more right-sided than are men. For handedness the difference, while statistically significant, is relatively small, with women more likely to be right-handed than men by about 4 percentage points (women 90 percent right-handers, men 86 percent). The difference is more than twice as large for footedness. About 86 percent of women are right-footed compared to 77 percent of men, which is a difference of about 9 percentage points. The same pattern shows up for earedness, with women more likely to be right-eared than men (65 percent versus 55 percent). This pattern differs in direction only for eyedness, as women are more likely to be left-eyed (69 percent of women are right-eyed as compared to 73 percent of males). Thus, for three out of four measures of sidedness, women are more right-sided than men.

With respect to the *strength* or *consistency* of sidedness, women also seem to be more strongly biased to the right and more consistent overall. Consider a person tested for handedness with a measure that involves ten activities. A person who uses the right hand to do all ten activities would be classified as consistently right-handed, while a person who performs seven out of ten tasks with the right hand would still be rated right-handed overall but be labelled a "mixed" or "inconsistent" right-hander. We find that right-handed women are 7 percent more likely to be consistently right-handed than are right-handed men. In fact, in terms of all aspects of sidedness—handedness, footedness, eyedness, and earedness—right-sided women are more likely to be consistently right-sided than are right-sided men.

Finally, we can look at the overall pattern of sidedness. If a person's dominant hand and dominant foot are on the same side, that person's handedness and footedness are called *congruent*. If all four measures of sidedness (hand, foot, eye, and ear) show dominance on the same side, the person has *totally congruent sidedness*. It appears that women not only are generally more right-sided, and more strongly or consistently sided but also tend to be more congruently sided. While 47 percent of all women are congruently sided for hand, foot, eye, and ear, only 41 percent of all men are.[12]

Although consistent differences exist between men and women in their patterns of sidedness, there is no easy explanation for these differences. However, these differences have certain implications for the nature of handedness that will be shown to be important later in this book.

Before leaving the issue of gender and sidedness, we might note that, just the left is usually considered to be evil or unlucky in language and religion, it is also usually considered to be the female side. This association probably arose because, in the realms of normal and natural activities, the male had greater strength and power. Through sympathetic reasoning, this fact led to the belief that the male must be symbolized by the strong and normally the right hand. As an example, the Bantu often use the term "the male hand" when referring to the right hand.

In ancient Egypt the right was always male and the left always female. The cult of Isis believed that the mother goddess was more important and powerful than her son Osiris. In the usual procession in honor of Isis, the worshippers are led by a priest holding an image of a left hand. Similarly, some Hindu sects in northern India divide themselves into left and right sects. The "left-hand" sect distinguishes itself from the right by the fact that its members worship *Sakti*, or the female powers of the Hindu deities.[19] In Buddhism, the right side is usually associated with the male principle and the left with the female. In the Cabala, the Jewish system of mysticism, Eve represents the left side of Adam, having been created from a rib taken from Adam's left side.

The association of sex with side was perhaps taken to an extreme when it moved from religion and philology to medicine. Two Greek physicians considered founding fathers of the medical profession were involved in this issue. Hippocrates (who gave doctors the Hippocratic Oath) and Galen (whose medical authority was virtually undisputed from the second through the sixteenth century) were both of the opinion that boys were products of the right ovary and girls of the left. In 1786, one Dr. Henke carried this belief a step further in his obstetrical textbook. To facilitate the expulsion of an ovum with the proper sex potentials, the worthy doctor "advised coition on the corresponding side when a child of that sex was desired."[20]

Despite the strong associations between masculinity and the right and between femininity and the left, we have seen that current scientific data suggest that men are more likely to be left-handed than women. Overall, women are more right-sided than men, and they are more strongly and consistently right-sided. Once the feminist movement has cleaned up the more obvious aspects of sexism in society, it might consider using this data to straighten out the sexist and sidist biases that still inappropriately classify women as creatures of the left.

3

Measuring Sidedness

To detect possible physical or psychological differences between left- and right-handers, an investigator must first determine who is a left-hander and who is a right-hander. For the non-scientist, this may seem at first to be a trivial problem. The average person would probably take it for granted that people can recognize their own handedness. If this is true, the investigator need only ask, "Do you consider yourself to be right-handed or left-handed?" What could be more straightforward?

The unfortunate truth is that this method does not collect accurate information. If you ask about handedness, the answer will usually indicate the hand used for writing.[1] For some people this information does not reflect their true handedness.

In the laboratory we have encountered numerous instances in which people reported their own handedness inaccurately. One man who confidently reported that he was a right-hander, when tested to see which hand he used to throw a ball, aim a dart, cut with scissors, and the like, performed every single action with his left hand. His only detectable right-handed activity was writing. At the end of the session we asked him, "Since you have done every test here with your left hand, we were wondering why you describe yourself as right-handed?" He replied, "I am right-handed, but I do some things with my left hand." "Some things" in this case, translated to "everything except writing."

That people sometimes misclassify their own handedness has been confirmed in a number of scientific studies. In one study, individuals determined their own handedness by answering the usual "Are you right- or left-handed? question. The researchers next determined experimentally which hand these people used in everyday activities. The results indicated that 7 percent of the group actually did *more* with their supposedly *nonpreferred hand* than with their preferred hand.[2] This means that the researcher must be sophisticated in measuring handedness to ensure accurate data.

Handedness Questionnaires

Questionnaires can measure handedness accurately. The trick is to ask people about very specific actions and activities such as "Which hand do you throw a ball with?" rather than about their concept of handedness. Researchers try to use questions that produce a high degree of agreement between what people say and which hand they actually use when tested.[3] We test each question in the laboratory to see if it is valid, because some items that appear to be useful don't work at all well. Questions like "Which hand do you use to hold a pitcher when pouring?" or "Which hand is on the top of the handle when you sweep the floor with a straight broom?" produce unreliable answers from too many people. Given a chance to demonstrate how they pour from a pitcher or use a broom, more than one out of every five people will not use the hand that they said performed this task. However, when the items are selected correctly, people are not only accurate but also very consistent in describing their behaviors, which means that we then get a good estimate of a person's handedness.[4]

Types of Handedness

Some researchers have suggested that there may be several types of handedness. Different type of handedness may be called for in different behavioral situations. Some types of handedness appear to be stable and consistent, and these are the ones that people accurately recall when asked. Others are weak or unstable and difficult to accurately recall.

Michael Peters, of the University of Guelph in Canada, has suggested that there is a distinct set of handedness patterns for behaviors and activities "that matter," as opposed to those for activities that "don't matter."[5] In certain instances, he suggests, we need the extra skill that using our dominant hand might supply, but in other instances that skill is irrelevant.

Another Canadian researcher, M. Philip Bryden of the University of Waterloo, who has been working on the issue of measuring handedness for many years, reached a similar conclusion. He has suggested that there are four types of handedness.[6] The first involves actions that require some skill (the situations where handedness "matters"). Such skilled actions include using a hammer, swinging a tennis racquet, throwing a dart, striking a match, and similar activities. If you use a needle to sew on a button, you are bound to hold it in your dominant hand. If you don't, you will find that the job takes much longer, is done less precisely, and it is more difficult to get the task done without doing damage to yourself. The same goes for writing. For such actions people know their handedness well, and they show strong, consistent handedness patterns.

The three other types of handedness all involve activities where handedness, in terms of the relative skill of the two hands, is not much of a factor. One of these types of handedness involves the *reaching actions*. To reach for a book or an apple on the table, it really "doesn't matter" which hand does the reaching. Both hands can manage the task equally well. There is no particular cost to using the nonpreferred hand, and there is no real advantage to using the preferred hand. Another form of handedness involves *power actions*, as in carrying a heavy suitcase. Although we might choose our strongest hand to begin with, that choice is not very stable, because we are inclined to switch hands a lot when we carry heavy loads and thus tend to use both hands. A third category is *bimanual actions*, two-handed activities such as swinging an axe. For these three classes of actions, people are less consistent and less strongly handed and more likely to use either hand than for the skilled actions.[7] For this reason, only skilled activities in which handedness matters reliably test for a person's handedness.

Measuring Your Own Handedness

You may feel that you know your own handedness pretty well, but, as we noted above, that impression can be misleading. To allow you to determine your own handedness I have provided a questionnaire based on items from studies that tested handedness by asking which hand performed skilled activities. Just follow the directions at the beginning and end. Be sure to answer every item.

Once you have answered the questionnaire, scoring it is easy. Notice the instruction to count the number of "left," "right," and "either" re-

sponses. Your final score is the number of "right" answers multiplied
3, plus the number of "either" answers multiplied by 2, plus the number
of "left" answers. This calculation is outlined at the end of the questionnaire.

A Handedness Questionnaire

Simply read each of the questions below. Decide which hand you use for
each activity and then put a check mark next to the answer that describes you
the best. If you are unsure of any answer, try to act it out to see which hand
you are using.

1. With which hand do you nor-
   mally write? ___✓ Left ___ Right ___ Either
2. With which hand do you draw? ___✓ Left ___ Right ___ Either
3. Which hand would you use to
   throw a ball to hit a target? ___ Left ___✗ Right ___ Either
4. In which hand do you use your
   racquet for tennis, squash etc.? ___ Left ___ Right ___✗ Either
5. With which hand do you use
   your toothbrush? ___✓ Left ___ Right ___ Either
6. Which hand holds a knife when
   you are cutting things? ___ Left ___✓ Right ___ Either
7. Which hand holds the hammer
   when you are driving a nail? ___ Left ___✓ Right ___ Either
8. In which hand would you hold
   a match to strike it? ___ Left ___✓ Right ___ Either
9. In which hand would you use
   an eraser on paper? ___✓ Left ___ Right ___ Either
10. Which hand removes the top
    card when you are dealing from
    a deck? ___✓ Left ___ Right ___ Either
11. Which hand holds the thread
    when you are threading
    a needle? ___ Left ___ Right ___✓ Either
12. In which hand would you hold
    a fly swatter? ___ Left ___ Right ___✓ Either

Total ___6___ ___4___ ___3___

Count the number of "left", "right" and "either" responses. Your score is the
number of rights multiplied by 3, plus the number of eithers multiplied by
2 plus the number of lefts. For convenience you should fill in the following

Number of right responses multiplied by 3 = __4__ 12
Number of either responses multiplied by 2 = __3__ 6
Number of left responses   = __6__ 6
                                                     1
Total   __24__

After calculating your handedness score, use the following guidelines to interpret your own handedness.

33 to 36	=	strongly right-handed
29 to 32	=	moderately right-handed (mixed right-handed)
25 to 28	=	weakly right-handed (mixed right-handed)
24	=	ambidextrous
20 to 23	=	weakly left-handed (mixed left-handed)
16 to 19	=	moderately left-handed (mixed left-handed)
12 to 15	=	strongly left-handed

About 72 percent of all people will be strongly right-handed, and about 5 percent of the population will be strongly left-handed. Although this questionnaire measures the strength of your handedness as well as the side of your handedness, there are times when researchers find it convenient to ignore the strength of handedness completely and to refer to each person as if he or she fell neatly into the category of right- or left-handed. For other purposes, researchers treat handedness as if there are three categories: strong (consistent) right-handers, strong (consistent) left-handers, and all mixed-handers form the third group. Which scoring system researchers use often depends upon what research hypothesis they are testing.

The Preferred Hand or the Better Hand?

If you ask most people what is meant by the "dominant hand," most will tell you that the term refers to the better or more skillful hand. Although the preferred hand (determined by something like the questionnaire in this chapter) is generally the more competent hand, this is not always the case. Handedness, as we have defined it, refers to the hand that you *choose to use*. The issue is choice rather than ability.

For instance, a device that measures the strength of a person's grip as a test of hand strength does not always show that the dominant hand is the stronger hand. Research shows that 13 percent of right-handers will have a stronger grip with their left hand.[2] For left-handers the inconsistency between strength and handedness is even greater. More than half of the left-handers tested (perhaps as many as 75 percent) may actually have a stronger grip strength with their right hand than they have with their preferred left hand.[8]

One might argue that hand skill, not hand strength, is what matters in handedness. The dominant hand is often more skillful at many tasks, but not at everything. One test, used to evaluate how nimble each hand is, asks people to manipulate small objects with a pair of tweezers. In such tests about 15 percent of right-handers usually do better with their left hands, while nearly 30 percent of left-handers do better with their right hands. Testing people on other types of tasks that require skill and accuracy, such as cutting, throwing, or tracing, we typically find that one out of every four people performs better with his or her nonpreferred hand.[9] Left-handers seem to have an edge in such skill-related tasks because, although left- and right-handers tend to do equally well with the dominant hand, left-handers tend to do better with their nonpreferred (right) hand than right-handers do with their nonpreferred (left) hand.

Part of the reason that the preferred hand and the most skillful hand are not always the same has to do with the many different types of hand skills. Each skill involves different muscles and perhaps different parts of the brain to control them. It is possible for one hand to be quite good at one set of skilled actions, while the other is superior for a different set of actions. Measurements of how skillful a hand is for any one task do not predict how that hand will do on any other task. As a case in point, one laboratory measure of the agility of hands is to see how fast a person can tap something like a telegraph key; another measure of hand proficiency is to see how well a subject can manipulate items with tweezers. For one out of every three people, the hand that can tap fastest is less efficient than the other hand at working with tweezers. Such findings show that the definition of the better of more dextrous hand depends upon the specific task under consideration. While for many tasks the dominant hand will be more skillful, for other tasks it will not.

An interesting indication of the inconsistency between handedness and the agility of the hands is found in some forms of finger movements. For most right-handers, the ability to flex individual fingers seems greater in their left hand than in their right. To test this ability, try to bend the middle finger of each hand so that it forms an exact right angle, while keeping the other fingers straight (as in part A of Figure 3–1). Now try to bend just the ring and small fingers into a right angle, again keeping the other fingers straight (as in part B). Finally, move the fingers of each hand so that a V-shaped separation is opened between the middle and ring fingers (as in part C). Right-handers find that these actions are usually done more easily with the left hand, but left-handers find the results less consistent.[10]

The lack of agreement between hand preference and hand skill should not be surprising. Remember that in the last chapter we found that the preferred eye is not always the eye with the best vision nor the preferred ear always the one with the best hearing. Similarly, handedness is not determined by conscious choice based upon careful consideration of the proficiency, strength, or agility of each hand for each task. People are no more logical in choosing a dominant hand in choosing their mates, the movies they see, or the food they eat.

Measuring Other Aspects of Sidedness

Just as questionnaires can measure handedness, they can measure the three other major aspects of sidedness: footedness, eyedness, and earedness.[11] With the three questionnaires that follow you can determine which foot, eye, and ear are dominant and also measure the strength of these tendencies. Each questionnaire uses a scoring procedure similar to

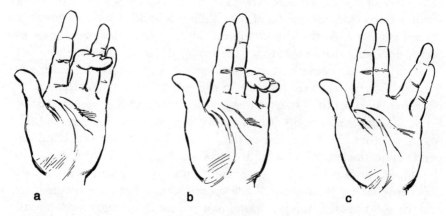

a   b   c

FIGURE 3.1: Most right-handers find these hand postures easier to perform with their left hand.

that used for handedness, although a different interpretive guide determines the meaning of the scores.

An Footedness Questionnaire

Simply read each of the questions below. Decide which foot you use for each activity and then put a check mark next to the answer that describes you the best. If you are unsure of any answer, try to act it out to see which foot you are using.

1. With which foot would you kick
   a ball to hit a target? ____✓ Left _____ Right _____ Either

2. If you wanted to pick up a pebble
   with your toes, which foot would
   you use? _____ Left _____ Right ____✓ Either

3. Which foot would you use to step
   on a bug? _____ Left _____ Right _____ Either

4. If you had to step up onto a
   chair, which foot would you place
   on the chair first _____ Left _____ Right ____✓ Either

   Total __1__ __0__ __4__

Count the number of "left", "right" and "either" responses. Your score is the number of rights multiplied by 3, plus the number of eithers multiplied by 2 plus the number of lefts as shown below.

Number of right responses multiplied by 3 = __0__
Number of either responses multiplied by 2 = __8__
Number of left responses   = __1__
                                             __9__

Total   _____

An Eyedness Questionnaire

Simply read each of the questions below. Decide which eye you use for each activity and then put a check mark next to the answer that describes you the best. If you are unsure of any answer, try to act it out to see which eye you are using.

1. Which eye would you use to look
   through a telescope? _____ Left ____✓ Right _____ Either

2. If you had to look into a dark
   bottle to see how full it was, which
   eye would you use? _____ Left ____✓ Right _____ Either

3. Which eye would you use to peep
through a keyhole?   _____ Left _____ Right _____ Either

4. Which eye would you use to sight
down a rifle?   _____ Left _____ Right _____ Either

Total   _0_   _4_   _0_

Count the number of "left", "right" and "either" responses. Your score is the number of rights multiplied by 3, plus the number of eithers multiplied by 2 plus the number of lefts as shown below.

Number of right responses multiplied by 3   = _12_
Number of either responses multiplied by 2 = _0_
Number of left responses   = _0_

_12_

Total   _____

An Earedness Questionnaire

Simply read each of the questions below. Decide which ear you use for each activity and then put a check mark next to the answer that describes you the best. If you are unsure of any answer, try to act it out to see which ear you are using.

1. If you wanted to listen in on a conversation going on behind a closed
door, which ear would you place
against the door?   _____ Left _____ Right _____ Either

2. Into which ear would you place
the earphone of a transistor
radio?   _____ Left _____ Right _____ Either

3. If you wanted to hear someone's
heartbeat, which ear would you
place against their chest?   _____ Left _____ Right _____ Either

4. Imagine a small box resting on a
table. This box contains a small
clock. Which ear would you press
against the box to find out if the
clock was ticking?   _____ Left _____ Right _____ Either

Total   _2_   _2_   _0_

Count the number of "left", "right" and "either" responses. Your score is the number of rights multiplied by 3, plus the number of eithers multiplied by 2 plus the number of lefts as shown below.

Number of right responses multiplied by 3 = _____6_____
Number of either responses multiplied by 2 = _____0_____
Number of left responses   = _____2_____

                                                                    _____8_____

Total   .   _____

Consult the following to interpret your scores for each form of sidedness.

11 to 12	=	Strongly right-sided
9 to 10	=	Mixed right-sided
8	=	Ambi-sided
6 to 7	=	Mixed left-sided
4 to 5	=	Strongly left-sided

If your footedness score is 12, you are strongly right-footed; if your eyedness score was 6, you are mixed left-eyed. Notice that no distinction is
made here between moderate and weak sidedness. For these aspects of
sidedness, researchers generally seem content with the categories of
strongly (or consistently) sided and mixed sided.

Strong sidedness in footedness, eyedness, and earedness is much rarer
than in handedness. For handedness, only 22 percent are mixed right-
or left-handed or ambidextrous. In contrast 46 percent of the population
are strongly right-footed and 4 percent strongly left-footed, while 50 percent show mixed right- or left-footedness. Similarly, 54 percent of all
people are strongly right-eyed and 5 percent strongly left-eyed, and 41
percent are mixed or ambi-eyed. Earedness shows the weakest form of
sidedness, with only 35 percent of the population strongly right-sided
and 15 percent strongly left-sided; the majority (60 percent) show a weak
or mixed ear preference pattern.[9]

Sidedness and Sports Performance

A good deal of research suggests that particular forms of sidedness may
predict whether an individual will excel in certain sports. My longtime
friend and research collaborator Clare Porac and I joined forces to conduct a fairly extensive research project to investigate this issue.[9]

We were interested in seeing whether sidedness could predict any aspects of a person's success in certain sports. Questionnaire methods to
determine sidedness allowed us to research this issue. We began by mea-

suring the handedness, footedness, and eyedness of 2,611 individuals who were active in fifteen categories of sports. To measure the sports proficiency of these people, we designed a rating system based upon how well each individual fared in actual competition. Points were awarded for the level of achievement as well: A person who had played on a national team was rated higher than someone who had been on a school or college varsity team, with extra points awarded for championships, international medals, records broken, and so forth.

The sports tested included the team activities of baseball, basketball, football, soccer, ice hockey, field hockey, and volleyball and the individual sports of bowling, boxing, figure skating, gymnastics, track, swimming, shooting, and archery. With such a variety of sports, we are dealing with many different talents. Some of these sports emphasize speed, others balance, ball throwing or hitting ability, aiming, or agility and strength. Our subjects varied over a broad range of achievement and accomplishment in their sports. Although some were national champions, Olympic medalists, and professional athletes, the skill level ranged down to that of the average weekend athlete. We hoped to find out whether a particular sidedness or a combination of sidedness preferences might be associated with more success in certain sports.

We first looked at handedness, asking "Does right- or left-handedness, considered by itself, make a difference in whether an individual will succeed at any of the sports that we measured? Common folklore suggests that there have been an unusually large number of great left-handed baseball players. As evidence, names such as Babe Ruth, Sandy Koufax, Ty Cobb, Casey Stengel, Reggie Jackson, Lefty Gomez, Lefty Grove, and Ted Williams are cited. James de Kay claims, "Almost half the major league batting stars, and at least half the pitching stars, are left-handed."[12] Upon examination, however, the idea that left-handers dominate baseball turns out to be a myth.

If we look at baseball players who serve at any position except that of pitcher, we find that 14 percent are left-handed, exactly the same rate for men in the general population. Among baseball pitchers, however, an unusually high percentage are left-handers. For instance, of 3,707 men who pitched in the major leagues up to 1975, 962, or a whopping 26 percent, were left-handed (although still far fewer than de Kay's "at least half"). This high percentage of lefties suggests that the people who hire major league pitchers believe that left-handed pitchers have some advantage over their right-handed colleagues.[13] However, to take this analysis one step further, we looked at the overall performance of left- and right-handed baseball players. We don't find any difference in baseball proficiency related to handedness in our sample. Left- and right-handed baseball players seem to be equal in ability and accomplishment over all of the positions on the baseball field.[9]

One sport in which we did find an advantage on the basis of handedness alone was boxing, lefthanders seem to have a clear edge over right-handers. The advantage probably comes from the fact that left-handers use an unfamiliar fighting stance that results in punches that come from directions and angles different from those used by a right-handed boxer. Because nine out of ten of a boxer's opponents will be right-handed, the boxer's reflexes and automatic defensive responses will be tuned to the typical style of the right-hander and will be less efficient against a left-hander. Left-handed boxers seem to be just as uncomfortable as right-handers when faced with another lefty in the ring, for the same reason. Left-handed fighters have also become accustomed to fighting right-handers and are just as handicapped when they face another lefty.

Another sport that has some elements similar to boxing and also seems to show a left-handed advantage is fencing. Records show that the top eight places in the Mexico games of 1979 for fencing were all won by left-handers. The same was true in the Moscow Olympics of 1980. In fencing, the number of left-handers increases among the higher rankings. The 1980 fencing records also show that among the world's top twenty-five fencers that year there was the amazingly high proportion of 48 percent left-handers. In the top ten for that year, 80 percent were left-handed. Presumably, the left-handed fencer has the same advantage as a left-handed boxer. His style and angles of attack are less frequently encountered, giving the southpaw the advantage of surprise, which can be converted directly into points in a combat sport such as fencing.

Handedness seems to be of limited use in predicting sports performance except in boxing and fencing. However, whether an athlete is a mixed-hander or consistently one-sided does seem to be important in some sports. Overall, being mixed-handed seems to result in better performance than being strongly handed for sports such as basketball, ice hockey, and field hockey. What these sports have in common is that they require active body movements and also an ability to respond to either side. In basketball it is important to be able to dribble with either hand. It is also important to be able to receive or pass the ball with either hand or both hands. In hockey, players must be able to respond to either side of the body. The good player must be capable of shifting his grip on the stick rapidly in order to power a shot from the right or the left, as needed. In addition, the very act of swinging a hockey stick requires the coordination of both hands. The fact that these sports involve action on both sides gives an advantage to the mixed-handed rather than the strongly or consistently handed player.

The situation is reversed for racquet sports such as tennis, squash, and badminton. Here our study shows that it is the strongly or consistently handed person that performs better overall. Although, as in hockey, the player must respond to either side, the racquet requires only one hand to guide and power it. Furthermore, while the grip shifts in hockey, the grip on the racquet remains quite constant and only the arm movements and the body stance change.

Footedness also plays a role in a player's success in one sport. It should be obvious why individuals that have mixed-footedness should do better at soccer. In this sport, one must be able to kick a ball with either foot. The strongly one-sided soccer player is at a definite disadvantage. For the other sports, however, footedness plays only a small role.

The strength of eyedness seems to be important in sports that involve aiming. It is particularly marked in the shooting sports, such as rifle and pistol shooting, and in archery. It is also important in bowling. For all of these sports, there appears to be an advantage to being strongly and consistently one-sided in eyedness behaviors, because the dominant eye is used for sighting behaviors (see chapter 2 on eyedness). The strongly eyed person always uses the same eye in sighting and aiming. The mixed-eyed person, however, sometimes sights with one eye and sometimes with the other. People are usually not conscious of which eye they are using in such sighting tasks, even though the two eyes have different lines of sight. In the eyedness demonstration related in the last chapter, the finger was on target with the dominant eye and off target with the nondominant eye. Consequently, if the sighting starts with one eye but shifts to the other, the result may be a misaligned shot. Such misalignment may cause cross-firing in the shooting sports and cross-laned balls in bowling. The strongly eyed person, however, is not subject to these problems, as the same eye is always used for aiming.

Up to now we have considered each aspect of sidedness as if it were a completely independent feature of behavior. The relationships between aspects of sidedness, however are also important for sports performance. If, for example, a person is both right-handed and right-eyed, we would say that person has *congruent hand-eye sidedness*. If, however, the dominant hand and dominant eye are on opposite sides, we would call that *crossed hand-eye sidedness*. Crossed and congruent hand-eye relationships are advantageous in different sports.

Congruent hand-eye preference is associated with better performance in the racquet sports, including tennis, squash, and badminton. When the dominant eye and hand are on the same side of the body, a larger field of vision covers the area of the environment in which most of the action is occurring. If, for instance, the player is left-eyed and right-handed (crossed sided), the hand swinging the racquet is out of sight from the dominant eye for most of its swing. Part of the view of the right side is blocked by the bridge of the player's nose. Because aiming is done with the dominant eye, any small corrections in the racquet's swing would come quite late. If the player is right-eyed and right-handed (congruently sided), the racquet appears in the field of vision earlier in the swing, leaving time to make minor adjustments to improve overall accuracy.

Individuals with crossed hand-eye preference seem to be much better at gymnastics, running, and basketball, because of the way in which congruent and crossed sided individuals position their bodies. When the dominant hand and dominant eye are on the same side of the body, its *center of gravity* (the balance point where the weight of the body seems to be concentrated) is shifted toward the dominant side. In sports such as gymnastics, the activities of tumbling, vaulting, and swinging from the rings or high bar, depend upon equal action from both sides of the body. A shift in the focus of the weight to the dominant side will add a slight tendency to twist to the body. Such twists away from perfect alignment, if large enough, mar the performance and result in lower scores for the exercise. Additional strength and skill would be needed to correct for such tendencies to turn. A person with a better-centered weight focus does not need to be so concerned about this problem. Generally, people with crossed hand-eye preference seem to have a center of gravity closer to the midline of the body, giving them better balance, and hence better performance in gymnastic exercises.

This same balance factor probably affects the performance of basketball players, who shoot straighter if their center of gravity is centered in the body so that they do not have to compensate for twists toward their dominant side. It also explains why people with crossed hand-eye sidedness are better at track events, particularly the races. In congruently sided runners, the weight is focused more toward the dominant side of the body, which produces a tendency to veer slightly from the chosen running line, This tendency to veer must be compensated for, either by expending more effort to run straight or by taking one or two steps sideways or diagonally to correct for the drift. Such corrective movements represent wasted activity because they move the individual from side to side rather than advancing the runner closer to the finish line. A few such steps can make a large difference in short races such as the hundred-meter dash, which is often won by fractions of a second. Such wasted motion over a long race costs the congruently sided runner quite a bit of time by lengthening the number of strides taken. For the crossed sided runner, with the focus of body weight more directly centered, the need for such sideways corrections is greatly reduced; and the runner can concentrate all the effort on advancing forward.

In baseball, again, we find that individuals who have crossed hand-eye preference tend to do considerably better than others. This advantage may have to do with the stance used by the batter. A right-handed batter generally stands parallel to the home plate with his left side, and hence his left eye, toward the pitcher. The bat is held to the right of his body, ready to swing around to the left. This stance is perfect for someone who is right-handed and left-eyed (crossed sided). As the dominant eye is usually used for sighting and aiming, having the preferred eye toward the pitcher should be an advantage. Certainly our data show that crossed dominant hitters do tend to do better in baseball.

It would be interesting to know if some of the great baseball hitters were crossed dominant. Unfortunately, the baseball record books report only the handedness and not the eyedness of players. However, two pictures that I encountered while browsing through a series of news photos provide food for thought. I was looking for pictures of great left-handed baseball players to illustrate an article I was writing. Most of the photos showed the players swinging a bat or throwing or catching a ball, but some informal photos showed these players in everyday activities. In one, the great left-hander Babe Ruth was looking through a telescope with his right eye. In the other, another star left-handed slugger, Ted Williams, was taking a photograph while sighting his camera with his right eye. Such sighting behavior is typical of right-eyed individuals. If these instances are typical, it suggests that two of the greatest hitters in baseball had crossed hand-eye preference, the pattern that our research indicates is most often associated with baseball excellence.

I have outlined some ways in which patterns of sidedness can influence performance in sports. Whether an athlete is strongly sided or mixed sided and has crossed or congruent sidedness alters the likelihood of success in certain sports. Being right-handed or left-handed is less important in sports, however, than in other aspects of your life.

4

Does Society Make
Right-Handers?

Having accurate ways to measure sidedness quickly and inexpensively has led us to some interesting research findings and to one major puzzling result that was to affect many years of my research life. Clare Porac and I were examining how handedness was related to the other aspects of sidedness. As this study required data from a large sample population, we collected sidedness information from people from all walks of life in the United States and Canada. We contacted various educational and community organizations, sports and recreation groups, senior citizens' associations, companies and unions, and the families of students enrolled in high schools, universities, and colleges. Meetings had to be held with some groups, and a very large mailing of questionnaires was also undertaken. When we had worked our way through the two-meter-high pile of data collected in this effort, we found that we had complete information from 5,147 people.[1]

Most of the data analyses dealt with the relationship between aspects of sidedness, as originally planned. However as our study used such a broad range of ages, with subjects ranging from 8 to 100 years of age, it gave us the opportunity to look at just how stable handedness is over a person's life span. Our original hypothesis (consistent with much of the reasoning of other researchers at that time) was that handedness was genetically determined. We expected to be able to confirm that a certain percentage of the population is left-handed and that this percentage never changes, whatever the age of the people that we measured. Unfortunately, we were in for a surprise.

What we found was that the percentage of left-handers in the population grew steadily smaller as we looked at older groups of individuals. This drop-off was really quite large. We found that 15 percent of the population at age 10 was left-handed. We had lost two-thirds of the left-handers at age 50, finding only 5 percent in the population. For groups aged 80 and older, less than 1 percent of the population was left-handed. This dramatic drop in the percentage of left-handers as the age of the people tested increases is shown in figure 4.1.

Since we collected this data, a number of other laboratories around the world have followed up on this work and have shown the same general pattern of results that we found.[2] Specifically, they report that in older groups of individuals left-handedness becomes progressively rarer. The point is not that there are *never* any left-handers who reach age 80, but rather that they are very scarce. For instance, from our data we find that at age 15 right-handers outnumber left-handers 7 to 1. At

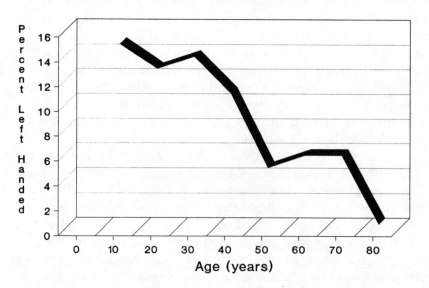

FIGURE 4.1: The decrease in the percentage of left-handers in older samples of individuals, based upon data from 5,147 people.[9]

age 85, however, right-handers outnumber left-handers by 200 to 1! Left-handers, then, in the oldest age groups, have gone from a modest minority to an almost invisible minority over a seventy-year span of time.

The intriguing question that immediately came to mind when I looked at this pattern of results was, "Why are the left-handers disappearing?"

There seemed to be two possible explanations for the data on disappearing left-handers. The first was that somehow the older left-handers had become right-handers. This could come about through several mechanisms. Any individuals whom we tested at 80 years of age grew up when left-handedness was not well accepted. They may have been forced by their parents and teachers to become right-handed. Now, of course, society has become more permissive about left-handedness, which means that left-handers are becoming more common. When we look at older people, then, we might be looking at people who had their left-handedness switched to right-handedness by parents or teachers who would not tolerate left-handedness. Because younger individuals are not subject to that pressure, we get more young left-handers and fewer older ones.

A variation of the learned right-handedness explanation is based on the fact that the world is set up for right-handers. The continuing pressure from engaging in everyday activities, such as using tools made for right-handers, just makes it easier for the left-hander to learn to function with the right hand. Over a lifetime the left-hander learns to do more and more with the right hand. Finally, when we come along to measure handedness in eighty-year-olds, the subjects now look like right-handers rather than like the left-handers they were at age 20. Both of these notions say that we don't find many older left-handers because they have learned to be right-handers.

A different explanation immediately sprang to my mind, however, Suppose that we don't find many older left-handers in our study because they are not there to find. In other words, suppose that they died at an earlier age. That would certainly give us the same pattern, with fewer left-handers in the older age groups.

The first time I mentioned this idea to any of my colleagues, it was met either with astonished interest or with skepticism. Interested colleagues immediately asked, "You are going to do further research to test that hypothesis, aren't you?" The skeptics were less kind. "Handedness simply doesn't have life and death implications," they suggested. "If it did we would have known about it before now." They would then proceed to bedevil me with stories about their maternal grandmother, who was a left-hander and lived to age 99. There would be the inevitable list of famous long-lived left-handers like Pablo Picasso, who lived to be 92; Charlie Chaplin, who lived to be 88; Benjamin Franklin, who lived to be 84; or Queen Victoria, who lived to be 82—all offered as counterexamples to my suggestion. Of course, I could respond with a long list of short-lived left-handers such as Babe Ruth, who died at 53; Jim Henson, at 57; Marilyn Monroe, at 36; Alexander the Great, at 33; and Billy the Kid (William Bonney), at age 22.

Such arguments from single examples, while useful and often successful as a debating tactic, do not make good science. Science has to be based on large enough sets of data that we can be reasonably sure that the conclusions drawn are valid and reliable for the whole population. Before I could seriously offer my rather morbid theory to the scientific community, I needed a lot of systematic measurements and a lot of solid data specifically aimed at determining whether my hypothesis were true.

In any event, I often found myself thinking about the gradual disappearance of left-handers and wondering whether there were solid scientific reasons that not being right-handed should lead to a reduced lifespan. The issue kept popping into my thoughts over the next several years, and I found myself more and more fascinated by the possibilities. "Where have all the lefties gone?" I wondered.

Theories of Handedness

In order to solve the puzzle of the disappearing left-handers I first tried to see if any of the existing theories of handedness might provide some clues. When I began research, two theories about the origin of handedness were dominant: first, that handedness was genetically determined, and second, that handedness was the result of education and social pressure. Other theories of handedness were discussed, but only these two seemed to have scientific credibility at the time.

Some of the other theories that were dismissed by researchers were actually quite exotic. One of my favorite whimsical theories of handedness was suggested by the Scottish essayist and historian Thomas Carlyle. We might call it the *Primitive Warfare Theory*. The notion goes that early right-handed warriors obviously held their weapons in their preferred (right) hand. The left side of the body was therefore turned slightly away from the opponent and protected by the shield held in the left hand. According to Carlyle, this posture is important because the heart, lying on the left side of the body, is protected by this particular fighting stance. The left-hander, of course, has to hold his shield on the right side of the body. Because the left side is exposed and forward, the southpaw is more likely to receive a fatal thrust to the heart. Because the right-hander thus gained a distinct edge over the left-hander for survival in battle, more right-handers lived to have more right-handed children while more left-handers died as a result of their wounds. In this way the population became predominantly right-handed.

The problem with this imaginative theory is that it works for only a limited historical period. Very early in human history, sticks and stones served as weapons and the shield was yet to be invented. If your major weapon and that of your opponent is a thrown rock, there is little advantage to either right-handedness or left-handedness. Later on, in the era of the bullet and cannon shot, shields were irrelevant and body posture not a concern, allowing no imaginable advantage to a right-handed warrior. Even for the era of the sword and shield, the Primitive War Theory works only if the warriors marched in a straight line, like toy soldiers, into a face-to-face conflict. Unfortunately for the theory, attacks in war come from all sides. Wounds to the head and back are also fatal, and death does not depend only on stabs to the heart.

More of a problem for the Primitive Warfare Theory is the fact that left-handed swordsmen were reputed to be fearsome fighters and seemed to enjoy a great advantage over their right-handed opponents. In a book on swordsmanship published in 1747, a Captain John Godfrey is quoted as saying, "I cannot help taking notice that the left-handed Man has the Advantage over the right-handed, upon an equal Footing. . . . In both Small and Back-Sword, I would rather contend with the right-handed Man with more Judgment, than the other with less."[3] Of course, if Captain Godfrey's observations are correct and if warfare is a major determinant of handedness by allowing survivors to pass on handedness genetically, then our population should have a majority of left-handers.

Another theory that I also classify as whimsy, first published in the scientific journal Mind in 1884,[4] we might refer to as the Nursing Theory of handedness. The article argued, "Nurses carry children on their own right arm, leaving the child's right arm a freer field of motion. They hug them on the right side, disturbing the equilibrium of bloodpressure." The deduced result of this behavior is right-handedness. There are a few problems with this theory, however. When 100 actual observations were made of the side on which mothers hold their children, it turned out that in 73 percent of the cases the child was carried on the mother's left arm, to leave the mother's own dominant right hand free to manipulate things.[5] Further, I examined a collection of 111 paintings of the Madonna and Child, reasoning that, as the artists were probably painting from live models or from a memory of a real person holding a child, the side on which the baby was depicted might indicate typical carrying positions. I found that in 76 paintings, that is, in 68 percent of the total, the baby was held on the left side. As in the case of the Primitive Warfare Theory, the Nursing Theory, examined closely, is found to predict that the majority of people should be left-handed.

As such fanciful theories of handedness are really scientific curiosities rather than accepted hypotheses, we won't consider them further here. However, two persistent theoretical themes of handedness offer some scientific plausibility. One says that handedness is controlled by genetic factors, and the other claims that social and cultural pressures have caused us to learn to be right-handed. We will turn our attention to the latter position first.

The *Learned Handedness Theory* seems to have the potential to explain the puzzling data showing a progressively smaller percentage of left-handers in groups of older individuals. The learned handedness explanation is quite simple: If individuals learn right-handedness from social, educational, and cultural pressures to use the right hand, then as they grow older, their right-handedness should grow stronger and more consistent. Subtle constraints on the use of the left hand probably continue to be applied throughout the life span. Those people who did not "properly learn right-handedness when they were young" (in other words, left-handers) should eventually succumb to the pressure toward right-sidedness by doing more and more things with the right hand. Thus when we come along and measure a group of 80-year-olds, we should find few left-handers remaining. Of course, many people we measure as right-handed are converted or switched left-handers who have finally learned to use their culturally accepted right hand instead of their socially unacceptable left hand.

Cultural Pressure and Right-Handedness

The idea that right-handedness is learned through the intervention of society is quite old.[6] Plato discussed the issue at some length in *The Laws*, where he speculated on the source of the pressure to become right-handed. Speaking in the voice of the Athenian stranger who is instructing poor dumb Cleinias, he says:

The Athenian: . . . There is a prejudice about which almost no one can do anything.

Cleinias: What prejudice?

The Athenian: That of believing that in all our actions there is a natural difference between right and left [hands]. . . . It is only the folly of nurses and mothers to which we owe it that we are all, so to say, lame of one hand. Nature, in fact, makes the members on both sides broadly correspondent; we have introduced the difference between them for ourselves by our improper habits . . . .[7]

The behaviorist psychologist John B. Watson took this explanation further, providing specific examples. He wrote:

Our whole group of results in handedness leads us to believe that there is no fixed differentiation of response in either hand until social usage begins to establish handedness. Society soon thereafter steps in and says, "Thou shalt use they right hand." Pressure promptly begins. "Shake hands with your right hand, Willy." We hold the infant so that it will wave "bye-bye" with the right hand. We force it to eat with the right hand. This in itself is a potent enough conditioning factor to account for handedness.[8]

Certainly, in Western countries and throughout the literate world, there has always been some social pressure toward using the right hand for most things. The action most frequently targeted for compulsory right-handedness is handwriting. One example comes from 1587, in the form of a Renaissance book called *The Petie Schole*, written by Francis Clement and considered one of the earliest handwriting books published in England. The student is instructed to "hold the pen in your right hande" and, to make sure that there is no mistake, a drawing of the right hand holding the pen is provided.[9] A left-handed writer is simply not a matter for consideration.

The conscious training of the right hand for writing, regardless of natural handedness, continued with great force until the middle of the twentieth century. Although vigorous enforcement of right-handed penmanship is less common today, it is still practiced in many places. There are many reports of extreme or harsh means that teachers have used to compel right-handed writing in naturally left-handed children. In some instances, children were whacked on the knuckles if they were caught writing with their left hand. In other instances, children had their left hands forcibly restrained during writing lessons.

Attempts to shift children's writing hands from left to right have become a crusade in some school districts. For instance, on 20 November 1922 in Elizabeth, New Jersey, a newspaper article was headlined, "Left-handedness is cured among pupils." Notice that the article treats left-handedness as a dread disease that requires a *cure*. The text went on to report, "An intensive campaign to cure left-handedness among pupils in local schools here has resulted in a reduction from 250 to 66 since 1919."[10]

According to a report published in 1933, teachers of penmanship were generally inclined to switch children toward right-handed writing, depending upon how "badly left-handed" the child was.[11] In 1950, the argument that left-handed children should be switched to right-handedness was still being aggressively offered. For instance, Gertrude Hildreth, a professor of education at Brooklyn College in New York, argued that the "best rule" was "not to let the child get well started in left-handedness for any skill he is likely to use steadily, that is eating, writing, sewing and using household tools and equipment." She goes on to say that the nursery school child "should not be permitted to make his own choices in handedness for basic skills." She advised that steps should be taken to ensure a pattern of right-handedness for actions and skills performed by most people with the right hand. Particular attention should be paid to skills that will be "consistently used through life and in which the environment favors right-handed patterns."[12] Even if left-handedness is already well established, Hildreth recommends retraining to right-handedness, although she advocates a sympathetic approach rather than the draconian procedures of punishment and restraint that she admits were still in use in some places.

Writing is one behavior where left-handers are often formally subjected to pressure to switch to right-handedness by teachers and the educational system acting quite openly and obviously. However, in other activities there is also pressure on the left-hander to become more right-handed. These pressures can be quite subtle and not readily visible. Parents, for instance, often (perhaps unconsciously) bias eating behaviors toward the right side. Mothers habitually place spoons in an infant's right hand and may remove a utensil held in the left hand and shift it to the right. During the 1800s some child-rearing books dictated that children should not be allowed to use a dinner knife or spoon with their left hands, often supporting this rule with dire descriptions of the social difficulties encountered by individuals who insisted on left-handed activity at the dinner table.

A similar pressure is apparent for reaching behaviors. Nurses in the mid–nineteenth century were instructed to correct any tendencies by their infant charges to reach for things with the left hand. If a child extended the left hand for some object, the nurse was to refuse to supply it until the "conventionally proper hand" was held out. The aim was to create a right-handed child because, as German anthropologist Robert Hertz wrote around the turn of the century, "One of the signs which distinguish a well-brought-up child is that the left hand has become incapable of any independent action.[13]

These actions are based on the presumption that handedness can be influenced by socially guided learning. This belief was widespread. A British doctor wrote in 1902 that, "from seeing young infants grasp objects with either hand indiscriminately and from the frequency with which one hears the admonition 'Not that hand—the other hand,' addressed to children somewhat more advanced in age," he could not "help thinking that right-handedness is not innate and that it is in most cases the result of teaching."[14]

If systematic pressure to become right-handed is effective and makes the majority of us right-handed, then right-handedness becomes the norm while left-handedness becomes a problem that we must explain. Why are there any left-handers? Certainly, the persistent pressure and downright coercion applied by teachers and parents should serve to eliminate all left-handed tendencies from the population.

One reason that left-handers persist in the face of compulsion, urging, and instruction to use the left hand was given by Abraham Blau. He was the chief psychiatrist at the New York University Clinic and worked at one time as a school psychiatrist in the Bureau of Child Guidance of the Board of Education of the City of New York. Blau was a firm believer that if left to their own devices the population would be evenly divided between left-handers and right-handers. In a forceful set of arguments he maintained that handedness was learned and that every child *should be obliged to learn to be right-handed* as society demanded. He suggested three reasons that someone might become left-handed, none of them were particularly kind to the left-hander or his or her family.[15]

First, he felt that a plausible explanation for left-handedness is that some people are simply too stupid to learn the right-handedness that society is trying to teach. He presented data to show that a higher percentage of left-handers is found in groups of mentally retarded individuals than in the normal population. He then equated left-handers with mentally defective children incapable of learning, saying:

> Because of the mental inadequacy of such children, they are also less adaptable and perspicacious to the common latent educational pressures and social training that in normal children results in dextrality. . . . Moreover, since the education for dextrality is gen-

erally indirect or tacitly inherent to the environment, the dull child tends to miss the cues in early infancy and childhood.

Blau's second explanation points to faulty educational practices. If parents and teachers fail to teach correctly, the child has a 50-50 chance of becoming left-handed:

> The origin of dextrality may be summed up as due to an encourage-ment of dextral tendencies. When this encouragement is absent, we have educational conditions for sinistrality, whether these are deliberate and intentional or accidental and unconscious.

Blau explains the fact that left-handedness sometimes seems to run in families by pointing out that left-handed parents must be failing in their duty to teach the child to be right-handed. They set a poor role model, and the child imitates the parents' left-handed activity patterns.

Blau's third reason for the persistence of left-handedness is that left-handers may be suffering from some form of personality defect, with their left-handedness being a symptom that this problem exists. Blau is quite specific in describing the *emotional negativism* that he thinks may lead to left-handedness:

> This theory, stated simply, is that sinistrality is the product of a con-trary attitude on the part of the infant and young child. In other words, sinistrality is thus a symptom or manifestation of an attitude of opposition or negativism along with such other signs as disobedi-ence, refusal to eat, temper tantrums, rebelliousness, etc. In place of a wish to comply with the social and cultural pressures toward the use of the right hand, there exists an active attitude of opposition, which manifests itself in the development of sinistrality. It is as though the child says: "Since you want me to use my right hand, I won't! I'll spite you by using my left!"[16]

According to Dr. Blau, if we believe that right-handedness is a learned pattern of behaviors then left-handedness must be evidence of an inabil-ity to learn, poor education, or a negative personality. Smarter, better educated, and nonneurotic people, according to the good doctor, were always right-handed.

The Ambidextral Culture Society

One offshoot of the theory that handedness is learned was a curious educational movement that began in England and later appeared in

America. This movement led to the founding of the *Ambidextral Culture Society*, dedicated to the promotion of equal use of both hands. There has been a long history of support for ambidexterity, at least in principle. Plato, for example, in the *Dialogues* made a strong case for the ambidextrous over the unimanual individual. He drew examples from both warfare and sports, noting that in wrestling, boxing, or armed combat the ambidexter, with the ability to respond to either side, with either hand, with equal skill would have a great advantage. Similarly, in France the author/playwright/philosopher Jean-Jacques Rousseau championed ambidextrality. In 1780 in *Emile*, which contained his ideas on child development and child rearing, he wrote, "The only habit the child should be allowed to contract is that of having no habits: let him be carried on either arm, let him be accustomed to offer either hand, to use one or the other indifferently."

When the Ambidextral Culture movement reached its peak, one of its most vocal advocates was the British author Charles Reade, who was active during the mid-1800s. He wrote what he called "novels with a purpose," which he used as a platform to attack the evils of Victorian society. One of his supporters described him as the "champion of the lunatic and the gaol-bird, and of other helpless and inferior members of the human race."[17] In 1878 Reade started to publish a series of letters, which were brought to the attention of the English public in the *London Daily Telegraph* and were then broadly circulated among American readers in *Harper's Weekly*.[18] These letters were not the reasoned arguments of a scientist or philosopher who might marshal scientific or educational data to support a case. Instead they were almost evangelical in their tone and style, with the zeal and passion of a missionary who senses the possible conversion of another heathen soul. For instance, on 19 January 1878 he wrote:

> In a word, Sir, I believe that "THE COMING MAN" is the "EITHER-HANDED MAN"—that is to say, neither "right-handed" nor "left-handed" but a man rescued in time from parroted mother, cuckoo nurses, and starling nursing-maids, with their pagan nursery rhymes and their pagan prejudices against the left hand; in short, a man as perfect in his limbs as his Creator intended.

Reade's letters attracted a lot of attention, particularly from one John Jackson, the author of several books on handwriting and the originator of the "system of upright penmanship," which is handwriting without a slant. In 1903, Jackson founded the Ambidextral Culture Society. Two years later he published a book that provided educational suggestions and a justification for the ambidextral movement. In one section he outlined the aims and beliefs that guided the movement with a tone and flavor that echoed the zeal of his predecessor, Reade:

Beliefs:

1. That two perfect and equally dextrous hands are better than one.
2. That the left hand *can* be cultivated to a much higher degree of dexterity.
3. That such an increase in dexterity will be fraught with great benefit to the person and with many blessings to the public.

"JUSTICE AND EQUALITY FOR THE LEFT HAND!"[19]

Within a short time, ambidexterity developed into something of an educational craze. There were many supporters for the movement. One of the better known advocates of ambidexterity was then Major General (later Lord) R. S. S. Baden-Powell, a hero of the Ashanti wars and the founder of the international Boy Scout movement, who wrote the introduction for Jackson's book. This introduction closes with two facsimiles of Baden-Powell's signature, one signed with each hand. Other well-known advocates of ambidexterity included Surgeon-General Bradshaw, the physician to the King, who said, "I am very much in favour of encouraging the use of the left hand for independent action." Lord Charles Beresford noted, "The utility of teaching Ambidexterity goes without saying." The list of supporters included the celebrated painter Sir Edwin Lanseer (who also taught drawing to Queen Victoria—herself a left-hander—and Prince Albert), the Countess of Jersey, the Reverend Dukinfield Ashley, and many others who added their voices to the call for an ambidextral society.

Comments appeared in learned journals about ambidexterity. For instance, the educational journal *Schoolmaster* commented, "The great convenience of being able to use the left hand with equal readiness will strike us all, and the only wonder is that we have never seriously considered the question before." Sir James Sawyer, a Fellow of the Royal College of Physicians, wrote to the *British Medical Journal* in 1900, "I desire to join in recommending the general culture and adoption of ambidexterity. . . ." Similar comments may be found in other leading medical, educational, and scientific journals of the time, such as the *Lancet*.

The reception was not all positive. The writing of Reade and Jackson was strident, argumentative, and full of an almost religious fanaticism for the cause of ambidexterity. It certainly seemed to invite both attacks and disbelief, and soon the predictable thunder sounded from the right. For instance, Dr. G. M. Gould wrote in the *Boston Medical Journal* about the "ambidextral cranks, sillies and mongers." Perhaps the most dedicated attack came from the eminent physician Sir James Crighton-Browne, who was also a Fellow of the Royal Society. In a lecture on "Dexterity and the bend sinister"[20] in 1907 he described the members of the Ambidextral Culture Society, saying:

> In this present movement . . . I fancy I detect the old taint of faddism. Some of those who promote it are addicted to vegetarianism, hatlessness, or anti-vaccination and other aberrant forms of belief. . . .

You might be wondering what happened to the Ambidextral Culture Society, especially in light of the massive stir that it seemed to cause in educational circles around the turn of the century. Two factors seem to have contributed to its demise. First, it simply had too many inflated claims. The benefits of ambidexterity were not obvious even to those who finally attained it, and it was turning out to be a more difficult thing to achieve than its supporters had suggested. Second, there was evidence suggesting that right-handedness was a natural consequence of normal development, perhaps genetic, perhaps wired into the organization of the brain, but certainly not always the result of the deliberate cultural practice of educating the right hand and suppressing the left hand.

Some relevant data were provided in 1890 by James Mark Baldwin, who was at the University of Toronto and later became the distinguished Professor of Philosophy and Psychology at Johns Hopkins University. He conducted an experiment on his own daughter to see whether learning played a part in the development of handedness.[24] The hypothesis was that if a child were left alone, with no pressure applied to determine hand use, the child should grow up to be ambidextrous as suggested by the supporters of the Ambidextral Culture Society. To make sure that there were no hidden influences, Baldwin's daughter was not carried in the arms, was turned over frequently while she slept, and items were placed directly in front of her rather than put into one hand or the other. Nonetheless, she developed into a consistent right-hander rather than an ambidexter.

Several other researchers conducted similar studies with similar results. For instance, the psychologist Helen Woolley repeated Baldwin's experiment with her own child, taking pains not to encourage either left- or right-handed activities.[22] Again the result was not an ambidextrous child. Instead, by 7 months the child was consistently reaching for objects with her right hand and by 15 months of age was uniformly right-handed for most of her activities. Woolley concluded that "right-handedness must be a normal part of physiological development, not a phenomenon explicable by training."

Such evidence was damaging to the ambidextral movement, showing that even with no deliberate influence on the behavior of children, they still grew up to be "lop-handed"—and right-handed at that! Dr. Crighton-Browne suggested, "Right-handedness is woven in the brain; to change the pattern you must unravel its tissues. My own conviction is that, as regards right-handedness, our best policy is to let well alone and to stick to dexterity and the bend sinister."[20]

It is perhaps just as well that John Jackson did not live long enough to hear Dr. Margaret Clark's conclusions after she reviewed all of the evidence that became available in the half century following the decline of his Ambidextral Culture Society. She summarized the situation by suggesting, "asymmetrical behavior is the normal mode of adjustment: therefore ambidexterity is abnormal."[23] It was probably bad enough for him to have heard Crighton-Browne quoting Holy Scripture and saying "Man's right hand hath gotten him the victory."

The Strictness of Parents and Teachers

Let me put our research goals back into the picture here. Remember that we were trying to find out why progressively fewer left-handers appear in successively older groups of individuals. We initially assumed that learning plays some role in the development of handedness and that society, operating through a number of agents such as parents and teachers, ultimately pressures every individual to become right-handed. There is a general feeling that our society has become progressively more permissive, and less strict about enforcing certain socially defined standards, over the last century. This permissiveness is supposed to be reflected in many ways. For instance, sexual behavior has become more casual. Dress codes have become less formal. Tolerance for other races and religions has increased. More important for our hypothesis, in the realm of child rearing, parents and teachers have become more supportive, less punishment oriented, and more tolerant of different behaviors in children. Around the turn of the century, in virtually every school in North America, the strap or some other form of corporal punishment was a common means of dealing with misbehaving children. Similarly spankings by parents were liberally applied. The old proverb "Spare the rod and spoil the child" was firmly believed and often recited. Today, of course, such actions are much rarer. A teacher in public school who strikes a child may be subject to civil or even criminal actions. Parents who strike their children frequently may be charged with child abuse. The end result is that less severe training procedures are imposed on children today than was the case seventy or eighty years ago.

The trend away from conservative constraints on behaviors is reflected in the way in which left-handedness is treated in schools. In the past, teachers frequently attempted to change handwriting tendencies from left- to right-handedness. I have received countless letters from individuals who described their own experiences in the classroom. People who were educated during the last twenty years or so often speak of having their hand slapped when they picked up a pencil in their left hand, or having the pencil forcibly taken from the left hand and placed in the right. However, in accounts from some older correspondents, whose education was in the 1920s and 1930s, the actions taken by teachers and parents were often more forceful. Several have written about having their left hand tied down during writing lessons. In some instances the left hand was kept tied down all during the day to enforce its inactivity for all actions, rather than just writing. One correspondent referred to the fact that his teacher balled his left hand into a fist with surgical tape to keep him from using it during writing and drawing exercises. Others have spoken of whippings, scoldings, ridicule, and public humiliation.

If older individuals were more explicitly subjected to pressures in childhood to use the right hand, this could explain the apparent disappearance of left-handers among them. We shouldn't expect to find many left-handers in older groups because their left-handed behaviors brought them such harsh treatment that they learned to be right-handers in self-defense. The correct interpretation of the vanishing left-hander data then says that we are looking not at an age trend, losing left-handers as they age, but at a historical trend that allows an increasing number of left-handers as society becomes more liberal and permissive over the years. As we come closer to the present, students who display a proclivity for the left hand are met with more tolerance or at least nonpunitive attempts to change handedness. This trend produces a gradual increase in the percentage of left-handers in younger groups.

Testing this proposed explanation involves using data collected by other investigators over the years during which this presumed liberalization of hand use took place. Suppose that we look at studies that attempted to determine the number of right- and left-handed adults in the population. If social and educational pressures present when a person is young determine whether the individual becomes right-handed, then measurements of handedness taken early in the century (when left-handedness was dealt with more forcefully and strictly) should show a smaller percentage of left-handed adults.

Looking at the scientific literature, we had to put certain restrictions on our data collection. First, we had to confine ourselves to studies conducted in North America and Western Europe, where the trend toward liberalization had been strongest. Second, because we wanted studies that used a similar measurement method for handedness, we restricted ourselves to studies that used a questionnaire procedure. We also required that several questions had been asked, to get a broad range of handedness behaviors. Thirty-four studies published between 1911 and 1978 met our requirements. When we made a scatter plot of the percentage of right-handedness reported, it looked like the graph in Figure 4.2.

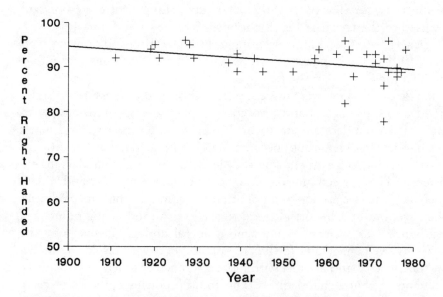

FIGURE 4.2: The percentage of adult left-handers has remained approximately the same over a period of nearly 70 years and that the strictness or permissiveness of society has not had much of an influence on left-handedness over recent history.

Despite some variability among the studies, most indicated that the percentage of right-handers was between 90 and 95 percent. A slight increase appeared in the proportion of left-handers in the more recent studies, as was shown by the best-fitting trend line, which I have drawn in. This slight downward trend might reflect the change in pressures on left-handers. Unfortunately, however, this decline was not large enough to explain the small number of left-handers observed in our older age groups. In our own data (see Figure 4.1), we observed that the proportion of left-handers dropped from about 15.5 percent to about one-half of one percent over a seventy-year age span, a reduction in the population's percentage of left-handers of about 15 percent. The historical survey data in Figure 4.2, however, show that, over the same time span, the percentage of left-handers in a young adult population has dropped by only 3.5 percent, about one-quarter of the amount necessary to explain our age trend data. This means that, although changing attitudes may have reduced the pressure on left-handers to become right-handers, they do not seem to have affected the overall number of left-handers in the general population very much. The small historical trend is not sufficient to explain why left-handers are so scarce in older groups.

Does Cultural Pressure Affect Handedness?

The data just discussed suggest that the pressure exerted by society toward right-handedness is not effective in changing handedness in the long run. However, even though attempts to turn native left-handers into right-handers are not so successful as most people believe, evidence suggests that some aspects of handedness can be learned. For instance, which hand a person writes with or eats with can be changed by the kind of deliberate intervention and education that left-handers are often subjected to in our society.

As we indicated earlier, probably the expression of left-handedness most often deliberately interfered with is handwriting. Many teachers routinely attempt to force children to write with the right hand regardless of their natural predisposition. Sometimes this pressure involves nothing more than taking the pencil out of the child's left hand and placing it into the right hand with a gentle, "Now hold it like this, Freddie." In some schools, however, more overt and aggressive actions are common. For instance, in many contemporary Catholic schools, where the left hand still has diabolical associations, the pressure placed on the child's writing hand may be more conscious and explicit and much more obligatory and forceful. Many of the letters mentioned earlier, those which spoke of tying the left arm down to prevent its use, had come from individuals who had attended parochial schools. One such writer reported that the nun teaching his class brought him up to the front of the classroom and announced to the entire group:

> Every time M——uses his left hand he is doing the Devil's work and placing his own soul in danger of damnation. Now class, it is your job to make sure that he doesn't do so. If you see him using his left hand you should report it to me at once. We will all be blessed if we can save him from becoming a tool of the Devil.

The class consequently became a veritable spy network, observing poor M——'s every behavior and reporting it to the nun. Each time he was caught using his left hand, he was brought up to the front of the class again, the hand was publicly slapped, and the classmate who had served as an informant was publicly praised for his or her diligence in saving M—— from the devil's grip. As might be expected, M—— eventually learned to write with his right hand, although he remained a left-hander for most of his other activities.

This pattern of force seems to have been quite common in the Catholic educational system. For instance, one sportswriter was describing Babe Ruth, the famous southpaw baseball slugger. He remarked on the Babe's good fortune on being "brought up in an institution where nobody had time to object to his complete left-handedness."[24] Actually, Babe Ruth was not completely left-handed, because some people had objected to his left-handedness in at least one area. Ruth had been officially classified as an "incorrigible," for which he spent most of his youth at St. Mary's Industrial School for Boys, a combination reformatory and orphanage in Baltimore. This institution was run by the Catholic Order of Xavernian Brothers, and according to the tradition in most Catholic schools, all boys were taught to write with their right hand. Although Babe Ruth threw a ball with his left hand and batted left-handed, through the intervention of his teachers he wrote with his right hand.

There is evidence that pressure for left-handers to change to right-handedness when writing continues today. For instance, Jean A. Laponce, of the University of British Columbia, surveyed 41,662 Canadian students in the 1970s.[23] He determined which hand each used for writing and whether they had been educated in public or in Catholic schools. Overall, his results demonstrated that individuals from Catholic schools were more likely to write with the right hand than their public-school counterparts. For males, the number of left-handed writers was 12.3 percent in public schools and 9.6 percent in Catholic schools. For females left-handed writing was found in 10.1 percent of the public school students and 7.4 percent of the Catholic school students. For every four left-handed writers in public school, he found only three left-handed writers in Catholic schools. Since there is no reason to believe that Catholics are genetically more predisposed to be right-handed than are non-Catholics, the difference is probably due to the direct pressure that Catholic teachers exert to mold left-handers into a right-handed handwriting pattern.

The effects of social pressure on the hand used for the handwriting can be shown by looking at another population of school children. In many Chinese homes, especially those that adhere to mainland Chinese traditions, it is considered improper for children either to eat or to write with their left hands. The effect of this social pressure on handedness was shown in a study that looked at the hand used for writing in 7,684 school children in Berkeley, California. This data showed that 9.9 percent of the non-Chinese children wrote with their left hands. However, when the researchers looked at the Chinese children, who supposedly were under greater pressure to use the right hand, only 6.5 percent used the left hand for writing.[24] For every five non-Chinese writing with the left-hand, there are only 3 Chinese who do. Again, social pressure seems to have reduced the amount of visible left-handedness, at least for one targeted behavior (handwriting) that was singled out for change.

The data suggest that for specific activities, such as handwriting, there may be some effect of learning on handedness. If this is the case, then perhaps the answer to why there are so few older left-handers might, in fact, be a lifetime of learning. During a left-hander's life continuous pressure promotes the use of the right hand for various activities. Although this pressure is often subtle and not aggressively applied, it is still there. Some comes from the fact that the natural left-hander sees everybody around working with the right hand, some from the fact that many tools and pieces of equipment are more easily used in the right hand, and so forth. This subliminal coercion causes the left-hander to do more and more with the right hand as he grows older. Eventually, according to this theory, when the left-hander does enough things with his right hand, he will no longer be classified as a left-hander. Thus older groups show fewer left-handers because, after seventy or eighty years of indirect pressure, those born as left-handers have finally learned to be proper right-handers. Of course, this explanation depends upon the presumption that handedness can be effectively switched. Is this presumption true?

The Switched-Handers

When we began to consider the possibility that the disappearance of left-handers was caused by a lifelong learning process whereby left-handers learn to be right-handers, we needed to determine how easy it is to switch handedness. Although many people offered opinions on this matter, we were surprised to find little work that looked at changing handedness. This lack of information meant that we would have to collect the data ourselves.

Our resultant investigation involved 650 young adults, and focusing particularly on 52 of them who had suffered attempts to switch their handedness from left to right.[27] A later study of 518 adults netted another 31 individuals with the same experience.[28] I'll combine the results of these two studies whenever possible for this discussion.

The first thing that we found was that attempts to change the handedness of left-handers were quite common. Approximately 55 percent of all left-handers remember situations in which attempts were made to switch them to right-handedness. In approximately two-thirds of the cases (64 percent), the attempts to change handedness were made quite early, usually before third grade (8 or 9 years of age). The most common activity targeted for change was writing, as we had suspected. Attempts to force left-handers to write with the right hand accounted for nearly half (46 percent) of all attempted changes in handedness. Because writing is singled out, it is not surprising to find that the principal agent of change is the teacher. In 28 percent of the cases the person trying to change the left-handed child's handedness was a teacher, while in 27 percent of the cases a parent tried to switch the child's handedness. For about 13 percent of the cases, an attempt also was made to change the hand used in eating; and in another 13 percent of the cases, the behaviors singled out for change involved sports activities. The most common method used to get the child to use the right hand was to switch the pen or the eating utensil from the left to the right hand, which happened in 44 percent of the cases. In one out of every four cases (27 percent), the parent or teacher resorted to verbal persuasion, arguments, appeals to logic, or fears of the devil to get the child to change. In one out of every five cases (20 percent), however, physical punishment was employed to enforce the right-handed use.

How successful were these attempted changes in handedness? Overall, left-handers were successfully shifted in only about two out of every five cases (41 percent). The greatest success came for handwriting, which was successfully shifted in 57 percent of the cases. Of the people who did successfully shift their handedness from left to right, it seems that the trick was to start the training process quite early. In 8 out of 10 of the cases where handedness was successfully changed, the process had begun before the child was in third grade. Beyond this time, the chance of success drops to about one out of five.

Gender may also be a factor in switching handedness. One study found that women were twice as likely as men to undergo a successful handedness change.[27] However another study failed to find any difference between men and women in successful switching, leaving the matter up in the air.[28]

A particularly interesting feature shows up in the most recent study on hand switching.[28] Even for people who rate themselves as successfully switched from left- to right-handedness, the measured handedness looks more like that of a left-hander than that of a right-hander. In other words, they still do more things with the left hand than with the right.

What is going on in cases of switched handedness can be seen very clearly from a study that looked at the handedness of 4,143 students from Taiwan.[29] As I mentioned, in Chinese culture social pressure enforces right-handed writing and eating habits; and the the practice persists among Taiwanese. The pressure for right-handed writing begins as soon as the child starts school and continues throughout the school years. Pressure for right-handed eating also begins quite early and is maintained in most traditional Taiwanese homes. Virtually all of the Taiwanese left-handers report frequent requests to change hand use from left to right. We had also observed in our own data that, if a child is pressured to switch *a specific behavior* and if that pressure is applied when the child is young enough (and probably if it is insistent enough), around four out of five times handedness will be successfully changed. This appears to be the case in Taiwan. Left-handed writing has been reduced in this population to an amazingly low level of occurrence, less than 1 percent. Left-handed eating is also quite rare, now in less than 2 percent of the population. This clearly indicates that changing left-handers to right-handedness has been successful—or does it?

Actually, this study shows that *handedness changes only for the specific actions singled out for right-sided pressure.* Let us compare the percentage of right-handers in the Taiwanese study to the percentage of right-handers in a British study of 2,321 young adults, whose handedness was measured for a number of common activities.[30] Let's make our comparisons for only those behaviors that are not usually subject to cultural pressure; hence we will leave out writing and eating, which we know draw most of the attention. When we do this we find that the British sample has 13 percent left-handed scissor users as compared to 14 percent in Taiwan. These are remarkably similar percentages of left-handedness for the "pressured" Chinese compared to the "non-pressured" English. The same degree of left-handedness is shown for hammering (12 percent left-handed for both), toothbrush use (18 percent left-handed for both), and striking a match (19 percent left in England and 21 percent left-handed in Taiwan). In other words, the successful effect of switching the writing or the eating hand from left to right has not carried over into any other activities. Only the specific behaviors that cultural and educational agents directly tried to influence have shown any real change. You can make a left-hander write with his right hand, but he will still brush his teeth, thread a needle, or throw a ball with his left hand. In other words, the individual will be a fairly consistent left-hander who now does one or two things with his right hand because of pressure from parents and teachers, much like Babe Ruth, the "complete left-hander" who nonetheless wrote with his right hand.

Learning and the Disappearing Left-Hander

We now have enough information to see if it is logical to suggest that the gradual disappearance of left-handers in older groups is due to either of the two learning explanations that we have discussed so far, specifically that (1) older individuals were more strictly treated and left-handers were coerced and pressured into becoming right-handers or that (2) as they grow older, left-handers gradually learn to become more right-handed.

The research we looked at gives us two sets of data that allow us to evaluate these hypotheses:

1. To begin with, it is true that society does pressure individuals to become right-handed. Although these pressures may have changed historically, the percentage of right-handers in the population seems to have remained fairly constant over the last eighty or ninety years, with about one out of every ten young adults being left-handed. It is unlikely that the reduced number of left-handers among older individuals has anything to do with less tolerance for left-handers several generations ago. Also, learning effects on handedness are quite specific. *Only the actions that are singled out for pressure or change become more right-sided.* The other, nonpressured, activities remain just as left-sided as they initially were. Furthermore, the data show that left-handers are generally pressured to become right-handed only for a few varieties of activities,

such as writing or eating. Thus it seems that, whether they were pressured to change handedness by teachers and parents or not, the number of left-handed adults doesn't seem to be influenced by such social factors over recent history.

2. In order to successfully change the handedness of an individual, you have to apply pressure when the person is quite young. If you try to switch handedness after the age of eight or nine years, your chances of success are quite slim, only about one out of five. For those who do show a successful change of handedness, it appears that the change is pretty much completed before adolescence and is *not a gradual shift* toward right-sidedness over the life span. In order to account for the gradual disappearance of left-handers in the older age groups we would have to presume that some such continuous learning gradually switches handedness, which just doesn't seem to happen.

If we believe these facts, then we are forced to conclude that we can't explain the decreasing number of left-handers in older groups on the basis of a simple theory of learning or social pressure. Something must be happening to eliminate left-handers in some other way. Perhaps we could shed some light on this puzzle if we step back a few steps, and ask some very basic questions such as, "If handedness is not learned, what makes a person left-handed in the first place?" We will begin to consider possible answers to this in the next chapter.

5

Is Handedness Inherited?

A few years ago, while on a trip to Scotland, I visited one of the castles built by the Kerr family. The tour guide was going through the usual commentary about the family's history, the antiquity of various pieces of furniture, and the significance of various obscure pieces of art by painters whose names she felt that we should recognize, but I knew that I did not. As we moved across the main floor, the guide began to ascend a spiral staircase that would bring us up a level and then stopped to say:

"You might notice that this staircase is a bit different from most other spiral staircases that you have seen. If you pay attention to the next few spiral staircases that you see in buildings in other places, you will notice that they tend to wind in a clockwise direction. This staircase, and in fact, almost all of the spiral staircases built in castles and manors owned by the Kerr family, tend to wind in an anticlockwise direction. The reason for this is that the Scottish Family Kerr, have a long history of left-handedness. An anticlockwise spiral gives an advantage to a left-handed swordsman defending against right-handed attackers trying to move up the stair. It looks like this . . . ."

The guide stopped and extracted from her pocket one of those collapsible pointers that speakers sometimes use. She opened it up, so that it looked like a fencing foil, and brandished it in her left hand downward toward the gaping group of tourists. Sure enough, with the anticlockwise bend, the left hand was free to move over the open railing. When she transferred her simulated weapon to the right hand, however, the central post obviously interfered with its action.

Everything about the Kerr family (or its variants Karr or Carr) suggests that left-handedness was a familial characteristic. Even the name Kerr, derived from the word *kier*, seems to confirm this. In Scotland the terms *kier-handit* or *ker-handit* are used as slang for left-handed. *Kier* also means "carry," and left-handers are referred to as *carry-handed* because a right-hander usually carries objects (such as a pail of water) in his left hand, in order to leave his dominant right hand free to manipulate things such as door knobs or gate latches. Thus the left-hander manipulates things with the hand that the rest of the world uses to carry things.

Another demonstration of the bend sinister in the Kerr family might be this bit of doggerel, by some anonymous author who clearly felt that left-handedness was a Kerr family trait.

But the Kerrs were aye the deadliest foes
That e'er to Englishmen were known,
For they were all bred left-handed men,
And 'fence against them there was none.

Apparently this legend of the left-handed Kerr family was taken seriously enough in Britain to cause a rather unscientific survey to be taken by the *Journal of the Royal College of General Practitioners* to check its accuracy. They invited doctors to send in information concerning the handedness of any of their patients with the family name Kerr. This call attracted a lot of attention from the press in both Britain and North America and resulted in a flood of responses. These came not only from doctors but also from individual members of the Kerr family. Most of the observations were not very well controlled in the scientific sense, and the definitions of handedness used by the various correspondents were probably quite variable (which, as we saw in chapter 3, makes a difference). If these data are to be believed, however, they revealed that 29.5 percent of the Kerrs were "left-handed or ambidextrous," as compared to only 11 percent of another family used as a comparison group.[1] While these data suggest that left-handedness may be more common among the Kerrs, notice that they still show that even among the Kerr family, there is a strong majority of right-handers. In the general population, 9 out of 10 individuals are right-handed, while for the Kerrs, 7 out of 10 are right-handers. Thus we have more left-handers in this family, but not all left-handers or even a majority.

In some respects the outcome of the study of whether left-handedness was inherited in the Kerr family is similar to the outcome that we usually find when we look for genetic contributions to handedness. The results are suggestive and seem to indicate some familial contribution. This might mean that handedness is inherited, but the result is much weaker than we would expect if genetic factors were playing a large role in determining handedness. The results of family handedness studies are always unclear enough that when I am asked the question, "Where does handedness come from?" I am uncomfortable about saying that handedness is genetically determined. However, I also have difficulty completely rejecting the possibility.

Even if learning or pressure from society could explain the predominance of right-handers, we would still want to know why left-handers exist in the population at all. The answer most commonly suggested has been that some percentage of people *are genetically programmed to be left-handers*. The genetic explanation for the existence of a small number of left-handers has a long history and seems to have been accepted by many scientists as an obvious truth. Yet when I began looking at the published data on handedness in families up to 1973 (the year that I turned to the problem), I was disappointed. Few people were gathering data to determine whether there was a genetic factor in handedness. Nearly ten years after our laboratory began to study this problem, the psychologist Philip Bryden was still able to say that "There is no wholly satisfactory study of handedness in families."[2] This statement is certainly true if a "satisfactory study" means one that proves unambiguously and convincingly that handedness is encoded in the genes and that the handedness of your parents determines your own handedness in predictable ways.

Evolution and Handedness

Before we talk about the interaction between genetics and handedness, I think that we ought to be clear about some things that tend to be glossed over in everyday discussions of genetics and inheritable features and traits. When scientists talk about inherited or genetic traits, they usually are looking at some feature that exists in several forms in a population of individuals. They are using genetic theories to try to explain why some individuals show one set of characteristics while others show a different set of characteristics. Eye color is an example of this. There are two dominant varieties of eye color in the population, namely, brown and blue. Whether you have brown or blue eyes can be shown to depend upon the eye color of your parents. If you get at least one brown-eyed gene you are brown-eyed, while to be blue-eyed you need two blue-eyed genes (one from each parent). In other words, brown-eyed and blue-eyed individuals are genetically different.

There are many such genetically determined characteristics that vary from individual to individual. These include: curly or straight hair, skin color, night blindness, hemophilia, tendencies toward schizophrenia, degree of intelligence (especially in the extremes, such as mental retardation), and some forms of personality disorders. These genetically determined traits allow us to predict the child's characteristics from the parents' characteristics. We can specify a gene or group of genes that determine whether individuals see colors normally or are color blind and can predict who is apt to have these characteristics. To assess the genetic contribution we ask questions such as, "If a color-blind man mates with a color-normal woman, will their children be color blind or not?" Particular mating combinations that produce specific characteristics in the children or in the children's children demonstrate that the characteristics are inherited. They allow us to determine the type of genetic coding or transmission we are dealing with. The factor that allows us to answer questions about the genetic mechanisms is that these traits exist in several forms, with different individuals in the population showing different characteristics (for example, both blue-eyed and brown-eyed people). I will call these characteristics *genetically variable traits*.

Another set of characteristics are also genetically determined but are seldom explored using standard measures of the parents' characteristics. As a human being, you have a series of genetically determined traits that distinguish you from other species. For instance, you have exactly two eyes, no more, no less. You were born with the ability to grow hair on your head and underarms, but not on the palms of your hands or the soles of your feet. Every human being has a thumb that can touch the tip of each of the other fingers on that hand. This *opposable thumb* is an important and uniquely human characteristic. Similarly, you have a set of hips arranged to be carried in an upright position, and the angle of insertion of your legs is such that you can walk upright. In addition, you are that rare monkey that has no visible tail.

All of these characteristics are part of your genetic heritage because you are human. These characteristics, however, can not be studied by looking at the characteristics of your parents. All human beings have no tail. We cannot ask the question, "What happens if a man with a tail mates with a women with no tail?" because the characteristic of not having a tail is species-specific trait. There are no humans with a tail. Yet all of these human characteristics are bound up in our genes. We are human because our genes provide us with programming that will allow us to develop the full set of characteristics that distinguish humans from other species of animals. These invariant but obviously genetically determined traits that are unchanging and found in all individuals I will call *genetically fixed characteristics*.

When we looked at how handedness (or pawedness) was distributed in the populations of cats and monkeys, we found that half of them were right-pawed and half were left-pawed. It is only among humans that we find that roughly nine out of ten individuals are right-handed. This right-sided bias looks like a unique human characteristic, and it may be a genetically fixed trait. How can we test this hypothesis?

If right-handedness is genetically determined, as a trait that is fixed in our species, then no matter how far back into history we look we should find that the majority of humans were always right-handed. Unfortunately, most histories do not include information on handedness. For information about very early handedness we cannot go back in time and ask Og the Caveman, "Which hand do you hold your club in when defending yourself from sabertoothed tigers?" However, residues from Og's behavior may provide us with the data that we need.

It is strange how often serendipity plays a role in science, or at least in science as I have come to practice it. Chance reared its helpful head while I was puzzling about how to determine whether handedness is a genetically fixed trait. I was reading a book about Benjamin Franklin. I have a fondness for history, since I like to tell stories. Histories and biographies are marvelous sources for interesting stories that one can insert into boring academic and administrative receptions in order to keep the conversation flowing and away from"more sensitive areas". This particular book explores the behaviors that led to Franklin's reputation as a womanizer who had been involved with a number of prominent ladies. The book contained a few illustrations, most made from life or created by people who had actually seen Franklin. One, made while he spent his eighteen-year sojourn in England, was a painting of Franklin playing chess with Lady Howe. I remember being bothered by that painting, although I couldn't quite discern why. Later on in the book, a drawing made during Franklin's stay in France showed him speaking with another lady. He was engaged in an animated discussion in which he had raised his cane and was gesturing with it like a sword. Again, there was something uncomfortable about the drawing. As I looked at it, I recognized what the problem was. In this picture, he was fencing with a cane that was held in his left hand. I flipped back to the painting of Franklin playing chess. Now I see what made me uncomfortable here. It was the fact that Franklin was moving the chess piece with his left hand. The pictures had looked wrong because I am so used to seeing people using the right hand for most actions that a painting that depicted left-handed activities just didn't seem correct. I later learned that the artists were accurate in their portrayals. Franklin was left-handed but had been forced to learn to write and eat with his right hand. It was always a frustration for him, and at one time it stirred him to write a piece entitled "A Petition to Those Who Have the Superintendency of Education," protesting the pressures placed on left-handers.

What nagged at me, however, was not that these drawings revealed something about Benjamin Franklin's handedness, but rather that my response to these pictures was that left-handedness in the pictures seemed wrong. It was at that moment that the flash of insight hit. You see, humankind is a very vain species and loves its own image. The validity of this statement is shown by the fact that Throughout history, cultures have produced numerous drawings and images of humans engaged in all sorts of activities. This practice goes all the way back to the *Paleolithic era* (the old Stone Age). Suppose that I am a Stone Age artist, about to make a picture of a recent successful bison hunt, where a group of us had encircled the beast and stabbed it to death with spears. I am of course trying to produce a picture that is an accurate representation of what I saw. Suppose that the majority of my fellow cavemen are *not* consistently right-handed. If, on the whole, half of the people use the right hand and half the left hand to hold tools and weapons, then my sense of aesthetics or correctness shouldn't be affected very much be which hand I place the spears in for my drawing of the hunt. I should be so used to seeing either hand in regular use that my drawings needn't consider handedness as a factor. However, if most of the people I see manipulate tools and weapons with the right hand, then I am likely to place the spears in my picture in the right hands of my characters. This need not be done at any conscious level, it is just that the picture will appear to me to be more "natural" and lifelike this way. Here was a key. We could estimate whether human beings have always been right-handed by looking at drawings of people using implements and determining which hand they were using in the pictures. The artist, by his placement of these objects in the picture, should tell us whether the people around him were, for the most part, right-handed or not.

Determining handedness from pictures is really quite simple. For instance, if you want to know whether Alice, of *Alice in Wonderland*, was

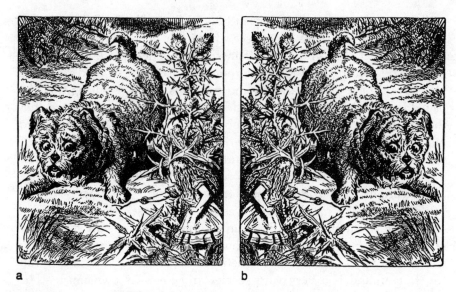

a   b

FIGURE 5.1: A) Right-handed Alice in Wonderland as originally drawn by
Tenniel. b) How Alice would look if she were left handed.

left- or right-handed, you need only look at pictures of her. For instance,
in part A of figure 5.1 we see Alice, now shrunk to the size of a mouse,
about to throw a stick for the big puppy in the garden. Notice that, in
the drawings by the English caricaturist Sir John Tenniel that accompanied the original edition of *Alice in Wonderland*, Alice is clearly tossing
the stick with her right hand. If she had been a left-hander, then Tenniel
would have had to draw her as we see in part B.

The next action that we took was to raid my university's collection of
art books and reproductions. We dug up pictures from European, Asian,
African, and American sources and then went through a careful selection procedure. We first eliminated any cases involving stylized mirror-
image drawings, where the whole point of the exercise was to create a
symmetrical pattern by making the left and right sides appear to be
mirror images of one another. Instead, we looked for cases where the
artist was trying to illustrate an actual scene. We also tried to make sure
that we had only one example from any one artist. In the end, we examined over 10,000 works of art and finally came up with 1,180 scorable
cases where there was an unambiguous picture of an individual using a
tool or a weapon with one hand.[3] The time period that these art works
covered was quite broad. The earliest scorable drawing was dated approximately 15,000 B.C., well back into the Stone Age. We extended
forward in time to 1950 A.D. An example of a scorable piece of art is

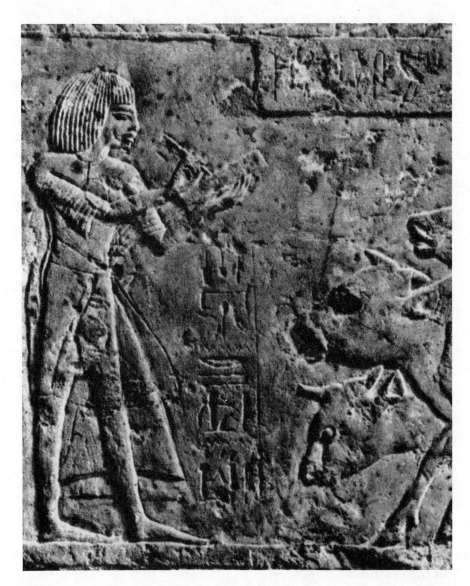

FIGURE 5.2: A right-handed scribe counts cattle around 2,500 BC in Egypt.

shown in figure 5.2. This is a bas-relief taken from the wall of a pyramid and was made around 2500 B.C. It shows a right-handed Egyptian scribe (or tax collector?) counting cattle arrayed in front of him. We know that he is right-handed because he holds his stylus in his right hand.

The results of this research indicate that handedness has remained relatively constant over a broad span of history. The average over the

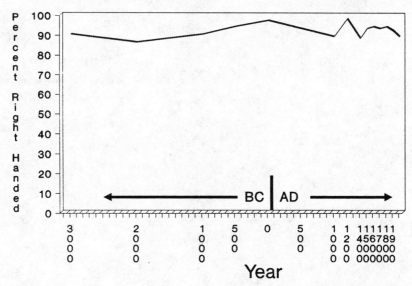

FIGURE 5.3: Right-handedness as shown in art works over a period of about 50 centuries.

more than fifty centuries we studied indicated that slightly less than 93 percent of all the people shown in drawings, paintings, and engravings are right-handed. There is virtually no change in the percentage of right-handers shown over time, as you can see in figure 5.3. In the earliest set of art works that we looked at (from 15,000 to 3000 B.C.), the distribution showed 90 percent right-handedness. In 1950, some 16,950 years after the earliest dated drawing, we find 89 percent right-handedness. Between these dates, except for some minor fluctuations, right-handedness continues at about the same level. It would seem that predisposition towards right-handedness is a genetically fixed and relatively invariant feature of the human species.

Since we conducted this study, we have learned of other data that suggests that right-handedness may go back considerably further. For example, one set of studies used a technique pioneered by the Russian anthropologist S. A. Semenov. Called *microwear analysis*, this technique uses a microscope to examine the working edges and surfaces of prehistoric tools. The polishing and wear patterns can help you to learn what a particular tool was used for, since a tool used to scrape hides will produce different patterns of wear than a tool used to scrape wood, bone, or stone. They also can tell you something about the hand that used the tool. Semenov examined Stone Age tools dating from 35,000 to 8000 B.C. and claims that about 80 percent of these were worn more heavily on the right side, suggesting that they were usually held in the right hand.[4] More recent work pushes this right-handed bias much further back into the old Stone Age. Tools recovered from an excavation at Clacton, in England, have been dated as created some 50,000 to 100,000 years ago. Using microwear analysis, it was found that some of the tools were apparently used in some form of rotary motion, accompanied by steady downward pressure. This pattern might be found in a tool used for boring holes or scraping out indentations in wood for use as a bowl. The wear patterns indicate that the rotary movements were *clockwise* in direction, which is the typical pattern of movement made by a right-hander. The anthropologist L.H. Keeley concludes, on the basis of this evidence, "The patterns suggest that the Clacton woodworkers of perhaps 200,000 years ago were consistently right handed."[5]

If we trace the evolutionary history of humans backward in time, the split between man and the apes probably occurred around 4 million years ago. The main characteristic by which anthropologists distinguish between man and the apes (or *pongids*) is the fact that the man-like *hominids* habitually walk upright on their two hind legs. The first evidence of a species that shows this form of upright walking or *bipedalism* was *Australopithecus afarensis*. The full-grown adult stood about 4 feet tall and had a pelvis that allowed it to stand in an upright posture. Its brain size was about 450 cubic centimeters, roughly the size of the brain of today's chimpanzee. The fossil remains of this species was initially discovered in South Africa in 1925 by Raymond A. Dart. Since that time evidence of its existence has been dated back some three and a half million years BP (before present times). When *Australopithecus* was originally discovered, it was widely hailed as the "missing link" between man and the apes.

The earliest species that was manlike enough to warrant the term *Homo* (meaning "man") in its name was *Homo habilis*. *Homo habilis* was taller than his predecessors, standing slightly under 5 feet tall as an adult. He still possessed the apelike jaw and skull shape of his ancestors. His most important evolutionary development, however, was his brain capacity, which ranged from 500 to 750 cubic centimeters, about half the size of our own brain. He had not yet discovered fire; however, he was an aggressive and skillful hunter. This creature appears to represent the divergence from *Australopithecus* that eventually led to modern humans. *Homo habilis* dates back to about one and a half million years BP.

Fascinating evidence suggests that, even back as far in evolutionary history as *Homo habilis* or *Australopithecus*, man may have been right-handed. This is the conclusion that is reached by N. Toth, who worked on stone flakes recovered from an excavation site near Koobi Fora in Kenya. These flakes were formed when early stone tools were shaped and sharpened by *Homo habilis*, some one and a half million years ago. The name *Homo habilis* actually translates to "handy man," a name given to recognize dexterity in fashioning stone tools. Microwear analysis suggests that these stone chips were created by right-handed tool makers.[6]

Perhaps the most fascinating evidence for right-handedness in our evolutionary predecessors comes from more than two million years ago. In the mid-1940s, Raymond Dart examined more than fifty specimens of *Parapapio broomi*, a baboon. Many of these had apparently been killed by murderous australopithecines. Although smaller than the baboon, *Australopithecus* did have one major advantage. The australopithecines apparently were weapon users. The habitat occupied by *Australopithecus* was probably open grassland, dotted with trees and near rivers or lakes that supplied water and some rich vegetation. *Australopithecus* was probably not intelligent enough to fashion stone tools or weapons; however, it appears that they did collect and use naturally occurring implements that could be employed for useful purposes. It appears that the australopithecine weapons were either naturally shaped rocks, bones such as the thigh bone of an antelope, or perhaps thick sticks that had fallen or were pulled from trees. These could be used as clubs to attack other species, such as baboons who might be competitors for food, without any further shaping required. When the skulls of baboons killed by *Australopithecus* were examined, Dart found that most of them showed damage to the front left. This is exactly the pattern of damage that would be sustained if a right-handed australopithecine were to swing a club at a baboon who was defensively facing his attacker. Just as an aside, it is interesting to note that Dart also examined the skull of an adolescent *Australopithecus*. This skull showed evidence that it had been struck just to the left of the point of the jaw, probably by a weapon. As the only weapon users of that time were australopithecines, it is likely that the killer was from the same species. Thus the earliest evidence of humankind's predisposition to murder members of his own species comes from the hands of a right-handed assailant.

All of this evidence—the historical art records studied by our lab that takes us back fifty centuries BP and the fossil record that extends our line of evidence some two or three million years into our evolutionary past—suggests that human beings have always been right-handed. Such evidence is consistent with genetic determination of handedness, at least at the species level. Thus we can conclude that right-handedness is a *genetically fixed* trait. What about left-handedness, though? Is it some form of genetic variation, some form of mutation, or some failure in the genetic coding for right-handedness? To answer this we must consider the evidence that there may be a *genetically variable* form of handedness that might explain why some people are left-handed while the majority are right-handed.

Is Left-Handedness Inherited?

The conclusion that we reached on looking at the evolutionary and historical evidence suggests that right-handedness is inherited, in the same way that the tendency to have five fingers on each hand or the structural characteristics that allow us to walk upright are inherited. In essence, the evidence suggests that right-handedness is one of the genetically fixed characteristics associated with being human. Many people, however, have suggested that tendencies toward left-handedness can be inherited as part of a genetically variable set of traits that make one individual different from another. This is clearly the rationale behind the interest in left-handedness "running in families" as in the Kerr family that we spoke of earlier. Thus the real questions becomes, "Are left- and right-handers different from each other at the genetic level?" The answer to this question, however, is neither simple nor clear. The reason for this lack of clarity has to do with the psychology of the scientist as well as the complexity of the problem itself.

When looking for a genetically variable trait in people, two methods of study are generally used. The first involves studying families of individuals to see if and how the characteristics of the parents are genetically passed on to the children. The second method involves the study of twins. Thus, if we were interested in the inheritance of eye color, we might use a family study to see what color eyes the children would have if both Mom and Dad are blue-eyed, or if one was brown-eyed, and so forth. We might use a twin study to see if identical twins are more likely to have the same eye color.

Both methods of looking for genetic factors have their disadvantages. The twin study technique is particularly difficult because it involves searching for pairs of twins, which are not all that common. Once the twins are found, a series of expensive blood tests should be done in order to determine the degree of their genetic similarity. Family studies are a bit easier, at least in terms of finding individuals to test. Families with children are quite common, and many are approachable and willing to participate in scientific studies. The problem associated with family studies is simply the amount of time and money that must be expended. These are very expensive studies to conduct because many families must be tested, often through field work, where you must go out to the family's residence to do the testing, rather than have them suffer the inconvenience traveling to your laboratory. Testing is often spread out over a long period of time or must be done in the evenings or on weekends when the parents are at home rather than at work. For example, our first family study took nearly three years to accumulate enough data to allow us to start analyzing the results. Perhaps it would be useful to take you through one of our own family studies of handedness to see what is involved and what the typical results of such studies are.

In 1976, Clare Porac and I took stock of the results of our first family study of sidedness.[7] The results had not been completely satisfying, although the data did look like that obtained by previous researchers who had looked at family patterns of handedness. The reason that the results were "not satisfying" is that the outcome was not clear. In terms of handedness, for instance, there were *hints* that *maybe* there *might* be *some* genetic involvement in the transmission of handedness. None of the results were clear enough to allow us to be sure, yet there were some *trends* in the data. In science a "trend" is probably best interpreted as a weak tendency for the data to confirm what you expected in the first place. A trend is just enough of a tendency to make you suspect that your hypothesis might be correct, but not enough to convince anybody else (except another "true believer"). A trend is to the researcher like bait is to a hungry fish. One has a tendency to snap at it before studying it carefully. I suppose that this was the case with us. The trend seemed to promise that a clear answer about whether handedness is inherited might be "just over the horizon." This hint, plus the fact that we had already spent three years of our lives on the question, served to convince us that the best course of action would be to conduct *another family study*. This time we would measure a larger sample of families, use more stable and more extensive measures, and find a much clearer answer.

Nobody scolded us about "investing good money after bad," or warned us that the reason that the results of our previous study might have consisted of merely "muddy" trends could be that the situation was more complicated than we thought it was. Besides, there was such a long tradition of belief in the inheritance of handedness and so many assertions in the scientific literature that handedness was genetically transmitted that it undoubtedly had to be true. We certainly entered this research project with the strong feeling that handedness was a genetically variable behavior trait and that our task was simply to do what no one else had done convincingly, namely, to *demonstrate* that left-handers came were created by some combination of their parent's genes acting to determine their handedness. It was just a matter of more precise measurement, wasn't it?

The task of organizing a family study is really herculean. This one involved contacting around 2,000 Canadian families in our immediate area. From this group we eventually ended up with 459 families from which we had taken data from the mother, the father, and at least one child.[8] The whole procedure took another three years. It also completely bankrupted my two research grants so that I ended up financing my next year's research by using money "borrowed" against future research funds from the university. What were the results of our expensive "rematch" with the question of the inheritance and handedness? The results were virtually the same as for the first study. We had "hints" and "trends." There was the very definite result that if your mother was left-handed your chance of being left-handed was approximately doubled. Dad's handedness didn't seem to matter that much.

These results are similar to the results that many other family studies of handedness have produced. In fact, I have surveyed the existing scientific literature and have found eleven family studies on handedness, published between 1913 and 1982, that had large enough numbers of families to make comparisons meaningful.[9] The results of this survey are shown in figure 5.4. Notice that if neither of your parents is left-handed, your chance of being left-handed is about one out of ten. If Dad alone is left-handed, your chances remain pretty much the same. If Mom alone is left-handed, however, your chances of being left-handed are doubled, so that the likelihood of your being left-handed is now two out of ten. If both Mom and Dad are left-handed, however, your prospect of being left-handed rises to between three and four chances out of ten. This is considerably higher than normal, but notice that even with two left-handed parents the probability that you will be right-handed is still twice as large as the probability that you will be left-handed. Even under these "genetically optimal" circumstances, the chance that you will be right-handed is still six or seven out of ten.

If you believe that left-handedness is genetically determined, this kind of data is enough to give you a headache. It certainly appears that if you

Parent and Child Handedness
(based upon 11 family studies)

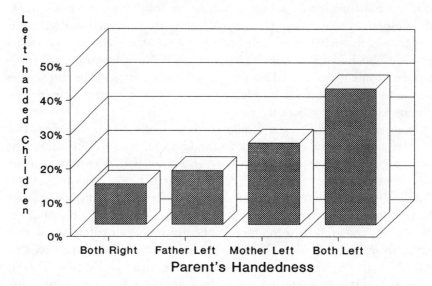

FIGURE 5.4: How handedness of children is affected by the handedness of their parents.

have left-handed parents, or at least a left-handed mother, your chances of being left-handed are increased, which suggests that there is some genetically variable contribution to handedness. Unfortunately, the change in the likelihood that you will be left-handed, especially when you have two left-handed parents, simply is not as large as the science of genetics would predict if we were dealing with a simple inherited trait. Let me show you why.

It is always best to start with the simplest case possible. Let's begin with a theory of genetic transmission of handedness based upon the sort of mechanism that you learned about in high school biology. You might remember your science teacher telling you about the Austrian abbot Gregor Mendel. He grew peas in his garden and carefully cross-pollinated them to see how certain characteristics (such as wrinkly vs smooth skin or normal vs dwarf size) were inherited. Unfortunately, this straight-forward application of genetics to handedness just doesn't work.

Suppose that we have two types of handedness genes, called R for right-handedness and L for left-handedness. This would be the simplest genetic system. All genes come in pairs, and everybody would then get one handedness gene from Mom and one from Dad to give the two handedness genes. Clearly, then if you have a genetic makeup of RR (that's a right-handed gene from each parent) you are right-handed, and a genetic makeup of LL (a left-handed gene from each parent) you are left-handed. What if you get an R from one parent and an L from the other? This RL (or *heterozygous*) case requires an additional assumption. Because there are so many more right-handers, we will assume that right-handedness is dominant, and all you need is one R gene to make you right-handed. If you have an RL gene pair, you will be right-handed and not distinguishable from an RR person, much as if you have one gene for blue eyes and one for brown you will be brown-eyed since the brown eye gene in dominant. Notice that, in this kind of genetic setup, the only way that you can be left-handed is if both of your handedness genes are L.

Our problems with this simple genetic model come about when we consider certain types of parents and their children. Suppose that both of your parents are left-handed, which can only be the case if each parent has two left-handed genes. If each parent is LL, when they come to transmit a handedness gene to you, the only type of handedness gene that they have to pass onto their offspring is an L. So with two left-handed parents you must have a genetic makeup that is also LL. If the straightforward genetic model is correct, you will, of course, also be left-handed. In fact, every child that these left-handed parents have should be left-handed. Unfortunately the data shown in figure 5.4 demonstrate that this is not the case. Even with two left-handed parents your chance of being left-handed is only around 35 percent, rather than the 100 percent that this simple genetic model predicts. If we take these data at face value, the idea of simple genetic transmission of handedness has failed.

A number of scientists have tried to salvage the idea of genetic determination of handedness by proposing more complex theories, or theories involving "neutral" or "wild card" genes rather than only genes for left or right-handedness. Such theories still require a lot of additional fiddling (called "parameter fitting" in scientific terminology) to make them fit in each case and have not proven to be very convincing.[10] Furthermore, they run into problems when we deal with the strongest test of any genetic model for any trait, namely, the case of twins.

Handedness in Twins

Twins are nature's gift to genetic scientists because they are, at least in theory, the perfect laboratory for studying the inheritance of any trait.

The important thing to recognize is that there are two types of twins. The first type are what are known as *fraternal twins*. Fraternal twins come about when two egg cells are fertilized simultaneously by two different sperm cells. Since different eggs and sperm are involved, these are really brothers and/or sisters growing together in the same womb. While they are twins, they are actually no different from any other pair of siblings genetically. On average, they will have 50 percent of their genes in common, and they might resemble each other just as family members do.

It is the other form of twins that are special. These are the *identical twins*. They begin as a single egg cell and a single sperm. After fertilization the egg begins to divide into cells as the growth process begins. At the first or second cell division, when there are only two to four cells in embryo, on some rare occasions the "glue" that sticks the cells together becomes unstuck, resulting in two separate embryos in the womb. Each of these new embryos can develop into a complete and intact human being. These two human beings now developing in the womb, however, are quite special. Because genetic material is duplicated in every cell, when these one-or two-celled embryos separate from each other, they contain identical copies of their original genetic codes. In other words, these two individuals, who will develop into identical twins, will have *exactly the same* genetic makeup. They will have 100 percent of their genes in common.

The differences between identical and fraternal twins are obvious. Identical twins are always the same sex (since sex is genetically determined), while fraternal twins may be the same sex or may be one male and one female. Identical twins will look virtually identical, with the same eye color, hair color, and even incredibly similar fingerprint patterns. They will usually be the same size and will age similarly, often with the same wrinkle pattern, and will even have similar IQs and personality types. Fraternal twins will be more similar to each other than to strangers, but no more similar than most other brother and/or sister pairs.

For the scientist interested in genetics, then, twins are the perfect test subjects. Anything that is genetically determined ought to be virtually the same in identical twins. Genetically determined features should be more variable in fraternal twins than in identical twins. Of course, fraternal twins ought to be more similar than unrelated individuals since they do have 50 percent of their genes in common, and ought to resemble each other in the way that siblings do. Actually we would expect fraternal twins to be more similar to each other than most brother and/

or sister pairs because they share an identical environment and identical growing and rearing conditions. After all, they grew up in the same womb and shared the same parents, home, food, school, friends, and other aspects of the environment. They are always the same age and have the same cultural and historical influences working on them. For the genetic researcher, then, looking for genetically variable traits, the perfect comparison would be between identical twins, who have genes that are perfect copies of one another and who have grown up in identical environments, and fraternal twins who, although sharing a common environment, have only some genes in common.

Now let us look at the case of twins and handedness. To estimate the effects of genetics on handedness, we have to look at the number of twin pairs that have the *same* handedness. For a simple genetic model where there are two genes, R for right-handedness and L for left-handedness, the prediction is quite easy. For identical twins, if one member of the pair has an RR makeup then the other does, too. The same goes for either RL or LL. Thus the prediction is that we should find that all identical twin pairs (100 percent) should have identical handedness. For fraternal twins, the predicted number of twin pairs with the same handedness is around 83 to 86 percent. As a comparison, we might look at random (nonrelated) individuals. If we randomly selected pairs of unrelated people off the street, the number of pairs predicted to have the same handedness would be around 78 percent.

A number of studies have looked at handedness in twins. I was able to find thirteen that met reasonable standards of scientific measurement, included both identical and fraternal twins, and supplied enough data to compute the number of twin pairs who had the same handedness.[11] These studies covered a period of time from 1933 to 1985. The results of this survey of studies are shown in figure 5.5.

One glance at figure 5.5 shows that we have a real problem with a simple genetic model. Where as we predicted that 100 percent of the identical twin pairs should have the same handedness, the data show that only 76 percent have the same handedness. For fraternal twins we predicted that around 83 to 86 percent of the twin pairs would have the same handedness, yet we find again that only 76 percent of the pairs have the same handedness. Both of these sets of values are virtually the same as would be expected on the basis of chance pairings of unrelated individuals, around 78 percent.

More complex models of genetic determination of handedness don't do much better at predicting the handedness of twins. They always end up predicting more twin pairs with identical handedness than the actual

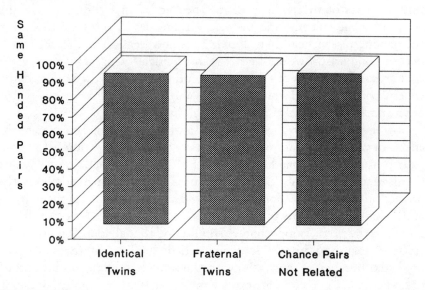

FIGURE 5.5: Number of same handed pairs of twins does not differ between identical and fraternal twins, and is the same as chance.

data ever produces. After considering some of these more complex genetic theories of handedness Michael C. Corballis, now of the University of Aukland in New Zealand, was forced to conclude, "On the grounds of parsimony, then, adding further assumptions to genetic model can only strengthen the case against it, and in favor of the much simpler hypothesis that the distribution of handedness among twins is simply a matter of chance."[12]

In other words, using the best naturally occurring laboratory available to test hypotheses that genetically transmitted variability exists in a trait, namely, the examination of data from twins, we fail to find any evidence for the inheritance of handedness.

Are Any Aspects of Handedness Inherited?

Consideration of the data on handedness seems to suggest that individuals who are right-handed do not differ in their genetic makeup from individuals who are left-handed. However, we should not immediately discard all notions of genetic variability in handedness. If we ignore the question of whether you are right- or left-handed and address ourselves to the question of just how *strongly* handed you are, the conclusions are a bit different.

In the family study conducted by our laboratory,[8] we asked whether being consistently or strongly handed, as opposed to being ambidextrous, was inherited. Here the results were much clearer, showing that an individual's consistency in handedness was related to that of both their mother and their father and that siblings also resembled each other in the strength of handedness. This result was confirmed in Philip Bryden's laboratory in Canada.[2] If your mother and father are ambidextrous or mixed-handed, you are more likely to be ambidextrous or mixed-handed. If your mother and father are strongly handed, although we can't predict on the basis of their handedness whether you will be right- or left-handed, we can predict that you will be strongly handed. Thus strongly left-handed parents may give rise to either strongly right-handed or strongly left-handed children. It is the strength, not the side, of handedness that is genetically variable.

I think that we can now safely specify how handedness is affected by genetic factors. In terms of *genetically variable traits*, the side of your handedness, that is, whether you are left- or right-handed, does not appear to be determined by your individual genetic makeup. The handedness of your parents has much less of an effect upon your handedness then most standard genetic theories would predict. Left- and right-handers do not appear to be genetically different.

Abandoning the idea that left- or right-handedness was a genetically variable trait was personally quite painful. I had spent years obtaining funding to conduct our family studies in handedness and Clare Porac and I had spent six years collecting, processing, and analyzing the data of our two family studies. I guess that I originally was a "true believer." I suppose that I really had accepted the idea that there had to be a relationship between the handedness of parents and of children. To give up a cherished hypothesis is as painful as losing a close friend. It leaves a void in your thinking that cries out to be filled, but filling it is not always easy.

Although the side of your handedness is not inherited, whether you are strongly handed or ambidextrous *is* a genetically variable trait. Children of ambidextrous parents are more likely to be ambidextrous.

It is clear, however, that right-handedness is *a genetically fixed trait*, carried in the genes and normally expressed as a characteristic of humans, much as having two eyes or having the ability to walk upright is.

The historical and evolutionary evidence suggests that all human beings probably carry the genetic coding to be right-handed.

This last conclusion caused me the most difficulty. If all human beings were genetically targeted to be right-handed, why do we have left-handers? Perhaps left-handedness should be looked upon as a failure to reach right-handedness, rather than as a different expression of handedness. Thinking in this way began to alter my outlook on the issue of how particular forms of handedness come into existence. Specifically, it caused me to reformulate the problem to ask, "What could have happened to make the expression of right-handedness run amok? If right-handedness is encoded in every human being's genetic makeup, doesn't it mean that something must have gone wrong to produce left-handers?" This was not a pleasant line of thought, and rather than pursue it immediately, I turned back to more basic considerations. Perhaps the answer to all of my questions would be clearer if I know more about what mechanisms control handedness and which specific neurological factors are involved. I began to consider the work suggesting that handedness is somehow involved with the organization of the brain. Perhaps it would be good to look at those speculations about "left-brained" and "right-brained" individuals, for any clues as to what controls handedness and therefore what could intervene to seize control from the normal right-sided pattern.

6

The Two Brains

It was one of those TV interviews that I occasionally allow myself to be roped into. The university encourages faculty members to participate in this sort of thing, under the questionable assumption that any publicity about research done on campus may provide a positive public feeling toward universities in general, and our university in particular. The president of our university believes that this may eventually help to win public support when the next round of government budget allocations (and cuts) inevitably arrives.

All that I had been told about this particular show was that it was nationally broadcast and that the interview would be done in typical talk-show style. I would be talking about left-handedness, and the specific question they wanted me to address was whether it is a good idea to try to switch the handedness of naturally left-handed children. I didn't know much about the show's host who was to interview me, as it was not a show that I normally watched, although I had been told that he was left-handed himself.

I arrived at the studio, had a cup of bad coffee, and stopped to have some makeup put on. (As I go progressively more bald, TV people seem more likely to claim that the lights glare on my rising forehead, and they cover it with a powdery stuff to remove the shiny surfaces.) I was then placed at the edge of the set and told how I was to enter, where I was to sit, and that the interview would last about ten or twelve minutes. My introduction was read by the host, who assured his audience that I was going to tell them "about the troubles that we lefties have."

He rose to greet me as I walked across the set, I shook hands with him and sat in my designated seat, and I looked at him, waiting for the interview to begin. Instead of sitting back down, however, he came around to the front of the set, stood in front of one of the cameras, and took off his jacket. Next, to my amazement, he pulled off his tie and unbuttoned his shirt. Underneath was a brightly colored T-shirt, which announced in large letters, "LEFT-HANDERS ARE RIGHT MINDED!"

While the audience cheered, I began to map out in my head the likely course that this interview would take. It would probably go the way that so many had gone before. . . .

"Dr. Coren, isn't it true that left-handers are more creative than right-handers because they use the right side of their brain, which thinks globally, instead of the lockstep, straight-line logic of the left side of the brain that right-handers use?"

"Aren't left-handers more musical than right-handers?"

"Why are there so many left-handed artists? . . . baseball players? . . . actors? . . . oddballs?"

"Isn't it true that there are more left-handed geniuses?"

"Don't left-handers have a better sense of humor?"

"Aren't left-handers more sensitive and emotional?"

"Is it true that left-handers are better lovers?"

Perhaps they would even trot out that quote from the eminent neurosurgeon from Los Angeles, Joseph E. Bogen, who reportedly said, "Right-handers are a bunch of chocolate soldiers. If you've seen one, you've seen 'em all. But left-handers are something else again!"

Where did all of this begin? Is there any truth to the notion that the brain organization of left-handers is different from that of right-handers? Even if so, does it make left-handers more likely to be sensitive, musical, artistic, caring, creative, smart, or athletic? Let's consider the actual history of research on this issue.

The Speaking Brain

Most people tend to think of the brain as a single structure. Actually, the brain is vertically divided into two parts, called *hemispheres*, which are tightly packed together inside the skull. If you removed the top of the skull and looked down on the hemispheres of the brain, they would look much like the halves of a walnut, packed together inside their shell.

These two halves of the brain are connected by several large bundles of nerve fibers, which provide the neural conduits by which the two hemispheres communicate with each other.

Anatomically, each hemisphere looks like the mirror image of the other, but, much like the hands, which are also physical mirror images of each other, the hemispheres function differently. The first evidence of these differences probably arose by courtesy of primitive military actions. A blow to the left side of the head would frequently cause paralysis to the right side of the body, so that the victim might not be able to move the right hand or leg. Damage to the right side of the head produced the opposite effect, with left-side paralysis. This suggested that there is *crossed* or *contralateral* control of the body, with the left hemisphere controlling the right hand and the right hemisphere controlling the left.

Around 1810 a new craze was sweeping the civilized world. It began with the work of Franz Joseph Gall, who was then in Vienna and later moved to Paris. He had the notion that particular parts of the brain were responsible for particular complex human characteristics such as *love, trust, courage, destructiveness,* and the like. This belief began when Gall was still a boy, when he had been struck by what he though seemed to be a relationship between the mental characteristics of his classmates and the shapes of their skulls. Years later, when he began his scientific career, he began mapping out the locations of these particular "brain centers" to try to verify his early impression. He reasoned that if a person showed a lot of a particular characteristic, let's say *hope*, the portion of the brain responsible for hope would expand, much like an exercised muscle. If this region of the brain were not well exercised, as in a depressive person with a permanent sense of *hopelessness*, then, like an unused muscle, the portion of the brain responsible for hope would shrink or atrophy. He next suggested that if a particular portion of the brain was well developed there would be a characteristic bump or protrusion of the skull at that place. If that region had shrunk there would be a hollow or indentation at that point. Gall collected instances of what appeared to be over- and under-development of areas of the brain as they were reflected in the shape of the skull. Thus measurements of the skulls of pickpockets in the local prison gave him the location of the part of the brain responsible for *greed*. Measures of the skulls of prominent religious people gave him the location of *veneration*, and of great political leaders gave him the location of the bump on the skull that indicated the location of *self-esteem* in the brain, and so it went. His measurements eventu-

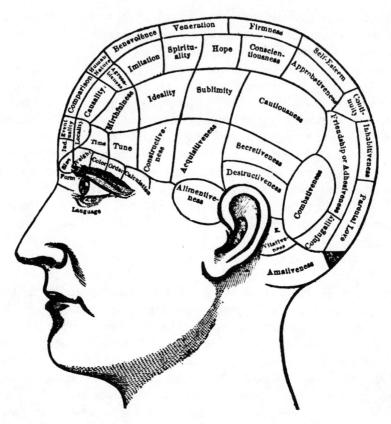

FIGURE 6.1: A typical phrenological map of the head, showing the location of various complex psychological characteristics.

ally led to the system called *phrenology*, which became quite popular in Europe and America. A typical phrenological map of the brain is shown in figure 6.1.

Phrenology was never generally accepted by scientists, even in its earliest days when its ideas might have been considered a reasonable possibility. Scientific opposition, however, did little to stop its spread. For instance, one of phrenology's most vocal advocates, Johann Kaspar Spurzheim, travelled through England and the United States, and received a warm reception from many physicians practicing in mental hospitals. In addition, an incredibly enthusiastic popular response made phrenology a veritable craze in its time; and Gall and Spurzheim and the Fowler brothers (who set up phrenological studios in the United States) became popular and wealthy. Although no scientific credibility has been given to phrenology, its appeal has lasted into our present century. Even today there are popular magazines devoted to phrenology, and phrenological charts are often prominently on display at the booths of fortune-tellers at amusement parks and fairs.

Phrenology did serve an important scientific function, however, It changed the thinking of psychologists, psychiatrists, and other scientists so that they began to think of the brain as the major controller of behavior. In addition, it focused researchers on the possibility that specific locations in the brain might be responsible for controlling specific behaviors. Out of this milieu, findings about the different functions of the two hemispheres emerged.

The first report of differences between the left and right halves of the brain was made in 1836. Marc Dax, a rather obscure country doctor, attended a medical meeting in Montpellier, France. In a long career as a general practitioner Dax had observed many patients who suffered from loss of speech ability. This condition, known technically as *aphasia*, had been recognized for a long time. There were even reports that have been traced back to Ancient Greece, which described a loss of speech after damage to the brain. What Dax had noticed, however, was that there appeared to be a systematic relationship between the loss of speech and the side of the brain that had been injured. After observation of more than forty patients with aphasia, he couldn't find a single case that didn't involve damage to the left hemisphere of the brain. On the basis of these results, he suggested that each half of the brain controls different functions, and the major function controlled by the left hemisphere is speech. It appears that Dax did not actually present a formal paper to the medical congress, but rather he distributed a report to a few medical colleagues attending the conference. Apparently his colleagues were not excited by these results and quickly forgot them. It was not until a quarter of a century had passed that the relationship between the control of speech and the left hemisphere was independently rediscovered.

The rediscovery was announced in August of 1861 by Paul Broca, who was already a distinguished neurosurgeon, anatomist, and physical anthropologist. He presented a paper to the Anatomical Society of Paris that described a patient called "Tan." This was not the patient's name, but because he was suffering from aphasia it was the only articulate sound he could make. Written communication was ruled out because his right hand was paralyzed, which meant that he could not write his name. Shortly after Broca observed Tan's speech deficit, Tan died. A postmortem showed that he had suffered damage to a frontal section of the left hemisphere. By 1863 Broca had examined eight additional patients, all of whom were aphasic with various degrees of speech difficulty and all of whom had brain damage in this region of the left hemisphere. This report stirred a great deal of interest and speculation about the likelihood that the left hemisphere was specialized for speech functions.

Broca also began to speculate about the relationship between brain organization for speech and brain organization to control the hand. He suggested, "Just as in the case right-handers, the left hemisphere directs the movements of writing, drawing and other fine movements, so do we speak with the left hemisphere."[1] But now he expanded the question to ask whether, if right-handers speak from the left hemisphere of the brain, what about left-handers? Here he theorized, "One can conceive that there may be a certain number of individuals in whom the natural pre-eminence of the convolutions of the right hemisphere reverses the order of the phenomenon which I have just described."[2] These individuals will be left-handers, of course. Thus, while the majority of people are right-handed but are "left-handers of the brain," left-handers will be "right-brained." Broca then suggested the rule that, in every person, the hemisphere that controls speech is on the side opposite to that person's preferred hand. *Broca's Rule* survived well into the twentieth century and is often stated as a fact by journalists and other people when the discuss the relationship between handedness and the organization of the brain.

Actually, Broca had isolated only one of the speech centers in the left hemisphere. This region, called *Broca's area* after its discoverer, is responsible for the organization and production of speech. Damage to this area results in a disruption of the patient's ability to *produce* speech; however, the patient's ability to *understand* other people's speech is unharmed. Another researcher, Karl Wernicke, discovered an area further back and lower in the brain, which seems to be specifically involved in the understanding of speech. Damage to this area (*Wernicke's area*, of course) results in a disturbance of the patient's ability to understand the speech of others. Such patients can produce words and sentences that sound like language but often are totally lacking in any comprehensible meaning. Both Broca's area and Wernicke's area are pictured in figure 6.2. They share two important common features. First, they are both vital to our ability to use language; second, they are both usually found in the left hemisphere of the brain.

Not long after the discovery that speech functions are usually in the left hemisphere, the concept of a *dominant hemisphere* became accepted. This notion of *cerebral dominance* probably comes from the British neurologist John Hughlings Jackson, who proposed the idea of a "leading" or dominant hemisphere. Specifically he wrote, "The two brains cannot

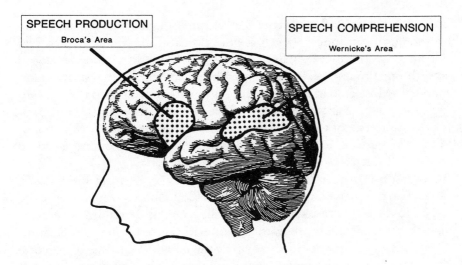

FIGURE 6.2: The speech control areas in the left hemisphere of the brain.

be mere duplicates. . . . For these processes [of speech], of which there are none higher, there must surely be one side which is leading." He finishes by concluding, "that in most people the left side of the brain is the leading side—the side of the so-called will, and that on the right is the automatic side."[3] Notice that there has been a very subtle shift of focus as we went from Broca to Jackson. Now the left hemisphere is not simply the hemisphere of speech, but rather the *controlling* hemisphere of the brain. This dominant hemisphere is responsible for the expression of will and perhaps for consciousness itself; it also controls our naturally dominant right hand. The localization of a global function such as the "will" in a particular part of the brain is an idea that would certainly have made Gall and the other phrenologists smile with a satisfied air of confirmation.

The Mirror Cracks

The first question to ask, then, is whether the brain of the left-hander is simply a mirror image of the brain of the right-hander, as Broca's Rule suggests. If so, we should find that speech centers in left-handers (and maybe their consciousness and their will) are located in the right hemisphere. This would certainly confirm Broca's speculations.

Some initial reports seemed to demonstrate the principle of mirror-imaged brains in left-handers. Some neuropsychological clinics did find some left-handers who suffered loss of speech (aphasia) after an injury to the right hemisphere, which is what Broca's Rule would predict. Unfortunately, there were also reports of left-handers who developed speech impairments after damage to the left hemisphere, just like right-handers. More embarrassing were cases in which damage to the relevant portions of the right hemisphere of left-handers, that is, to the regions of the right side of the brain that would correspond to Broca's area or Wernicke's area in a mirror image of the right-hander's brain, produced no speech disruptions.

A reason for this puzzling pattern of results comes from Juhn Wada, a psychiatrist at the University of British Columbia in Vancouver, Canada. He developed a technique that allows us to determine where the speech control centers are in the brain, without requiring us to wait for brain-damaged patients to show up at the clinic. Wada has been working with patients who have chronic epilepsy. When this disease can not be controlled with drugs, surgery is often called for. It is important to determine in which hemisphere of the brain the patient's speech functions are located, to prevent damage to these important centers.

Wada's testing procedure uses a drug called *sodium amytal* to literally shut down one side of the brain. To do this, a small tube is inserted into the carotid artery. There are actually two carotid arteries, one on each side of the neck. The carotid artery on the right side provides the major source of blood to the right hemisphere of the brain, while that on the left provides the blood for the left hemisphere. By selection of the appropriate carotid artery, injections can be used to carry chemicals directly to only one side of the brain. The drug sodium amytal is a barbiturate, part of the same chemical family used in most powerful sleeping pills. Injecting this drug into the carotid artery puts the brain to sleep, but because each artery supplies blood to only one hemisphere, only one half of the brain goes to sleep for any one injection.

Watching this test is really quite a dramatic experience. In the beginning the patient is lying down. The neurosurgeon asks the patient to hold both arms up in the air and to count backwards from 100 by threes. As the patient begins intoning "100 . . . 97 . . . 94 . . . 91 . . . ," the drug is injected through the tube in the artery. The effects occur in less than half a minute. First, the arm opposite to the side of the sodium amytal injection begins to droop and finally falls limply to the patient's side. This serves to confirm that each arm is controlled by the hemisphere on the opposite side. More importantly for the neurosurgeon, it confirms that the drug has reached the target hemisphere of the brain and has, in effect, turned its conscious activities off.

At about the same time that the arm is going limp, the patient's count-ing will stop. If the drug has reached the hemisphere that controls speech, the patient will remain silent for as long as the drug is active. Typical doses used in this sort of test will result in a speechless interval of 3 to 5 minutes. If you ask the patient questions or request continued counting, you do get some response indicating that the patient is not totally unconscious. Such patients will appear to be paying attention to you, will follow you with their eyes, turn their head, move an arm toward you, or even open and close their mouth. The important thing is that no speech is produced, and the patient doesn't seem to fully understand spoken instructions like, "Wave your left arm up and down." If the drug has reached the hemisphere that doesn't control speech, the initial pause in the patient's counting will last only around 15 or 20 seconds and then the patient will continue counting: "88 . . . 85 . . . 82 . . . ." If you now interrupt the count and ask a few questions, the patient responds with little difficulty and follows spoken instructions with ease. Wada's test, then, allows you to rapidly determine which hemisphere controls an individual's speech functioning.[4]

There is another technique that allows us to test which hemisphere controls speech. It involves a process sometimes use to treat severe symp-toms of psychological depression: An electric current is passed through the brain of the patient, using a set of electrodes attached to the scalp. The result is a series of convulsions that look much like an attack of epilepsy. For reasons not fully understood as yet, this procedure often produces dramatic improvement in severely depressed individuals. This procedure is not without costs, however. Most obvious are periods of confusion and loss of memory after treatment. At the National Hospital in Queen Square, London, an alternate procedure has been under study. Instead of passing the current through both sides of the brain at once, the current is applied to only one hemisphere at a time, alternat-ing sides on each successive treatment day. It has been suggested that this alternation does not change the effectiveness of the treatment for depression, but it does reduce the risk that memory may be impaired. Not only does this procedure reduce unwanted side effects, but it also provides a means for testing which side of the brain has the speech control. Immediately after the treatment with electric current to one hemisphere, as soon as the patient appears to be aware and capable of responding, some very simple questions, really tests of language compre-hension, are given. The side of the brain that received the therapeutic shock will be only semiconscious and somewhat disoriented for several minutes while the side that did not receive the shock is relatively unaffected. If the patient can answer the questions, then language is present in the side of the brain that has *not* been treated.[5]

The data from both the sodium amytal and the shock experiments not only confirmed some hypotheses about the way in which the two hemispheres of the brain function but also provided some surprises. It confirmed that most people have their language functions controlled by the left hemisphere of the brain. It also showed that a minority of people did have their language control in the right hemisphere. One of the surprises was that there were some people who had language functions on *both* sides of the brain.

It is when we try to relate language control in the brain to handedness that things start to break down. While virtually all right-handers (97 percent) have language in their left hemisphere, we do not find the mirror-imaged brain that we expected to see in left-handers. As can be seen in Figure 6.3, seven out of ten left-handers also have language in the left hemisphere! Only two out of ten left-handers follow Broca's expected rule, with language in the right hemisphere, while about one out of ten has language on both sides. Although clearly more left-handers are using the right or both sides of the brain for language than are right-handers, to say that left-handers have mirror-imaged brains is not correct. The vast majority of left-handers are as left-brained for language as their right-handed counterparts.

Speech Dominant Hemisphere

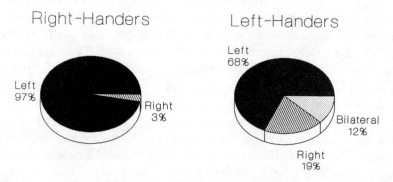

FIGURE 6.3: The side of the brain that controls language ability for both left- and right-handers is usually the left hemisphere.

The Silent Brain

Let us leave the "speaking hemisphere" and look at the other side of the coin or, more accurately, the other side of the brain. For many years the right hemisphere of the brain was referred to as the "minor" hemisphere. The second-rate reputation for the right side of the brain came about because a relatively small injury to the left hemisphere could cause massive disruptions of vital speech abilities, yet much larger injuries to the right hemisphere didn't cause any thinking or functioning impairments that were immediately obvious. This result was interpreted as meaning that the right hemisphere served to process only minor, automatic, supportive and unconscious functions.

A hint that special functions were associated with the right hemisphere of the brain was provided by John Hughlings Jackson, mentioned earlier. In 1876, he reported his observations of a patient who had developed a tumor in the right hemisphere. This patient, whose vision seemed quite normal, still had problems interpreting visual stimuli. He had great difficulty in recognizing objects, patterns, and even people. He also had problems with his spatial orientation, which showed up as a difficulty in recognizing familiar places. This led Jackson to suggest that the right hemisphere was the "leading side" for "visual ideation and thought."[3] Unfortunately, this idea seem to have been ahead of its time, and little attention was paid to it or to other reports of similar right-hemisphere deficits. Neuropsychologists were far too involved in searching for various mental functions in the "dominant" left hemisphere and had developed a tendency to ignore the right hemisphere.

Shifts in scientific outlook usually occur in two ways. The first is a slow accumulation of evidence that eventually forces researchers to change their thinking. The evolution to a new way of thought is often quite subtle, and only upon looking back over the history of the research can one notice the change of orientation. The second is a dramatic experiment or the introduction of a new research technique that sweeps away existing concept and replaces them with a new way of looking at the problem. Both processes played a role in altering our view of the right hemisphere's functions.

First, the slow accumulation of clinical evidence began to suggest that the right hemisphere might be specialized for spatial and perceptual thinking. For example, one large-scale study conducted in the 1930s examined more than 200 patients who had suffered brain damage. The magnitude of the task and the dedication this research project required are apparent from the fact that each patient was given more than 40 different tests and that testing time averaged around 19 hours for each person. Damage to the left hemisphere showed up quite clearly in poor performance on any form of test oriented toward verbal abilities, as we would have expected. However, damage to the right hemisphere did not go unnoticed.

A number of the tests measured spatial ability and the ability to do perceptual (nonverbal) thinking in assembling puzzles, copying forms, drawing figures with appropriate spatial relations, looking at incomplete patterns and either identifying or completing the figures and the like. It was here that the individuals with damage to the right hemisphere showed the greatest problems.[6] Many other studies showed similar patterns of results.

Two tasks that might cause problems for an individual with right-hemisphere damage are shown in figure 6.4. In A, the task is to synthesize or fuse the parts together to be able to identify the object from the incomplete form given. With the right hemisphere intact, it is easy to recognize the dog in this figure. In B the task is different. Here the individual must recognize the objects whose outlines are intertwined. The person with normal right-hemispheric function should see a bottle, hammer, tea cup and saucer, handbag, and so on. With a damaged right hemisphere, separating and identifying these items becomes extremely difficult or impossible. In fact, right-hemisphere damage produces such

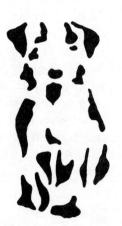 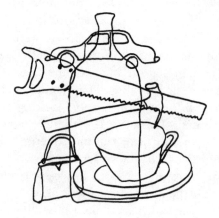

FIGURE 6.4: Part A is a task that requires an ability to fuse parts of a figure together, in order to recognize an object, while part B requires an ability to separate objects from one another. Patients with right hemisphere damage do poorly on both types of task.

reliable deficits in this kind of task that versions of this very figure are part of clinical tests now used by neuropsychologists to diagnose the nature and extent of the problems when damage to the brain (particularly the right hemisphere) is suspected.

The dramatic experimental breakthrough came when a new surgical technique for treating some forms of epilepsy was introduced. Epileptic seizures are caused by a sort of electrical storm that spreads across the cortex of the brain, causing many millions of neural cells to fire. The typical pattern of convulsions identified as a seizure happens when this wave of electrical activity sweeps over the centers that control various parts of the body, causing violent spasms and an eventual loss of consciousness. It had been discovered that when some patients with epilepsy have seizures, both hemispheres of the brain become involved, each amplifying the action of the other and contributing to the seizure. Some clinical observers had noticed that, if an epileptic had suffered damage to the pathways that connect the two hemispheres, the frequency and severity of the seizures were often reduced. This led to the introduction of the so-called *split-brain operation*, which involves cutting a band-like connection between the hemispheres called the *corpus callosum*. Corpus callosum literally means "large body," which is not an understatement, as this particular pathway involves over 200 million nerve fibers that allow the two hemispheres to communicate with each other. In addition, the surgery sometimes includes cutting some smaller connecting links between the sides of the brain, called *commissures*, that provide additional links between the hemispheres.

The first complete split-brain operations on humans, that is, one in which the corpus callosum and all of the commissures were cut, was done by two neurosurgeons in Pasadena, California, Philip Vogel and Joseph Bogen. They began a series of these operations (technically called *commissurotomies*) on about two dozen patients whose epilepsy had been shown to be untreatable using other techniques. In virtually all of these cases, the medical benefits, in terms of control of the epileptic seizures, were quite dramatic. Furthermore, the operation did not appear to have any noticeable effects on the personality, intelligence, perceptual ability, or motor performance of the patients.

Bogen and Vogel were practicing medicine not far from the California Institute of Technology, where Roger Sperry was doing neurophsychological research. Sperry had developed the split-brain operation for animals in the early 1950s. He recognized that this procedure gave researchers the opportunity to test each hemisphere of the brain separately. He also realized that such testing in human beings might provide the definitive answer as to whether there were any differences between the abilities of the two hemispheres. Therefore, Sperry's laboratory began extensive tests on the patients whom Vogel and Bogen had operated on, using techniques that ensured that each hemisphere of the brain was tested separately. The results of this testing changed our way of thinking about the brain, and won Sperry the Nobel Prize in 1981.

Sperry and another creative associate, Michael Gazzaniga, developed some ingenious techniques to allow testing of the right and left hemispheres one at a time, which involved some clever means of presenting visual information. Getting the answers from the two hemispheres also involves special considerations. When you talk to the patient, for example, you are talking to the left hemisphere. If only the right hemisphere knows the answer, it can't use the patient's voice to answer. The patient's hands, though, can provide the answers. The left hand is directly connected to the right hemisphere, and it can be used to select objects, draw, or point. This means that we can still find out what the right hemisphere is thinking about, if we are inventive enough.

Tests of split-brain patients have confirmed the fact that the right hemisphere is specialized for various visual spatial abilities. A right-handed split-brain patient retains the ability to write but is unable to draw with the right hand. The left hand can still draw, but it cannot write coherent sentences.

Differences between the visual and spatial abilities of the left and right hemispheres became more obvious as tasks were made more complex. For instance, although both the left and the right hemispheres could identify a previously seen pattern when it appeared among a group of other patterns, the left hemisphere generally failed when the pattern was shown upside down or flipped on its side. The right hemisphere seemed to have the ability to solve such problems, which involve mental manipulation and rotation of the pattern.

One striking example of the dominance of the right hemisphere for manipulation of spatial patterns comes from a black-and-white film made by Michael Gazzaniga and Roger Sperry. They were testing a patient known only as W.J. He had been the first patient operated on by Vogel and Bogen in their series of commissurotomies. The test was a fairly standard test of people's spatial ability, known as the *block design* or *Koh blocks* test. Figure 6.5 shows an example of this test. Notice that a pattern has to be constructed from a set of cubes. Each cube is made up of two solid red sides, two solid white sides, and two red-and-white sides, split along a diagonal line running from corner to corner. The pattern always fits into a square outline involving four, nine, or sixteen

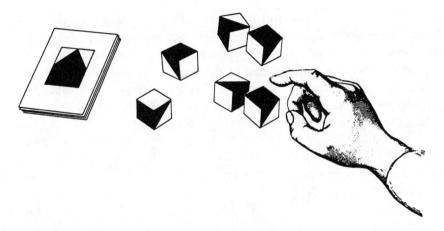

FIGURE 6.5: The block design test involves arranging a series of blocks to match a sample pattern.

blocks, but the lines marking off the edges of the individual blocks are not shown on the test pattern that the person must match. The person being tested must decide the number of blocks to be used as well as the particular location and orientation of each.

I remember sitting in an auditorium in New York City and watching a grainy bit of black and white film that Michael Gazzaniga had brought to illustrate a talk. In the first portion, the split-brain patient W.J. is shown a pattern and quickly assembles the blocks needed to match it with his left hand under the control of his right hemisphere. When the same task is given to his right hand (that is, his left hemisphere) his behavior changes dramatically. He hesitates, moves slowly and unsurely, and is clearly making some major errors in his attempt to assemble the pattern. As W.J.'s frustration level increases, suddenly from the lower edge of the screen his left hand darts into the picture to make a grab for the blocks and to try to assemble them. Only a quick movement from Gazzaniga, grasping W.J.'s hand and gently but firmly removing it from the table, prevents the left hand from taking over. The left hand, of course, was impelled to step in because the right hemisphere, which knows that it is proficient and can do this kind of task, was getting frustrated and annoyed watching the bumbling actions of the right hand, controlled by the spatially inept left hemisphere. In the end, the patient resorted to sitting on his left hand to stop this sort of interference!

One fascinating hypothesis suggests that the right hemisphere's greater ability to process and mentally manipulate visual images may form the underpinnings for other, more complex functions. For example, individuals with damage to the right hemisphere often report that they no longer dream. This is also mentioned by split-brain patients; however, it is important to remember that when talking to a split-brain patient you are speaking only to the left hemisphere. Perhaps this statement from the left hemisphere should be interpreted as meaning that the left hemisphere does not dream. It is possible that the right hemisphere still does, although it can't speak about it. This is sensible since dreams are predominantly a sequence of thoughts dominated by visual imagery.

The Singing Brain

Visual thinking and spatial ability are not the only things at which the right hemisphere seems to be the most skilled. Music appears to be a right-brain function as well. In numerous examples, individuals whose injuries to the left hemisphere have resulted in major speech disturbances have still retained the ability to sing quite clearly, with good pitch and in tune. One example, which received a good deal of publicity at the time, involved the popular singing duet of Jan and Dean. Jan Berry and Dean Torrence were part of the surfing-music craze of the early 1960s, with a number of hits with titles such as "Surf City." Another of their successful songs, "Dead Man's Curve," somewhat prophetically described a dangerous stretch of highway that was the location of many drag-racing accidents. Jan Berry suffered a motorcycle accident going around a curve on just such a road. Tragically he sustained injuries to the left hemisphere of his brain that left him with severe speech difficulties. His conversational speech was halting, stilted, slurred, and limited. Yet, he was still able to sing his hit songs well enough that he and Dean could go on tour together, performing before enthusiastic audiences, most of whom did not know that Jan was suffering from aphasia due to left-hemisphere damage. With his right hemisphere intact, he was still capable of performing his music to his former standard.

Another example, in a classical vein, comes from the French composer Maurice Ravel, who created orchestral masterpieces such as *Bolero* and *Scheherazade*. At the peak of his career, he developed aphasia due to some form of left-hemisphere damage, which severely impaired his spoken and written language abilities, although it caused no noticeable intellectual weakening. It also did not handicap Ravel's musical thinking ability. According to one report, "Recognition of tunes played before our musician is generally good and prompt. He recognizes most of the works he knew, and anyway he recognizes perfectly his own works. . . . He immediately notices the slightest mistake in the playing. . . ."[7]

Unfortunately this story does not have a happy ending. Although Ravel retained perfect clarity of musical thought, recognition of notes and musical dictation are language-like activities. Because the left hemisphere is necessary for these skills, Ravel could not write down or dictate the musical notes, and thus the productive part of his musical life was brought to an end.

The Feeling Brain

Another interesting suggestion about the "minor" hemisphere's functions is that the right hemisphere may be more involved in the recognition of emotions. For example, it is well known that damage to the left hemisphere of the brain causes what is sometimes called a *catastrophic reaction*. This is a highly emotional condition in which the patient cries, shows intense anxiety, swears, and refuses to cooperate with the medical personnel, denouncing the testing situation as "useless." This passion presumably has come spilling out of the intact right hemisphere. An interesting observation is that all this emotion usually comes forth without any mention of the obvious complaint that the patient should make, namely, that his or her right side is paralyzed.

Damage to the right hemisphere of the brain produces a different reaction, sometimes called *la belle indifference*, an indifference reaction, including denial of the symptoms. In one case I observed, the patient seemed to be blind to the fact that he was paralyzed on his left side. He told a few sorry jokes when we spoke about how he was feeling. I asked him, "Can you move your left arm for me?"

"Oh, sure," he said, "only I'm a little tired now and don't feel like moving it right now." He than lapsed into one of his attempts at humor: "Of course, if Miss Wilkinson [his nurse] comes over here I might not be so tired." All of this was said with a flat, unemotional tone and little facial expression and in marked contrast to the implied sexual content of the words.

I persisted a bit asking "Do you have any problems moving or anything like that?"

"Not really. I'm not really sick, you know, other than the side effects of these drugs that they give me which make me too tired to do much moving at all." It seemed as if, with the right hemisphere inactive, the patient was unresponsive emotionally and refused to face any emotion-laden situation.

Other evidence suggests that the right hemisphere of the brain perceives emotions more accurately than the left. In one study a group of patients with right- and left-hemisphere injuries were read some fairly neutral sentences such as, "The boy is walking the dog." Although the words expressed no emotional content, the sentences were read with an emotional intonation. The tone of the voice reading the sentence was varied so that the voice sounded happy, sad, or angry. Patients with both right- and left-brain damage understood and recalled the verbal content of these sentences with equal ability. Yet there was an important difference in their ability to recognize the emotional tone of the words. To test for emotional recognition, the patients were shown pictures of four faces, one expressing sadness, another happiness, a third anger, and the fourth indifference. When asked to point to the face whose emotion was the same as the emotion in the sentence they had been read, patients with right-hemisphere damage did much more poorly than patients with left-hemisphere injuries.[8] This suggests that the right hemisphere is more intimately involved in emotional processing than is the left hemisphere.

The Picture Blurs

A lawyer friend of my mine always complains that researchers and scientists have "one too many hands" for his needs. The problem seems to be that whenever scientists are called to provide expert testimony and information, either in court or in public hearings, as a lawyer he wants a crisp, straightforward opinion and summary of the data. Much to his dismay, however, scientists first present a set of facts that lead to a conclusion A, and then insert the caution that "on the other hand, conclusion B does have some evidence in its favor." This "other hand" is one too many for my lawyer.

You may guess that there is also an extra hand, which I am now going to reveal, to locating functions in the hemispheres of the brain. A reasonably accurate but short description of the functions of the hemispheres of the brain would say that the left hemisphere handles language functions and several other functions that are language-like, while the right hemisphere handles functions not easily translated into language, including spatial abilities, music, and perhaps emotion. *On the other hand,* things are really not quite so clear as this division would suggest.

To begin with, the right hemisphere is not completely devoid of language. Split-brain studies have shown that it can certainly understand much of what is said to it and may even have some reading ability. For example, one study of split-brain patients showed the ability of the right hemisphere to comprehend language and to go beyond given information in a logical manner. Patients were asked to retrieve particular objects hidden in a bag, with the left hand. In one case the patient was asked to take out of the bag "the fruit monkeys like best" and immediately retrieved the banana. Remember that the control of the left hand and the touch information coming from the left hand are completely processed in the right hemisphere.[9]

Under the appropriate conditions, the right hemisphere may even be able to produce language, although this language is pretty simple, compared to the abilities of the left hemisphere. Right-hemispheric language tends, for instance, to have really rotten grammar, with lots of the "little words" missing. Thus the left hemisphere might say, "I have put the book on the table," while the right hemisphere might laboriously spell out ". . . book . . . table . . . ." This resembles the language of a young child, but it is still language.

Similarly, the left hemisphere does have some spatial ability. In the split-brain subject the right hand, connected to the left hemisphere, can still point out directions and locations and indicate spatial relationships such as "above," "below," "beside," and even "left" and "right." It doesn't draw perspective or other aspects of three dimensions very well, and its representations of complex scenes aren't very good. Much as the right hemisphere handles language, however, the left can do simple spatial tasks. If you present the left hemisphere with a simple figure like a square or a triangle, the right hand can copy these quite adequately and orient them properly. The left brain can also recognize some complex patterns that it has seen before when they are shown among a group of unfamiliar patterns.

Just to add some more fingers to the "other hand", many abilities seem to involve both hemispheres. For instance, I pointed out that musical abilities seem to be in the right hemisphere, but that is only half the story. The ability to sing the proper notes (pitch) and to convey emotional shading in the music (intonation) are certainly right-hemisphere functions, but complex rhythm is a left-hemisphere function. The right hemisphere's rhythmic ability is limited to "keeping the beat" in a simple repetitive manner, especially when both hands are involved. You can demonstrate this for yourself by tapping out a steady beat with one hand while tapping out a more complex one (try the familiar *boom-da-di-ya-ya-boom-boom* rhythm) with the other. Most people find that this easy when the right hand handles the complex rhythm and the left the beat, but often leads to a garbled mess of taps and thunks when the left hand is given the complex series and the right marks the time.

An example of how the left hemisphere interacts in musical production comes from Ludmil Mavlov, who studied the case of a musician who suffered a stroke that damaged his left hemisphere and left him aphasic. In addition to language problems, it left him completely unable to deal with rhythms. He could imitate single tones and melodies, but they lacked proper rhythm. This loss of rhythmic ability was so complete that it make no difference whether the rhythm that he was to try to imitate was described to him by sound, sight, or touch.[10] As music, as we know it, involves all three qualities, pitch, intonation, and rhythm, to say that music is in the right hemisphere is, clearly to oversimplify the situation. Perhaps we should say that the right hemisphere is "more important" in music, with two out of three elements controlled there.

Our discussion of music brings up the final "hand," which is that normal brains do not operate as isolated hemispheres. Remember that the corpus callosum connecting the two hemispheres contains over 200 million nerve fibers. That gives an opportunity for a lot of communication between the hemispheres. There is plenty of evidence that such communication takes place continually. In the intact brain we *can* talk to the right hemisphere quite fluently, because the right hemisphere conveys its information to the left hemisphere, which in turn, converts the information to language. Looking at the "other hand," it seems as if there is more of an overlap between the functioning of the two hemispheres than has generally been pointed out in popular discussions.

Our next task is obvious: to connect a left and a right hand back onto this double brain. Our goal is to see whether having a left hand attached to a hemisphere with different functional skills than the hemisphere attached to the right hand means differences in the behavior of left- and right-handers. First, we may have to clear up some basic misunderstandings that seem to have filtered into most people's minds about handedness and brainedness, but which are often treated as "common knowledge."

7

Psycho-Neuro-Astrology

S omtimes being a scientist is more of a burden than remaining bliss-fully ignorant of the facts. As one of Christopher Hampton's charac-ters says in *The Philanthropist,* "You know very well that unless you're a scientist, it's much more important for a theory to be shapely than for it to be true." Scientists are more likely to hold to the words of the fictional Sherlock Holmes, who said, "It is a capital mistake to theorize before one has data."[1] Give a theory to one of us, and we immediately start to evaluate the facts that support it. This makes us appear to be cautious, dull, tedious individuals, especially when the newest intellec-tual fads and theories are discussed. Caution also robs us of feelings of insight and enthusiasm that the nonscientist often gets from reading the science pages of the local newspaper describing the latest new theory of the mind or the newest "cure" for cancer, Alzheimer's disease, the com-mon cold, or dishpan hands. While theories fly where they want to, the facts seem to crawl along with their bellies to the ground. Unfortunately scientists must first catch the facts before they can look to the sky. The nonscientist walks with his head held high and his eyes riveted on the theory, only occasionally pausing to catch his balance when he trips over the obstinate and disconfirming facts that litter the ground and seem to be always getting in the way. The nonscientist has much more fun and is often more optimistic and enthusiastic than the scientist craw-ling along with his nose to the ground.

Right now an immensely popular movement has caught the attention of educators, artists, management advisors, and the general public. Its stated goal involves "unlocking the elusive qualities of the right hemisphere." This movement has so gained in momentum that in everyday conversation one may hear comments such as, "Perhaps this problem will require a little bit of creative right-brain thinking to solve it." In a article subtitled "Fad of the Year," Daniel Goleman, a psychologist and associate editor of *Psychology Today,* was moved to ask, "Is our romance with the right side of the brain too hot not to cool down?"[2] This *right brain movement,* based upon a particular set of theories about the operation of the brain, has expanded to include a set of beliefs about differences between left- and right-handers.

Let's look at this movement and the tenets underlying it. We will start with our eyes on the theories flitting about in the sky, but, as I am a scientist, I will ask us eventually to glance back at the facts on the ground. The typical beliefs have been pulled together by many writers. Often the "data"—or, more accurately, the mixture of data, conclusions, and speculations—are presented with a fervor that rivals that of many charismatic religions. It usually begins with a comment such as that of astronomer and Pulitzer Prize-winning popular science writer, Carl Sagan, who said, "In my opinion the claims of borderline science pall in comparison with the hundreds of recent activities and discoveries in real science, including the existence of two semi-independent brains within each human skull. . . ."[3] The discussion usually proceeds to indicate that the two brains inside our heads correspond to our left and right hemispheres. Each of these brains has a different way of knowing and dealing with the world: its own mind, so to speak.

The basic belief of the *Two-Mind Theory* is that the left hemisphere is the brain for language, science, and mathematics. It is the hemisphere that *analyzes,* abstracts details, and plans step-by-step procedures. The left hemisphere counts, verbalizes, marks time, and is responsible for any rational statements, based upon logic, that we might formulate. The left hemisphere is sequential and linear in its thinking and can use and manipulate symbols. Thus, the left hemisphere knows that "if A is greater than B, and B is greater than C, then A must be greater than C." The left hemisphere is the objective, dispassionate, analytical mind, capable of deductive and inductive reasoning, and little else. It is the cold, hard mind of the scientist, the lawyer, the accountant, and the boring drones of regimented society.

The right hemisphere, however, is quite different. Its mode of knowing involves *synthesis* rather than analysis, which means seeing the whole picture, how all of the parts go together, rather than extracting details. The right hemisphere is responsible for "the mind's eye." It is the source of our visual imagery, our dreams, our fantasies. When you use a meta-phor you are using the skills of your right hemisphere. This part of the brain handles ideas that are too complex to describe verbally. While the left hemisphere thinks in a straight line, the right hemisphere flits from idea to idea, sometimes processing several ideas at one time. The right hemisphere is operating when we create new combinations of ideas, so it is the source of our creativity, the basis of the "Aha!" response. Our aesthetic sense belongs to the right hemisphere. Our sense of art, form, line, and space are right-brain activities. Our appreciation of music, tone, and harmony also belong to the right hemisphere. Further, we must not forget feelings in this discussion of intellectual abilities. Emo-tion and empathy are all controlled, processed, and appreciated in the right brain. The right hemisphere is the soft, empathic, sympathetic, creative, and insightful mind of the artist and musician, the intuitive problem solver, the compassionate educator, the sensitive philosopher, and the driving force behind all of the people who bring color, joy and innovation to society.

A model of the brain, according to this Two-Mind Theory, would contrast the rectangular and regular qualities of the left brain to the free-form, sparkling qualities of the right brain, much like figure 7.1.

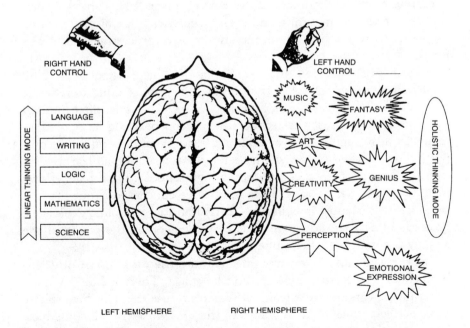

FIGURE 7.1: The Two Mind Theory conception of the organization of the functions of the hemispheres of the brain.

The Duelling Minds

Most of the people offering the Two-Mind Theory of the brain are non-scientists in various fields of endeavor. They are usually educators, management counsellors, self-help advisors, and the like. For this reason the theory is offered not as an isolated set of facts for study, but rather as the basis for direct action. The two-minders generally begin their programs with a diagnostic. They ask us to consider first those individuals who fail to show much interest or skill in music, art, or visualization and those who lack creativity or empathy. We are told also to consider those individuals who are logical and precise, who feel comfortable when the world is orderly. Such folk are not simply people who have a different life-style, a different set of tastes, habits, or cognitive skills. The two-minders assure us that these poor people are instead victims of a brain imbalance, suffering from either overreliance on or overdevelopment of their left hemisphere. Furthermore, they place the blame directly on society and our educational system.

A professor of music education wrote about the sorry results of our left-brained educational system. In the *Music Educator's Journal*, he stated that our conventional educational system has developed the left hemisphere "to the detriment of the 'whole' person." This professor says that this tends "to minimize and even atrophy right-hemisphere thinking which is responsible for music and creative processing of stimulus input."[4]

In *Today's Education*, we find a similar point. The principal of the University Elementary School of the Graduate School of Education at the University of California, Los Angeles, wrote "The [scientific] findings . . . powerfully suggest that schools have been beaming most of their instruction through a left-brained input (reading and listening) and output (talking and writing) system, thereby handicapping all learners."[5]

In the *Journal of Creative Behavior*, a high school English teacher presents the view that there is "little need to be concerned about the left-brain abilities of most individuals. The traditional schooling experience provides more than adequate practice in developing the power of the already dominant left hemisphere."[6]

But the two-minders do not offer us only the dark vision of a left-brained world, overrun by logic and language. There is hope. We are told that we can and *must* train individuals to use the right hemisphere more actively. Imagine the benefits of this training. Art will come blossoming forth because, we are assured by art professor Betty Edwards of California State University at Long Beach, "A new way of seeing will

be developed by tapping the special functions of the right hemisphere."[7]
In addition we are told that problem-solving abilities will be enhanced
and creativity will be magnified and enriched. An educator writing in
the *Gifted Child Quarterly* merrily speculates that "Since creativity . . .
might be further developed in the right hemisphere, a new major thrust
in education, which might educate the whole brain of the child, could
evolve out of current efforts to stimulate early right hemisphere functioning."[8]

To help you tap and educate your right hemisphere, there are countless books and popular science treatments such as *Drawing on the Right
Side of the Brain, Whole-Brain Thinking, The Right Brain, Writing the Natural Way: Using Right-Brain Techniques to Release Your Expressive Powers,
The Aquarian Conspiracy, The Psychology of Consciousness, Educating the
Right Brain, Unchaining the Right Brain, The Other Side of the Mind, Teaching for the Two-Sided Mind*—and the list could go on for pages. Alternatively, if reading is not your preference, you could send for tapes adver-
tised in the *New York Times* that promise "brain—mind expansion" and
are "7 levelled or tracked—3 hearable by the left brain and 4 unhearable
by the left brain—bypassing your resistance to positive change."[9]

Numerous programs and workshops are available to help you expand,
amplify, and intensify your right-brain processing. Some are quite expensive and intense. One, which begin in 1975 and has virtually
achieved cult status since, is *Neurolinguistic Programming*. It is aimed at
educators and virtually any individual interested in self-improvement.
If you want extra use from your right hemisphere, which in turn will
allow you to solve your business and management problems, programs
such as *The Neuropsychology of Achievement* or the *Applied Creative
Thinking Workshop* are available. If you want a direct educational application, your might try the *Neuro-creativity Workshop*. And these are
merely the tip of the iceberg.

Left Hand, Right Brain

Up to now we have concentrated on the way in which the right hemisphere is treated in the current two-mind theory thinking. What about
the hands? Within this theory the relationship between the hands and
the hemispheres is not overlooked. Many references are made to handedness; some are direct and unambiguous, others are more subtle and
oblique. For example, Edwards is quite typical when she writes, "Keep
in mind that these phrases generally speak of hands, but because of the

crossover connections of hands and hemispheres, the terms can be *inferred* also to mean the hemispheres that control the hands."[7] She makes it specific when she says, "This, then, is the right-hemispheric mode: the intuitive, subjective, relational, holistic, time-free mode. This is also the disdained, weak, left-handed mode which our culture has generally ignored."

According to the two-minders, some methods to "unchain the right hemisphere" involve simply listening to music and looking at art. It is, I suppose, nice to feel that the current generation of kids, whose heads appear to have become permanently fixed between a pair of tape-recorder earphones, may actually be increasing their creativity. Some practitioners of the right-brain view suggest greater use of television, although I fear that that approach might kill off both hemispheres.

Some two-minders have decided that the hand-brain connection might be one of the more expedient means of releasing the right hemisphere's talents. For example, one right hemisphere-oriented educator is the state coordinator of gifted education for the New Mexico Department of Education. His work is published in the ERIC Clearinghouse of Handicapped and Gifted Children under the auspices of the Council for Exceptional Children, which is a publication source that is often regarded as authoritative and has its documents widely distributed to school systems throughout North America. He recommends no fewer than thirty-six specific activities "to stimulate right-brain processes," some of which are relaxation, guided fantasy, and photography. However, he also counsels right-handers to switch to their left hands to perform everyday activities for periods of time. He argues that this will serve to stimulate the right hemisphere of the brain.[10] Do you think that he would be equally accepting of a suggestion that left-handers who are having difficulty with reading and mathematics would be helped by switching some of their activities to right-handedness?

Another example deals directly with art. Ann O'Hanlon of Mill Valley, California, is an art teacher. She reports that in teaching a summer art class to a group of Catholic nuns she was upset by their rigid and ineffectual performance. To try to release their creative right hemisphere, which "sees things differently," she had them switch to their left hands for drawing. She claims that the result was better art. O'Hanlon has never, in her memory, asked a left-hander to change to the right hand, so it is clear that we are referring to an improvement caused by switching to the left hand (right-brain) of right-handers.[11]

All of this left-hand-use therapy is based upon the presumptions that the two halves of the brain think differently and that one hemisphere is under-used and requires exercise. It presumes further that by using one hand or the other we can alter our mode of thinking. Let us consider the actual facts of this matter.

Science, Myth, and Rumor

The suggestions I've described in the previous section are based upon a theory of the operation of the brain's hemispheres that is quite different from the theory described in the preceding chapter. When we spoke of the function of the hemispheres in the last chapter, we spoke only of language and language-like processes in the left hemisphere and of some visual and spatial (perhaps musical) functions in the right hemisphere. Next to the Two-Mind Theory version of brain function shown in figure 7.1, that description seems rather impoverished. Was I holding back the "good stuff" from my account? Not really.

The differences between the scientific picture of the mind presented by neuropsychologists and the popular concept of brain function described by the two-minders are predictable. These differences do not have to do with neuropsychology at all, but have to do with social psychology. Let me digress from discussing the Two-Mind Theory to explain an important phenomenon: how scientific data are dealt with in the public domain.

The two pictures of the mind, one held by scientists and the other by the popularizers of science and the general public, differ because of processes that affect what happens when facts are transmitted from one person to another by word of mouth, in other words, the processes that take place when rumors and gossip are spread. The only difference is that here we are not dealing with the social psychology of the rumor, "Helen is now 'sleeping around'" but the social psychology of the dissemination of scientific information.

The psychologists Gordon Allport and Leo Postman studied what happened when information was verbally transmitted from one person to another.[12] They used a procedure much like a party game called *Whispering Down the Lane*. In the party game a group of people sit around in a circle. One person reads a short paragraph to himself and then whispers it (from memory) into the ear of the person to his side. This second person tries to recall the message exactly, and then whispers it to the next person in the group, and so it goes around the circle. The last person recites, out loud, the message that he has gotten, as precisely and completely as he can. The person who started the process then reads the original paragraph. The content of the starting statement and the final version (after it has been transmitted through many people) is usually quite different, and the differences are often quite amusing, hence the charm of the game.

Allport and Postman found that as information was passed from person to person, there were some systematic biases, or distortions, that crept in. One was due to a process that they called *levelling*, which means that details tend to get lost as information moves from one individual to another. Details are important in science, but not so important when you are just trading information with other people. The problem with details is that they tend to slow up the communication process; so rather than let the conversation bog down, details tend to be omitted. The transmitted information becomes shorter until it reaches the form of a pointed or snappy "slogan."

The opposite of levelling is *sharpening*. When passing on information, you usually engage in some form of selection of the information that you want to tell. By omitting some material during the levelling process, you increase the emphasis on what remains. When trying to convey the essence of an interesting scientific finding, you will probably emphasize what you see as the main point of the results. At the same time you will look for phrasings that will make your description of the information more lively and memorable. When you find such a wording, it will become part of the final slogan form of the message.

Finally, we have the process of *assimilation*, in which the individual alters the material slightly to fit into his or her own set of beliefs or interests. Thus, in passing on some information, a teacher might emphasize the educational implications, and a stock broker might emphasize the economic implications. Such emphases are often in the form of conclusions or speculations. However, when they are passed on, the communicator's conclusions are treated as if they were part of the original set of facts.

Let me give you an example of how such influences have come to distort our picture of the relationship between handedness and the brain.[13] I was attending a national scientific meeting that included a symposium on the different functions of the two hemispheres of the brain. One of the papers delivered at that session was by Doreen Kimura, an innovative Canadian psychologist from the University of Western Ontario in London, a city in the province of Ontario, not far from Toronto. Her paper used a particular form of hearing test that she helped to introduce as a means of testing the functions of the two halves of the brain. Normally each ear sends its information to both hemispheres of the brain. There is a difference, however, in the quality and nature of the connections between the two ears and the two hemispheres. The left ear has a better connection with the right hemisphere than with the left hemisphere while the right ear has a better connection with the left hemisphere than with the right. Technically speaking we would say that the *crossed connections* are stronger, and probably faster, than the *uncrossed connections*.

A special hearing test that makes use of these differences in the connections between the ears and the hemispheres is called a *dichotic listening test,* where the Greek root *dich* means "two" while *oti* refers to the ears. The reason for this label is that the two ears are given different information to listen to at the same time. In Kimura's study,[14] one ear was listening to a particular melody while the other ear was listening to a different melody. The college student volunteer subjects were asked to select the melody or melodies that they had heard from a series of test melodies that they listened to afterwards. Kimura's findings were that the melodies heard by the left ear were usually more easily recognized than those that were presented to the right ear. As information from the left ear is more speedily and efficiently processed in the right hemisphere, it seemed reasonable to conclude that the right hemisphere processes the melodies a bit better than the left. This finding is consistent with some of the clinical data from brain-injured musicians discussed in the last chapter. Kimura's conclusion was conservative, in the manner of most scientists' conclusions. She suggested that because the left-ear performance was superior in the dichotic listening task, her data could be interpreted as indicating that *recognition of melodies is better in the right hemisphere.*

At major scientific meetings, especially those held in large cities, it is not unusual to find members of the press attending. Science reporters from newspapers and magazines and even representatives from radio and television will attend sessions on topics that the public might be particularly interested in. This was certainly the case for this meeting, and a few days later an article appeared on the science page of the *New York Times,* which claimed, in part, that "Doreen Kimura, a psychologist from London, Ontario, has found that musical ability is controlled by the right side of the brain." The first thing that the reader should notice is that there has been some levelling, which shows up in the loss of detail. Notice that the article no longer mentions that the task was actually melody recognition. Some sharpening and assimilation have also taken place. The reporter clearly speculates that melody recognition is probably related to musical ability. Now we find that instead of report-

ing that the findings are associated with the ability to recognize simulta-
neous melodies, the reporter's conclusion, "musical ability," is reported
as the actual data of the experiment.

I fear that I was annoyed at this overextension of scientific findings
and did a bit of public groaning to my colleagues and students. This
probably sensitized them to such reports, and about a week later I found
in my mail a syndicated newspaper report that a colleague had clipped
out for me. It announced, "London psychologist, Dr. Doreen Kimura
claims that musicians are right-brained!" The text of the article seemed
to be based upon the *New York Times* report, since some of the phrases
used were the same. However, notice that the report had continued to
become more distorted. It shows more levelling (notice that Kimura is
from London, not London, Ontario), and several distortions have been
introduced. Now we are presented a conclusion about the brain organization *of musicians*. This is clearly a conclusion drawn by the journalist
who wrote the article after reading the *New York Times* account. Kimura
would never have said this, as she did not even test musicians in her
study but used university students who were asked to recognize melodies. Notice that the bit about musicians is passed on as if it were Kimura's own conclusion or research finding.

I suppose that my next encounter with this piece of data should have
been predictable. About a month or so later, I opened an envelope
stuffed into my mailbox by a student, one who had heard me storming
through the halls waving the previous article and bemoaning the way
in which scientific information tends to get distorted by the media. In
the envelope was a neatly clipped article from some glossy magazine that
began, "An English psychologist has finally explained why there are so
many great left-handed musicians. Dr. Doreen Kimura has found. . . ."
As I looked at this article, snippets of commentary stored in the crazy
quilt of my memory began to surge forward: Erwin Know, the great
American editor commenting, "Everything you read in the newspaper
is absolutely true except for the rare story of which you happen to have
first-hand knowledge"; the American political writer Norman Mailer's
comment, "Once a newspaper touches a story, the facts are lost for ever
. . ."; or the British writer C.K. Chesterton's suggestion, "Journalism is
popular, but it is popular mainly as fiction. Life is one world, and life
seen in the newspapers another." It is certainly the case that science seen
in the newspapers is a world apart from science as I know it. This article
appeared to be based on the syndicated article, which was based on the
New York Times article. As that second article omitted "Ontario" from
the location of her university in "London, Ontario," it would at least

explain why Kimura had now lost her Canadian identity and become English. The reporting of the scientific facts are even worse. Kimura's work never said anything about handedness, as she had only tested right-handers. She certainly said nothing about the handedness of musicians. All of this is simply sharpening, assimilation, and conclusions drawn by the journalist. The writer clearly recalls that the left hand is controlled by the right hemisphere of the brain, and from this infers that left-handers must have better musical abilities because by inference from the previously distorted reports, musicians are right-brained. Remember, the only fact that Kimura actually reported is that *melodies received by the left ear are easier to recognize in a group of right-handed university student volunteers!*

What happened to the Kimura data is probably typical of what happens when scientific information dealing with special abilities in the hemispheres and their relationship to handedness are reported. I had been allowed to see this one emerge so clearly because my colleagues and students followed it for me in the press (perhaps because it amused them to see me with steam flowing out of my ears).

I think that the process that occurred with Kimura's findings is characteristic of what has happened to shape the public's belief in the Two-Mind Theory of brain operation. It begins with an interesting finding, which is then picked up by the radio and TV, who quickly reduce it to a 30-second report with an 11-second quote from the scientist. This process will virtually force the results to be quickly levelled and formed into something like a slogan. Next the findings appear on the science pages of the *New York Times, Globe and Mail, Wall Street Journal,* and *Washington Post.* Sometimes these initial reports are already biased in the direction of oversimplification, as the journalists working in the print media may well have been alerted to the story by seeing it on TV and thinking that there "might be a feature story here." Next, the results are widely covered in popular science magazines like *Psychology Today, Science Digest, Omni,* and so forth. In the case of the reports on the specialized functions of the right and left hemispheres, the research findings (or what had become of them) were soon being propagated with almost religious zeal in public conferences, workshops, and educational journals. They even began to appear in standard supermarket outlets in articles in *Family Circle, Cosmopolitan, Atlantic Monthly, Glamour, National Enquirer,* and *Reader's Digest.* Each time the data were discussed, ideas become more speculative and more distant from the actual research. Conclusions, inferences, and fantasies introduced by one writer simply get passed along as facts by successive writers. After a while, the neuropsychologist is no longer even visible in the communication chain. The journalist quotes an investment manager who refers to a discussion by a management professor who based his discussion on comments by an educational counsellor who reported material given at a workshop, in which the speaker discussed an article written by a journalist based upon discussions with. . . . And so it goes.

The end result of this passing on of scientific data from one source in the mass media to another is not the transmission of scientific fact, but the popularization of scientific rumor. When these rumors grow older, they turn into scientific myths. When the myths have been around long enough, they become "accepted truths," which show up in conversation and writing in sentences that begin with, "As everybody knows . . . ," or "Scientists have shown that . . . ," or "The well-established fact that you probably learned in school that. . . ." The problem is that the well-known facts may have nothing to do with the reality at all. They are simply distortions of the original facts, often overgeneralizations or speculative conclusions that have been repeated so many times that they are no longer questioned. There may be a kernel of truth in the scientific myth, as it started with some basis in fact, but the gap between the current version and the actual data may be tremendous. When you look at something like Figure 7.1, you are looking not at a scientific summary of the data, but rather at a drawing based upon the scientific myth currently told and believed in by the "Cult of the Two Minds."

If I am correct, why has this idea persisted? Why haven't scientists debunked this myth? Scientists who have tried to clean up this situation have found that the truth is often unpopular, and the contest between agreeable fantasy and boring fact is quite unequal. For example, Michael Gazzaniga's book, The Bisected Brain,[15] which described the results of testing the separated hemispheres of split-brain patients, probably served as the source for many descriptions of the "two brains" that followed. For instance, Robert Ornstein's tremendously popular book, The Psychology of Consciousness,[16] extracted much of its neurophysiology from Gazzaniga's book. Ornstein went on to tie left and right hemisphere function to more mystical ideas such as the pre-Confucian Chinese concepts of yin and yang, the Hindu notions of buddhi and manas, and contemporary conceptions such as the phenomenologist Claude Levi-Strauss's distinction between positive and mythic. It is in this form that the book achieved its popularity; it is probably greatly responsible for the wide acceptance of the notion that differences in the function of the two hemispheres are responsible for differences in abilities and thinking styles that affect behavior in all areas of everyday life. The interesting feature of this history is that, less than ten years later, Gazzaniga and a colleague, Joseph LeDoux, wrote another book based on research on additional patients with the split-brain operation. In this book, called *The Integrated Mind*,[17] he sounds a loud and clear caution that the two hemispheres are not so separate in their functional abilities as the general press and public seem to think. The book points out that there is a lot of overlap in the way in which the two hemispheres operate, and there is little evidence that tremendous differences in thinking styles, so entrenched in the public mind, are really characteristic of the left and right hemispheres. In other words, the Two-Mind Theory of figure 7.1 is wrong, according to the conclusions of one of the very researchers whose data served as the starting point for the development of this new scientific myth.

Further cautions came from the psychologist Michael Corballis, who went so far as to write an article called "Laterality and Myth," published in the psychological journal with the largest circulation of any in the world.[18] Corballis speculated that there must be some carry-over from philosophical and cultural feelings about "right" versus "left," such as those that we discussed in chapter 1, that lends itself to the sorts of overstatement that characterize the two-minders and the right-brain thinking advocates. He warned that the kind of overgeneralization and overextension of the data that seems to be part of the public's concept of the issue is not justifiable, given the data that scientists have collected.

The whole move toward "educating the right brain" has also drawn concerted attacks from scientists. Educational psychologists Hardyck and Haapenen worried about the way in which the educational establishment had swallowed the Two-Mind Theory of thinking and were building programs upon it. They cautioned that research on specialization of the two hemispheres of the brain as yet provides "no scientific basis . . . for any reorganization of curricular, teaching or testing programs within contemporary educational practice."[19]

What were the results of these words of caution and the evidence against an exclusively right- or left-brain mode of thinking? The public is bigger, stronger, and more vocal than the small band of scientists pursuing the truth. As the eminent jurist Oliver Wendell Holmes said, "Truth is the majority vote of the nation that can lick all of the others." The multitudinous voices of the press and the enthusiastic two-minders drown out the weak voices of the dissenting scientists. The warnings of Gazzaniga, Corballis and the others have been ignored, and reference to them virtually never occurs. People quote Gazzaniga's first book freely and ignore Gazzaniga's later evidence that contradicts it. As Voltaire wrote, "Error flies from mouth to mouth, from pen to pen, and to destroy it takes ages." I suppose that is why there are still books on phrenology in the bookstores, even though scientists abandoned that concept over a century and a half ago.

The two-brain view of the mind is not going to go away by itself, as too many people have too much at stake to let the truth work itself out quickly. Individuals who are the modern equivalent of the snake-oil salesman of the mid-1800s are busy peddling their expensive programs, workshops, books, tapes, and other wares to schools, to business and industry, and to the insatiable consumers of mental-health "quick fixes," "miracle cures," and "mind-expanding experiences." What can we expect of these people, who seem to be motivated more by greed than by a search for scientific truth? Those out for the newest psychological gimmick know that the two-mind theory sells. They can point to Edward's book, *Drawing on the Right Side of the Brain*, and tell you that it has sold more than 1,250,000 copies and has been translated into ten foreign languages. It may well be a good book on drawing instruction, but much of its popularity probably depends on the two-mind gimmick, with its semiscientific justifications. The royalties on this book have probably amounted to more than the total funding distributed this year for neuropsychological research on left- and right-brain functions by many funding agencies. As long as authors, information peddlers, and program hucksters continue to be rewarded by school administrators, corporate officers, mental health workers and private citizens who have more dollars than sense, the two-minders will continue to tell you about the hidden creativity in your right brain and how to shed the chains of logic that confine the left-brain and all left-brain thinkers.

Phrenology, Astrology, or Neuropsychology?

One source of appeal for the Two-Mind Theory should not be overlooked; it concerns the natural human desire to predict and explain the behavior of oneself and others. Many systems that attempt to do this have been tried, and some have persisted over many centuries. Such systems convey a certain comfort and provide some meaning to otherwise unpredictable behaviors. Take astrology, as an example. "Well I wouldn't worry too much about Herman's behavior. He's a *Taurus*, you know, and they're all stubborn." How about palmistry? "I would expect that of Harriet. Remember how her head line merged with her life line, well, that's the sign of a really cautious person, you know." Add to that phrenology, where character is read from the bumps on the head; graphology, where personality is predicted from handwriting patterns; physiognomy, where the shape of the head or face is used to predict behavior; or moleosophy, where the location of moles predicts the qualities and traits of the person. Each of these systems began with claims of some sort of scientific basis for its predictions. That these scientific underpinnings have failed to be confirmed does little to dim the popularity of these systems. Any explanation for a behavior, even if it is wrong, is more comforting than no explanation at all.

Comfort is not the only appeal of such systems. They also give us labels to describe other individuals that we know. As a species, we act as if we have a pressing need to categorize and label the things and people in our environment placing every person into some sort of group or category, which we then label. Finally, we use labels to describe and predict the way in which we believe people will think and act. Typical labels and categories include introverted versus extroverted, liberal versus conservative, bright versus dumb, artistic versus scientific, mystical versus rational, and so forth.

At varying times the labels that are in vogue change. In the 1960s there was the separation of patterns of thought, phrased in terms of contemplative Eastern thought versus that shaped by authoritarian Western religious influences. More recently excitement focused on a division of people on the basis of holistic versus linear thinking. Now the argument is based upon left versus right brain. It is interesting that this new division does not shed the old ones, but merely absorbs them. "Right brain" has absorbed the Eastern and the holistic, and the "left brain" has absorbed the Western and linear thought patterns. The new system, however, has translated the old religious (hence philosophical) metaphor to one that appears to be scientific and hence more acceptable in our contemporary technologically oriented world.

Once it was accepted that the two hemispheres of the brain were different, people had a neuropsychological "reason" to explain why some people are logical and others are not. It "explained" why brother Joe, the left-hander, was so "wonky" and unpredictable, while brother Fred, the accountant, was so boring, logical, and right-handed. "You see, it has to do with the difference between the right and the left brain. . . ."

To claim that behavior differences are based on the organization of the nervous system confers a certain scientific aura to the statement and seems to provide at least some feeling that individual differences are predictable. Like astrology, however, left- versus right-brain explanations give something to everybody. The right-hander can look down on the southpaw. After all, right-handers know that they are left-brained thinkers, which means that they can feel superior because of their greater logical thinking ability, their clear-cut linear thought patterns, their better language skills, and their agility in symbolic thinking. The left-hander can, in turn, look down on the right-hander. Left-handers know that they are right-brained, which means that they are more creative, musical, artistic, sympathetic, caring, and perceptive.

Unfortunately, as in astrology, there is selective reporting, observing, and remembering. Many of the categories of behavior are fuzzy to begin with. Furthermore, when the data fit, they are used to show that the theory works; however, when the data don't fit, they are dismissed, forgotten, modified, or replaced with confirming instances. Haven't you heard conversations like

"Bill is just like all *Gemini* people, he's very talkative."

"Well Sally is a *Gemini* too, and you know how quiet she is."

"Yeah, but Sally does crossword puzzles all the time, so she must be good with words like all *Gemini* people."

You could almost directly substitute "left brained" for "Gemini" and reproduce conversations describing people according to the Two Mind Theory. There is always some way in which the interpretation can be shaded to fit.

Why let the miserable facts, which indicate that left and right-handers have much the same brain organization, interfere with such fine fantasies. Somehow, true believers among the two-minders don't seem to hear or believe you when you point out to them that seven out of ten left-handers have their language control in their left hemisphere just like right-handers. They still believe Broca's Rule that left-handers have a dominant right hemisphere, even though Broca himself came to doubt its truth long before he died. Researchers have measured the electrical activity of the brains of lawyers (who all two-minders know are left-brained) and compared it to the activity patterns in sculptors (known to be right-brained). Using sophisticated EEG measurements of the responses of the two hemispheres, no differences were found! The supposedly left-brained lawyers and the supposedly right-brained sculptors had exactly the same patterns of electrical activity, with the same distributions across the two hemispheres.[20]

Goethe warned, "We are so constituted that we believe the most incredible things; and once they are engraved upon the memory, woe to him who would endeavour to erase them." A sign in my colleague's office reads, "Don't bother me with facts; my mind is already made up." So it is with the *Two-Minds Theory*. It is the new astrology which claims that it will allow us to predict how people think. We might call it *Psycho-Neuro-Astrology*. With a name like that, who could disbelieve it, except for some boring, plodding, linear thinking, left-brained scientist?

Think Left, Think Right

We mentioned that phrenology, although not scientifically sound, did serve to stimulate some research on the localization of specific abilities in specific regions of brain. In much the same way, the Two-Mind Theory has stimulated interesting research, despite the fact that the theory itself is suspect. Enough hullabaloo has been raised about the left- and right-brain modes of thought and their association with handedness that some neuropsychologists decided to test the issue experimentally. The persistent popular belief that the thinking patterns of left- and right-handers differ has caused researchers to wonder whether some of the two-minders' claims might confirm casual observations of left- and right-handers in everyday life. The question is whether handedness is related to *cognitive style*, the psychologist's way of saying "typical way of thinking."

One method to investigate cognitive style involves naturalistic rather than laboratory research. It starts with the idea that people tend to gravitate toward doing the things that interest them the most and the things that they are best at. A person who hates to draw and is very bad at it will not be likely to decide to become an artist or an architect. People who are good at using words and language might be expected to become writers, actors, or teachers, while those who have good spatial ability and can visualize things well might become photographers, artists, engineers, or sculptors. In psychological terms this translates to the prediction that people will tend to select an occupation consistent with their cognitive style.

Starting with the idea that occupational choice and cognitive style may be related, some investigators have asked whether there is any difference in the occupations selected by left- and right-handers. Such a difference might mean that there are different modes of thinking for the two handedness groups. Because this research was stimulated by the broad generalizations of the Two-Mind Theory, researchers began with one of the two-minders' basic assumptions, that left-handers are more likely to show what has been called a right-brained mode of thinking (whatever the underlying physiological truth), while right-handers would show what is presumed to be left-brained thinking.

My own laboratory did a bit of research on this issue, but more because the data were available than as a deliberate investigation. We had been collecting data on the handedness of university students for several years to answer other research questions. We had already analyzed one particular set of data and submitted the findings based upon it for publication. We were in the "clean-up phase" of the research, meaning that I was preparing to finish the documentation of the computer files on this study and place the results in our permanent archives. Virtually all of the data that we have collected over the last 20 years is now processed this way and permanently stored. If any questions arise about the results, if some interesting comparisons have been overlooked, or if other researchers would like access to this material, it is always available. When the data is archived, we prepare a complete listing of every measure that it contains and where it is in each file, how the measure was taken, what the specific scores in the file represent, and so forth. Earlier in my career I was not so compulsive about this sort of thing, trusting to my memory and some casual notes. Then one day, a former student of mine, Howard Erlichman, who had become a faculty member at the Graduate Center of the City College of New York, contacted me about his research, which overlapped some research that I had done several years before. He had noticed an inconsistency in a data table and wondered whether I could check the original data for the correct value. Much to my chagrin, I could not reconstruct the original files. I had forgotten some of the details of the data placement and coding. I never could answer his question, which left me quite embarrassed and uncomfortable but taught me a lesson. I now know that, no matter how intimately one knows the data when working on it, within a year or two the memory inevitably fades, details are forgotten, and the data may become irretrievable. As I was preparing the archive records for the current study, I noticed that for a large number of students tested we had recorded the subject that they were majoring in at the university. I pointed this out to Clare Porac, who agreed that it might be interesting to see whether left-and right-handers tended to major in different subjects.

We didn't expect to find anything of interest, but as the statistical analyses would require only a small amount of computer programming and very little working time, it seemed like an interesting diversion. We started out by classifying 497 university students into two groups according to their academic majors. The first group included students who were studying languages or literature and hence should have good linguistic skills (left-brain thinking?). The second group required much less in the way of language skills and included those majoring in the graphic arts and the sciences (right-brain thinking?). We were somewhat surprised to find that there were some differences in the handedness patterns of the various majors. Right-handers were much more common in the language-based majors and left- or mixed-handers were much more rare. In fact, for every two left- and mixed-handers that we found majoring in language-based subjects, we found three left- or mixed-handers majoring in the nonlanguage subjects.[21]

Other researchers have been more systematic, setting up their experimental procedures from the beginning to look at the question of handedness and occupational choice. Most of these started with the observation that there appear to be a large number of famous left-handed artists, including Leonardo da Vinci, Raphael, Hans Holbein, Paul Klee, and Pablo Picasso. To see if handedness was associated with artistic skill, one study compared 103 art students at the Massachusetts College of Art and the Boston University School of Fine Arts to 87 undergraduate liberal arts students at Boston University.[22] They found that among the art majors 47 percent were left-handed or mixed-handed, while only 22 percent of the more general students were.

Another interesting series of studies looked at architects. it appears that an unusually high percentage of students of architecture are left-handed. The same holds for the architecture faculty, with 29 percent of the faculty being left-handed. Furthermore, left-handed architecture students seem to do better. For example, of 405 right-handers who entered the architectural program in college, only 62 percent eventually graduated, while 73 percent of the 79 left-handers successfully finished their architectural degree.[23]

Let's take the relationship between left-handedness and spatial ability one step further. Several games require good spatial skills. One of the best known of these is chess, where the ability to recognize patterns and geometrical relationships is vital. There is some evidence that there is an overabundance of left-handers among chess players in general and among chess masters in particular. The oriental game of *go* also requires the ability to recognize constantly changing patterns. When handedness is determined among championship go players, we again find that there are more left-handers than in the general population.[24]

While the data on spatial abilities and handedness seem to be consistent with the two-minders' beliefs, they certainly don't confirm the Two-Mind Theory. First, the differences between right- and left-handers in terms of their occupational choices and general spatial ability are not very large. Even in the most artistic occupations, left-handers are still a definite minority. One certainly cannot deny the success in art of many right-handers, including Rubens, Titian, van Gogh, Mondrian, Rembrandt, Rodin, and about seven out of ten of all other famous artists. Conversely, many left-handers have excelled in more literary fields, including H.G. Wells, Peter Benchley, James Michener, and Lewis Carroll. The ability of handedness to predict thinking style or specific areas of ability is at best weak and only suggestive.

The parallel situation with musical ability indicates that the relationship between handedness and ability is far from cut-and-dried. Two-minders often point to such southpaw musical stars as Jimi Hendrix, Paul McCartney, or Cole Porter for confirmation of their theory. In favor of their contention is the fact that when we systematically look at samples of professional and accomplished amateur musicians we do find more left- and mixed-handers than we tend to find among groups of nonmusicians. In this case, however, it is hard to determine whether the difference is based upon differences in ability. If we test musicians on the *Seashore Test of Musical Talents*, often used as a measure of musical ability, we find no difference in talent shown between the left- and mixed-handers compared to right-handers. The only place where left-handers seem to show any definite musical advantage is in pitch recognition, where they are required to identify and match the tones of musical notes.[25]

How about creativity? According to the Two-Mind Theory, left-handers are more right-brained and hence more creative. Although many famous people were both creative and left-handed, it turns out the left-handers do not show superiority in this realm when they are systematically tested. In our lab we tested 704 people, using two different tests of creativity. In one, people had to find alternate and novel uses for common objects, while in the other people had to group objects together in novel and creative ways. Left-handers and right-handers showed no difference on these tests, suggesting that handedness is not related to creativity.[26]

Although the evidence in favor of the Two-Mind Theory is based upon distortions and oversimplifications of the neuropsychological data, there certainly are some differences between left- and right-handers. We will look at some more interesting differences, remembering that these differences, even when found in the direction predicted by the two-minders, are usually small. More important, in many cases the predicted differences don't hold up under systematic laboratory testing. Several major scientists in the field have suggested that there is no such thing as a left-handed/right-brain mode of thinking as opposed to a right-handed/left-brain mode of thinking. In terms of abilities, too many right-handers seem to do well at what are supposed to be activities requiring right-brained thinking and too many left-handers do well at what are supposedly left-brained tasks. Finally, even at the level of brain organization, too many left-handers are left-brained for language for brain organization to be predictable on the basis of handedness. Contrary to the slogan on the talk show host's T-shirt, only three out of ten left-handers are right-brained.

How can the real differences in the behavior and the abilities of left- and right-handers be explained? The next few chapters will move us closer to an explanation.

8

Is Left-Handedness
Pathological?

We scientists, like everyone else in any society, grow up with a set of attitudes that have been shaped by our culture. Although we try to distance our theoretical or research thinking from the political and cultural attitudes that surround us, we are still influenced by them, sometimes in very elusive ways. The early American psychologist William James warned "A great many people think they are thinking when they are merely rearranging their prejudices."

Scientists, just as all nonscientists, have grown up in a world that has a set of vague prejudices against left-handers. Perhaps the subtle influence of such cultural biases first stimulated the hypothesis that there might be something psychologically or physically "wrong" with left-handers. A lifetime's exposure to indirect cultural insinuations that left-handers are "damaged goods" might nudge a scientist's thought processes so that he or she might want to check out the possibility that left-handers arrived at their left-handedness because of an injury or impairment that prevented them from becoming right-handed. For instance, one philosophical note dated back to 1686 refers to left-handedness as a "digression or aberration from the way which nature generally intendeth"[1]

The general tone used by early theorists who suggested that left-handedness might be some form of pathological occurrence was captured in a popular science article in *McClure's Magazine* in 1913.[2] The article notes, "A sound and capable stock, like a right-handed one, breeds true generation after generation. Then something slips a cog, and there appears a left-handed child, a black sheep, or an imbecile." The article makes it clear that "slipping a cog" refers to some form of damage or injury that results in the development of left-handed tendencies. It continues:

An adult brain, wrecked on the educated side by accident or disease, commonly never learns to do its work in the other; the victim remains crippled for the rest of his days. But a child in whom the thinking area on the other side is still uncultivated, hurt on one side, can usually start over again with the other. A shift of this sort carries the body with it, and the child, instead of being permanently disabled, becomes left handed.

Although this may sound extreme, the article was based upon intriguing scientific evidence that seemed to support the conclusion that something pathological or defective was associated with left-handedness. This line of evidence (extending back to the turn of the century) was based upon a series of experimental studies that found that the percentage of left-handedness was much higher in various groups of individuals with psychological problems. For instance, when researchers looked at groups of retarded individuals, epileptics, criminals, or schizophrenics, they often found a much larger proportion of left-handers than in groups of normal individuals. Such observations soon led researchers to the presumption that, if left-handedness was so frequently associated with abnormal conditions, then left-handedness itself might be an abnormality. The controversial British psychologist Cyril Burt concluded, "If it is even safe to treat left-handedness as a sign or symptom, it should be regarded rather as a mark of an ill-organized nervous system."[3]

The suggestion of a link between left-handedness and some form of affliction still is found in contemporary scientific circles. Today, perhaps more than ever, scientists appear to support the view that left-handedness may be a form of "deviation from the normal." The argument begins by accepting the conclusion that right-handedness is a genetically fixed characteristic of our species. A child born with 11 fingers would be considered to be suffering from a pathological condition, not that such a child could not survive in our world but rather that such a child differs from the pattern we have come to accept as normal for a member of the human species. To explain such a deviation we might look for some form of genetic abnormality or, more likely, some set of problems, injuries, or complications that affected the mother during pregnancy or perhaps cropped up during the birth process. Just as a deviation from the genetically fixed number of fingers might lead to speculations about pathological factors, the deviation from the genetically fixed characteristic of being right-handed has led some scientists to suggest that some form of pathology causes an individual to be left-handed.

Even though some researchers feel that left-handedness might be the result of pathology or injury, few researchers would dare to suggest, even in theoretical speculations, that all left-handedness results from damage the individual has suffered. The majority of left-handers do not show any visible evidence of injury or pathology. Most left-handers perform competently, and many have become prominent in their fields. The ranks of famous left-handers include authors, artists, musicians, actors, lawyers, doctors, scientists, and businessmen. At least five presidents of the United States were left-handed, starting with James Garfield and including Harry Truman, Gerald Ford, Ronald Reagan, and George Bush. While one might disagree with their politics or aspects of their actions in office, none appeared to be obviously brain damaged or suffering from any discernible pathological condition that would impair their everyday performance.

In the face of evidence for and against pathological factors, most researchers have adopted an *Alternate Form Theory* of left-handedness, which maintains that there are two alternate types of left-handedness, according to their causes. The first type of left-handedness comes about through the operation of some form of pathology; in the second type, left-handedness is created by naturally occurring genetic or physiological factors. Early in this century the geneticist H. E. Jordan suggested that left-handedness "is not necessarily a stigma of inferiority"[4] He wanted to distinguish between "pure" (presumably genetically based) left-handedness, "which constitutes the bulk of the left-handed population," and the subset of abnormal left-handedness that results from some neurological or psychological problem. His viewpoint has generally been accepted by modern theorists, as today it is common to distinguish between presumably genetic left-handers and an additional group commonly designated as *pathological left-handers*. Is there evidence to support the suggestion that any aspect of left-handedness is pathological?

Pathological Left-Handedness

Over the past fifteen or so years, a team of researchers from the Neuro-psychology Department of the Neuropsychiatric Institute at the University of California at Los Angeles has been working on the concept of *pathological left-handedness*. This team, led by the psychologist Paul Satz, has included a number of collaborators such as Donna Orsini.[5] Basically this team has been able to show that in groups of individuals with known brain injuries or even in groups of individuals with suspected brain injuries, the number of left-handers is much greater than is found in groups of normal individuals. Their guess is that many of these surplus left-handers, if allowed to develop normally, would have become right-handers. Their presumption is that the pathological conditions associated with their brain injuries probably also have altered their handedness and increased the number of left-handers.

These researchers give some typical case histories to illustrate their point. For example, they discuss a case of a 16-year-old woman who suffered a head injury at age $2\frac{1}{2}$. Following the injury there was a major seizure. The patient then lapsed into two days of unconsciousness, which were followed by five days of an inability to speak, suggesting a left-hemisphere injury. She also switched her handedness at this time, from right-handed to its current status of left-handed. The UCLA group reported a number of other case studies that also linked left-handedness to brain damage, including the following four cases: (1) A 37-year-old nurse, the product of a very difficult birth involving prolonged labor and breathing difficulty, was clearly left-handed. (2) An 18-year-old man had a history of repeated physical abuse, including head injuries, and neglect and was now obviously left-handed. (3) An 11-year-old left-handed boy may have arrived at his left-handedness through a fairly difficult breech birth. He also may have suffered neurological damage, as he was extremely underweight at birth, which increased his vulnerability to neural injury. (4) A 34-year-old woman whose birth history included prematurity and possible toxemia (exposure to poisons or toxins from an infection in her mother) and who was also a member of a pair of twins was also obviously left-handed. The UCLA team describes other cases that, according to their analyses, represent individuals who have become left-handed because they suffered some form of pathological condition.

Obviously, left-handedness is not the only symptom shown by these patients. They often suffer from a variety of other problems. Some have movement difficulties, seizures possibly due to epilepsy, symptoms of psychological depression, and in some cases subnormal IQs. As the description of pathological left-handedness slowly emerges, it appears that such left-handedness is usually found in conjunction with other problems and abnormalities.

Many reports, covering a period from around 1900 to the present, find left-handedness associated with a broad range of difficulties, running the gamut from juvenile delinquency through psychopathology. For example, the British educational psychologist Hugh Gordon looked at handedness in 3,298 normal children and compared them to 4,620 children in schools for the retarded in the regions of London and Middlesex. He found in the normal elementary schools that 7 percent of the students were left-handed, while in the schools for the retarded, 18 percent were left-handed. These numbers mean that, among the mentally retarded, left-handers are two and a half times more common. Gordon anticipated current scientific thought about this issue in suggesting that many of the retarded left-handers may have been natural right-handers who "had been driven to the use of the left hand by some defect of the left hemisphere. . . ."[6]

Other symptoms of major psychological difficulties are found more often in left-handers. More left-handedness is found among schizophrenics than among the normal population. In addition, left-handed schizophrenics tend to suffer from a more severe form of the disease than do right-handed patients. The most serious type of schizophrenia is usually associated with a loss of brain cells and an enlargement of the fluid-filled areas in the brain called the *ventricles*. In left-handed schizophrenics these ventricles are larger than in right-handed schizophrenics. Furthermore, left-handers suffering from psychopathology tend to do more poorly on most neuropsychological tests, suggesting that their psychological problems are more pronounced.[7]

For many left-handed patients, clear signs of brain damage are visible. Quite often these injuries are more pronounced on the left side of the brain than on the right. Just such a left-hemisphere injury might be expected to shift an individual from a natural right-handedness to left-handedness.

Might I be ignoring the possibility of *pathological right-handers*, who are "natural" left-handers who arrived at right-handedness because of injury to the right hemisphere of the brain? Such individuals seem to be much rarer than their opposites for a variety of circumstances. One interesting finding is that the left hemisphere (which controls the right hand) seems to be more vulnerable to injury than the right hemisphere.

For instance, a common symptom of major damage to one side of the brain is partial or full paralysis of one side of the body. This one-sided paralysis (called *hemiplegia*) seems to be much more likely to occur on the right side of the body. Various researchers have found that right-sided paralysis may be up to four times more likely than left-sided paralysis, suggesting that the left hemisphere of the brain may be up to four times more susceptible to damage than the right hemisphere. If damage to the left hemisphere causes naturally right-handed individuals to develop into left-handers, this bias might predict that pathological left-handers are four times more likely to occur than pathological right-handers.[8]

Data suggesting that the left hemisphere is more vulnerable than the right appear in a number of other research investigations. One such study looked at over four thousand EEG records for patients in whom an injury had occurred to one side of the brain. The EEG registers electrical activity in various regions of the brain. The data here demonstrated that damage to the left hemisphere was nearly two and a half times more likely than damage to the right.[9] Even in the developing fetus, the pattern repeats itself. If a fetus is deprived of oxygen during pregnancy, left-brain damage is much more likely than right-brain damage. Any injury to the left hemisphere makes it less likely that normal right-handedness will develop.

A number of specific physiological factors may make the left hemisphere more vulnerable to injury.[8] The blood supply to the left hemisphere is a bit less in volume, which means that, under conditions of low oxygen availability, the left side of the brain would be starved of oxygen more quickly than the right. This problem seems to be worsened by the fact that the left hemisphere seems to require more energy for its normal metabolism than does the right, burning the available oxygen more quickly. During the birth process, the most common position of the infant's head during delivery allows compression of the skull in a manner that places the left side of the brain at greater risk of having its blood supply, and therefore its oxygen, temporarily stopped by pressure on the head and arteries.

Some factors that involve the development of the brain also might selectively affect the left hemisphere. According to psychologists Michael Corballis and Michael Morgan, during pregnancy both hemispheres of the brain do not mature at the same rate. The growth pattern is such that the right hemisphere develops somewhat earlier. The left hemisphere catches up later and then continues to grow and develop long after the right hemisphere has ended its period of rapid growth.

The fact that the growth of the left hemisphere takes place over a longer time period than that of the right hemisphere means that the left side is vulnerable to damage for a longer period.[10] Later damage could switch a person away from genetically programmed right-handedness.

Another variation of the uneven development theme was proposed by the late Norman Geschwind, the James Jackson Putnam Professor of Neurology at Harvard University, and his associates, particularly Albert Galaburda of the Harvard Medical School.[11] According to their hypothesis, the left hemisphere is more subject to difficulties caused by a hormonal imbalance during pregnancy. The problem has to do with either an increased concentration of the male sex hormone, testosterone, in the womb or heightened sensitivity to testosterone in the growing fetus. Because of the action of testosterone, the development of the left hemisphere is delayed and retarded. This abnormal development of the left hemisphere results in a shift toward left- or mixed-handedness. This same left-brain abnormality may also lead to other psychological problems, including dyslexia, attention deficit disorders, learning disabilities, and mental retardation.

All of these theories and experimental results have one common thread, namely, that the left hemisphere seems more vulnerable to injury or abnormal development, whatever the reason. Damage to the left hemisphere may well be the cause of shifts away from right-handedness. In other words, the scientific consensus seems to be that at least some left-handedness may be pathological. The major candidate for the pathology that converts a natural right-hander to a pathological left-hander appears to be some form of neural injury, most likely associated with the left hemisphere of the brain.

Birth Stress and Handedness

If you read with a eye toward finding patterns or common threads in a set of arguments, you might have been struck by a consistent reoccurring theme in the case studies of pathological left-handers presented by the UCLA Neuropsychiatric Institute group. This has to do with the large number of cases that report birth problems or difficulties during pregnancy as part of their medical histories. The importance of pregnancy and birth problems in determining an individual's later health and psychological well-being has been recognized for a long time. As far back as 1729, the obstetrician James Blondel was specific in pointing out the relationship between what happens during pregnancy and the welfare of the developing infant. He described a number of pregnancy-related factors that could harm the child while it was still in the womb. These factors included "distempers of the parents . . . , great falls, bruises, and blows the mother receives, . . . the irregularity of her diet, . . . immoderate dancing, . . . excess of laughing, frequent and violent sneezing, and all other agitations of the body. . . ."[12]

In 1861, William John Little suggested in a paper before the Obstetrical Society of London that the birth process itself and the events surrounding the delivery are responsible for a number of deformities, mental problems, and subsequent health problems. Little thus shifted the emphasis from the whole period of pregnancy to the "few minutes surrounding birth." Although his ideas did not achieve universal acceptance, their discussion served to focus the attention of researchers on the process of childbirth (specifically, on labor and delivery) as a period when many injuries and other forms of pathology may happen.[13]

Our major interest, of course, is with handedness. However, before we look at the relationship between handedness and birth problems, we have to understand two things. First, a continuum of problems emerges from birth and pregnancy complications. Although some impairments from birth stress might be quite major and visible (such as mental retardation, physical deformity, or obvious psychopathology), others may be quite slight, almost "invisible" impairments that seem to have only trivial effects. All individuals who have suffered injury or damage during the birth process may be referred to as *reproductive casualties*.

Second, when looking at handedness, researchers interested in reproductive casualties often use a definition of handedness that I hinted at previously but have not explicitly set forth. According to this definition we refer to two classes of handedness, *right-handedness* and *non-right-handedness*. Under this system, to be right-handed you must be consistently or strongly right-handed for virtually all of your activities. Non-right-handers, then, include left-handers and also include all of the mixed-handers who do some things with their left and other things with their right hand. For example, in the handedness questionnaire presented in chapter 3, there were twelve specific activities. To be classified as right-handed under the system discussed here, you might be required to do eleven or twelve activities with your right hand (a score of 33 or higher). Notice that this is what we have called "strongly right-handed." An individual who does nine or ten of the twelve items with the right hand would still be classified by some researchers as "non-right-handed."

This very strict definition of handedness has been useful in some research. The idea is that the fixed, genetically programmed normal human being is not only right-handed but very strongly right-handed for almost all activities. Other researchers have been more permissive in their definitions in terms of the strength of right-handedness needed for an individual to be classified as "right-handed." For convenience, when I refer to left-handers, at least in this part of the discussion, I will usually mean non-right-handed people, which includes the mixed-handers as well as the consistent southpaws.

Around the turn of the century, psychologists such as Charles Woodruff were already exploring the possibility that non-right-handedness (which he defined as ambidexterity and left-handedness, of course) resulted from problems during pregnancy and childbirth. This was based upon his observations that there appeared to be some relationship between left-handedness and nervous instability or neurosis, which he thought were also birth-related problems. Other researchers noticed that birth complications were associated with epilepsy, schizophrenia, and learning disabilities such as dyslexia. They also noticed that there were more left-handers in each of these afflicted groups than in equivalent normal groups. The logical conclusion involved very little deductive work. As birth complications cause all of these difficulties, and all of these difficulties are also associated with an increased percentage of left-handedness, it seems rational to suggest that birth complications might also be the cause of left-handedness. In fact, some researchers began to refer to left-handedness as a permanent "disability" that resulted from birth-related trauma.[13]

Science, like all other aspects of life in any society, is subject to trends and fads. Between the turn of the century and around 1950, a gradual consensus developed from the kind of indirect evidence that I've just described. This consensus was that left-handedness was probably caused by some of the same birth- and pregnancy-related difficulties responsible for so many other psychological abnormalities. Then, for some reason more related to the type of research considered "fashionable" at the time, there was approximately a twenty-year dormant period, during which issues of handedness and birth stress virtually disappeared from the current scientific literature. Interest had developed in the issue of how the two hemispheres of the brain were specialized for certain skills. Other reasons may have had to do with the development of new techniques to look for genetic factors in human behavior or with the search for new neuropsychological diagnostic procedures for brain injuries. These issues attracted the attention of many neuropsychologists. Relative to other specialities in psychology, a limited number of clinical neuropsychologists engage in research; when research interests drew many off to other problem areas, there simply weren't enough researchers to keep experimentation on the issue of handedness going strongly. All of this, however, changed in the early 1970s.

Paul Bakan, a research neuropsychologist at Simon Fraser University in Canada, published a series of short, provocative articles that eventually led to one of the most heated controversies in the area of handedness. In 1973, Bakan and his collaborators[14] conducted some research that (like most interesting ideas) seems obvious in hindsight but had not been attempted by anyone else. Up to that time, researchers had noted that individuals with major psychological difficulties were often both birth stressed and left-handed. If much of left-handedness is caused by some form of birth stress, than a history of birth stress ought to be found in otherwise normal left-handers. Bakan's study involved giving a questionnaire to university students, asking them whether their own birth had been associated with any items on a list of birth or pregnancy complications. When he tabulated the results, he found that left-handed and mixed-handed individuals were twice as likely as right-handers to report such complications, which seemed to support the notion that pathological factors might account for left-handedness. Actually, his early statements were a bit stronger than that. He literally went so far as to suggest that *all* left-handedness might be the result of birth-stress-related injuries to the brain and associated structures. An interesting additional finding of his research was that the ability of birth stressors to cause left-handedness was much greater for males than for females.

The response to Bakan's report of his findings was immediate and vigorous. Many laboratories were moved to investigate the relationship between handedness and birth stress using different techniques. The results of these follow-up investigations were inconsistent, with some researchers confirming the birth stress and left-handedness relationship and others not.

The controversy over whether a possible link between birth complications and left-handedness became quite heated. At one scientific meeting, the discussion among some researchers seemed more like an exchange of insults than a mutual sharing of information. I remember one neuropsychologist (who had not been able to confirm the expected association between handedness and birth stress) standing up at one symposium and shouting, "Anyone who suggests that all left-handers are brain damaged must be brain damaged themselves!" At the time I couldn't quite understand this emotional outburst, as the issue seemed to me one of whether the facts stated were correct or not. I later learned that this neuropsychologist is himself left-handed, and then the pieces began to fall into place. When one proposes pathological causes for left-handedness, of course, it is a short step to suggesting that anyone who is left-handed must also be pathological. If the suggested injury might be damage to the brain or associated neural centers and pathways, one is obviously saying that left-handers must be brain damaged. In the everyday (nonscientific) use of our language, we apply terms like "brain damaged" to individuals whom we want to insult, to suggest that they are dumb or acting in an illogical or insane manner. Under these circumstances, left-handers naturally may feel themselves under attack. As a researcher used to the quiet obscurity of the lab and the relatively civilized interactions of the scientific journals, this was all quite new to me. I certainly hoped that I might never draw that sort of heated commentary, but unfortunately, it was only a matter of time until I would be in a similar position.

Our own lab was drawn into the controversy as to whether left-handedness might be the result of some sort of birth-stress-related injury. In thinking about the research results on this question, it dawned upon me that some of the inconsistency in the available research findings might be due to the way the data were collected. Remember, the procedure introduced by Bakan and picked up by most researchers following up on his original investigation involved asking individuals whether they had themselves experienced any of a set of birth complications. Clearly, one's information about one's own birth must be second-hand. The only way to get information about this stage of existence is to be told about it by your mother or someone else who was there. In some families there is a free exchange of such information, but in other families one does not talk about such things (and certainly not to the children). Many individuals wouldn't know whether their own birth was simple or complicated. On the other hand, mothers will certainly know the conditions surrounding the births of their children, as they experienced the pregnancy and delivery and interacted with the obstetricians and hospital personnel. For this reason we decided to contact mothers directly, rather than to rely on an individual's self-report about his birth history. The people whose handedness we are interested in were required to provide only handedness information, and their mothers provided the information on birth conditions.

We conducted several studies involving very similar measurement procedures that all produced data supporting the assumption of an association between birth complications and left-handedness. Let me describe a typical study from this series. In this particular investigation,[15] we began by contacting around four thousand families. We asked each mother to tell us the birth histories of their children and also gathered data on the handedness of their offspring. In the end, we had 1239 usable cases in which each mother indicated whether their offsprings' births had been associated with several potential birth stressors or signs that some form of birth stress might be present. These were:

1. *Premature birth*. An infant born before the full nine-month development period is considered to be at risk and often shows neurological damage. Once outside the womb, the brain and neural tissues develop more slowly and are more susceptible to various sources of injury. Generally speaking, the more premature the child, the greater the risk factor.

2. *Prolonged labor*. The longer the period of labor and the longer the child is in the birth canal, the greater the risk of problems. Much of the danger has to do with the mechanical aspects of the birth process such as increased pressure on the child's head and body, which may restrict blood flow and the availability of oxygen.

3. *Breathing difficulty*. Sometimes the report tells of a "blue baby," as blood that is short of oxygen takes on a bluish cast and gives a blue pallor to the baby's skin, especially around the fingers and toes. According to Bakan, it is the consequences of breathing difficulty, namely *hypoxia* (which means "low oxygen"), which then serves as a major cause of damage during birth. The symptoms of hypoxia can be caused by problems other than the breathing difficulty itself. Anything that restricts air intake or the flow of blood from the lungs to vital parts of the body can starve organs of oxygen. For instance, extended pressure on the arteries around the head when labor is prolonged may sometimes induce "blue baby" symptoms.

4. *Low birth weight*. When babies are born weighing less than about six pounds, they are at risk for a variety of problems. Often, low birth weight is a sign that the infant is suffering from malnutrition or has not fully matured. It may also be a sign that the mother's health is weakened, perhaps because of drug or alcohol use, smoking, or other factors. The lower the infant's birth weight, the more likely we are to find a variety of neurological complications. Low birth weight is often associated with premature births, where it is a sign of immaturity and incomplete development.

5. *Breech birth*. Normally, babies pass through the birth canal head-first. Some, however, are rotated so that their feet point toward the vaginal opening, the "breech" delivery position. The breech position

always leads to delivery complications and usually requires turning the child, possibly with some form of implement or instrument. The process of manipulating the child's position, the resultant slow delivery, or the unusual pattern of pressures incurred in the birth canal can damage the vulnerable young nervous system.

6. *RH incompatibility.* Individuals have different blood characteristics. The blood typology based on the ABO system discovered by Karl Landsteiner in 1900 divides people into four blood groups according to the presence or absence of certain blood *antigens.* An antigen is a substance that produces some form of sensitivity or tissue response. Incompatible antigens can cause allergic-type reactions or may cause the immune system to respond. In the ABO system people are classified as having Type A blood if their red blood cells have the A antigen, Type B if they have the B antigen, Type AB if they have both A and B, or Type O if they have neither. Another important antigen is the Rhesus antigen, named after the rhesus monkey in whose blood it was first isolated it is called the *Rh factor.* Among human beings, 84 percent have this Rh factor and are called "Rh positive," while the remaining 16 percent lack this factor and are called "Rh negative." Rh antibodies do not occur naturally but may develop under certain unusual circumstances. When an Rh negative woman is pregnant with an Rh positive baby, we refer to the condition as an *Rh incompatibility.* In some such cases, blood leakage from the baby to the mother causes her to develop antibodies that may progressively destroy the blood of the growing baby, causing great neural and other tissue damage. In less severe cases, the baby is born prematurely, or the baby may be born with anemia, which deprives the developing infant of the oxygen needed for normal brain and nervous system development.

7. *Instrument birth.* The most common instrument is a special set of forceps, which are clamped around the infant and used to rotate a baby out of the breech position or to ease the infant out of the birth canal when the mother's contractions are not strong enough to deliver the child. Although instrument deliveries often speed up and simplify the birth process, in many instances they are a sign of problems in the ability of the mother to deliver the child naturally, and we consider instrument births as a sign of a risky birth. The instruments themselves can damage the infant's tender nervous system through excess pressure and restriction of blood flow, much like prolonged labor.

8. *Caesarian delivery.* In this process a surgical operation is performed on the mother to remove the child, rather than allowing her to attempt

to deliver it in the normal manner. It gets its name from Julius Caesar, who was supposedly "cut from his mother's womb." Caesarian deliveries are usually attempted only by doctors who feel that delivery through the birth canal is too risky. Caesarian deliveries serve as an indicator that the pregnancy or birth process is suffering from problems.

9. *Multiple birth.* This refers not to a possibility that an individual may be born more than once but rather to the case when an individual is one of a set of twins, triplets, or quadruplets. This is considered a risky birth condition. To begin with, the mother's nutrients have to be shared by more than one developing child, which may explain why twins are typically lighter in weight than singletons. The birth process is usually more complicated and certainly takes longer than usual, especially for the infant who is last out of the birth canal. Even more important is the fact that members of a twin pair are suffering from being "beaten up" more than the single child. Sharing a womb with another infant means that when your partner kicks, swings his arm, or twitches his body, you are the one who is kicked, punched, or shoved. All of this mechanical banging on the developing child can cause neural damage and may affect the integrity of the infant's nervous system.

When we looked at the results of our study, some interesting facts emerged. Most important, we found that when mothers reported that a birth was stressful or complicated by one of the problems listed above, there was an increased likelihood that the child would be left-handed. The effect was much larger for males than for females. The fact that male children are more likely to be affected is consistent with a lot of evidence that runs against the *macho*, tough and invulnerable male image. When it comes to birth complications, males are much more vulnerable to neurological damage than are females. Male infants were most likely to be left-handed if their birth involved prolonged labor, breech delivery, low birth weight, Caesarian delivery, multiple births, or Rh incompatibility. Females were more likely to be left-handed when their birth involved prematurity, prolonged labor, breathing difficulty, or multiple births.

This particular study went further than most previous studies, because it looked at other aspects of sidedness, namely, *footedness, eyedness,* and *earedness.* These aspects of sidedness were measured much the way that we described in chapter 2. It appears that all four aspects of sidedness are affected by birth stress. When individuals suffer from various birth and pregnancy complications, they are not only more likely to be left-handed but also more likely to be left-footed, left-eyed, and left-eared.

As in the case of handedness, however, the effects tend to be stronger for males than for females.

In recent years several large and well-controlled experimental studies have looked at the issue of birth complications and handedness. As the data have begun to accumulate, the case for a relationship between left-handedness and birth stress has become much stronger. Better measures (such as hospital reports) have been used, and larger groups of test subjects have been tested, as in the following examples of recent work.

On recent study looked at a group of children who were born very prematurely and had an extremely low birth weight. The normal human pregnancy is about 38 weeks in length. As these infants were born between 26 and 29 weeks (6 to 7 months) after conception, they were quite premature. These infants also weighed less than 1000 grams (less than 2 pounds) when born. Researchers kept track of this group of children until they were about four years old, which is old enough to consider handedness reasonably set. For this group of prematurely born children, an amazing 54 percent were found to be left-handed, about five times more left-handedness than found for children born under more usual conditions at more usual birth weights.[16]

In general, premature children show reduced percentages of right-handedness even when their birth weight is not extremely low. One typical study found that premature children were nearly twice as likely to be left-handed or mixed-handed as compared to children delivered after a full-term pregnancy.[17]

Another recent piece of research had left-handers report whether they had experienced any of a list of twenty-three birth or pregnancy problems. Left-handers were approximately twice as likely to report two or more of these birth complications than were right-handers. This study added some new stress factors to the list used in our lab. They found that left-handedness was much more likely in a person whose mothers had high blood pressure during their pregnancy. If labor was very short or had to be chemically induced, the number of left-handed children was also increased.[18]

Some other psychologists have looked directly at obstetrical records to find an association between handedness and birth complications. The neuropsychologist Murray Schwartz, from the Victoria General Hospital in Halifax, Nova Scotia, used the *Apgar* scores recorded by the obstetrical nurse within the first minute after birth. Apgar scores are based upon several observable indicators of infants' health and physiological well-being. The infant's status on each item is graded on a scale from 0 to 2, with higher scores meaning better. The items used are:

1. *Heart rate.* In the normal infant this should 100 beats per minute or more.

2. *Breathing pattern.* There should be an obvious breathing pattern accompanied by a good strong crying response in normal infants.

3. *Muscle tone.* In the healthy child there should be active and obvious movements of the arms and legs.

4. *Responsiveness or irritability.* When the sole of the infant's foot is scraped, pinched, or stuck with a needle, the normal infant should respond with a cry.

5. *Color.* The infant's skin should be pink, with no sign of blue on the face, hands, or feet.

Low scores on this Apgar rating scale have been shown to be associated with a poor physical status. Low scores also have been found to be associated with a higher likelihood of neurological abnormalities. Schwartz found that the Apgar score taken one minute after birth predicted the infant's later handedness. Children with low Apgar scores, who are the children that are at highest risk of some form of neurological problems because of birth complications, are more likely to be left-handed than children who are apparently normal, with a high Apgar score.[19]

Other investigators have looked at more indirect indications that an increased risk of birth complications is associated with an increased likelihood that the child will be left-handed. One such study, done in my laboratory, was based on the well-known fact that the age of a mother is strongly related to the chance of birth and pregnancy abnormalities. If we eliminate very young mothers, say, 16 years old and younger, we find that as the mother grows older the chance of problems during pregnancy or delivery steadily increases. In mothers in their middle thirties and older, the incidence of various pregnancy problems is much higher then in younger mothers. Older mothers are more likely to deliver prematurely, to have miscarriages or stillbirths. Children of older mothers are at higher risk for a range of physical and psychological problems, from mental retardation (due to problems such as Down's syndrome) to bodily malformations (such as webbing of the toes or other more extreme deformities). The safest age range to have a child is when the mother is between 17 and 24 years of age. Each year after the age of 24 is associated with greater risk of birth complications. Each year after the age of 35 increases the risk of some form of birth problems by about 20 percent. Based upon the knowledge that children of older mothers are at greater risk of pregnancy and birth problems, the experimental prediction becomes quite obvious. If our hypothesis that left-handedness is produced by injuries due to birth or pregnancy complications is correct, then older mothers should be more likely to have left-handed children than younger mothers. Furthermore, the number of left-handed off-spring should increase steadily with an increase in the mothers' ages.

To test this prediction we collected data over a period of approximately five years. By the time we had finished we had tested 2,228 college freshmen for their handedness and determined how old their mothers were at the time of their birth. We used the safest childbearing ages (17 to 24 years) as a reference point for our comparisons. What we found was that as the mother's age increased, the likelihood that she would bear left-handed offspring increased. The rate of increase was quite startling, as you can see in figure 8.1. Notice that if the mother is 35 to 39 years old when she gives birth, that child is 69 percent more likely to be left-handed. If the mother is over 40 years old, the likelihood of left-handed offspring is 128 percent higher than if she had been in her early twenties when she gave birth. These data, although indirect, strongly suggest that pathological problems resulting from birth complications may be one cause of left-handedness, at least in some individuals.[20]

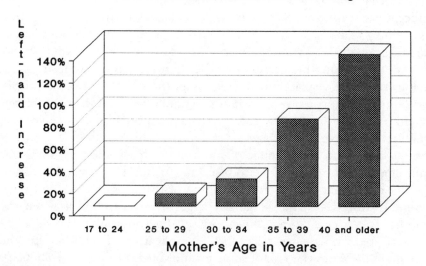

FIGURE 8.1: The risk of the child being left-handed steadily increases as the mother's age at the time of delivery increases.

Other indirect evidence points in much the same direction. For example, in one study Bakan looked at the children of mothers who smoke. Smoking tends to reduce the oxygen that the developing fetus gets and places the infant at risk for a number of birth-related problems, such as low birth weight or breathing difficulty at birth. Because of this, Bakan reasoned that mothers who smoked during pregnancy should have more left-handed children. In fact, this is exactly the result that he found.[21]

During the last twenty years, studies like these have continued to be conducted. As the measures became more reliable and the researchers used more innovative methods, the conclusion became clearer. A couple of years ago, Alan Searleman, Clare Porac, and I assembled all of the studies we could find that looked at the direct link between birth and pregnancy problems and left-handedness. We concentrated on data which had appeared in the scientific literature since the mid-1970s, feeling that this would give us the precision of more modern scientific methods of data collection and the advantage of the powerful statistical techniques that have developed in recent years. We were hoping to establish a reasonable overview of modern knowledge available about this issue. In thirty of the thirty-three comparisons we looked at, we found that if a birth stressor was present, there was a reduced percentage of right-handed individuals. In some instances, the shift was away from strong right-handedness to a weaker form of right-handedness or toward mixed-handedness. However, in most instances we saw an increase in the number of left-handers in the birth-stressed group.[22] Since that survey, several new pieces of research have appeared, virtually all of which seem to confirm the conclusion that left-handedness is often associated with birth complications and may be the result of some form of neural damage or injury.

Let's be quite clear about one thing, however: I am *not* saying that all left-handers are brain damaged. I am not saying that every left-hander is some form of neurological cripple. What I am saying is that left-handedness appears to be associated with the presence of certain abnormal or pathological conditions, such as birth or pregnancy difficulties. Before the left-handers reading this go into a panic, please remember that pathologies come in all degrees of severity. If you have a cavity in a tooth or if you have athlete's feet or are near-sighted, you are suffering from a pathological condition. The word *pathology* sounds ominous but can vary from a minor problem to a major disability. The present state of our knowledge suggests that, for a certain percentage of people, left-handedness may be caused by pathological conditions or may indicate the presence of pathological conditions. In many otherwise normal people, these pathologies may be no more consequential than a hang-nail, or flat feet, except that they have altered the way in which the brain's control of handedness is organized.

Scientifically, the interesting question becomes, "Why do certain pathological conditions and left-handedness go together?" The answer to this question does not require additional knowledge about the physiology of the brain or the nervous system. The answer comes from a bit of razzle-dazzle having to do with rare traits or infrequently encountered qualities in general. Left-handedness turns out to be only one special case of this mechanism, as you will see in the next chapter.

9

The Sign of the Left

We have shown that left-handers get a "bad press" from the cultural attitude that "different is bad." Left-handers, with their distinct pattern of hand use, are certainly seen as different by the right-handed majority. Perhaps, at least at the subconscious level, this feeling stirred researchers to look for links between pathological conditions and left-handedness. Whatever the initial motivation, we have already seen data that suggests that, for many people, left-handedness may have come about from some form of birth-related injury or pathology. Yet the data discussed in the last chapter is only the tip of the iceberg. Recent research shows that left-handedness may serve as a *sign* or a *marker* indicating the presence of other psychological and neurological problems in the individual. This conclusion is based upon findings that the percentage of left-handers seems to be much higher in groups with an assortment of psychological and physical problems. To give just a brief list,[1] left-handers are more common in groups of individuals with a history of:

- alcoholism
- allergies
- attempted suicide
- autism
- bed-wetting
- brain damage
- chromosomal damage
- criminality

- depression
- drug abuse
- emotionality
- epilepsy
- homosexuality
- immune disorders
- juvenile delinquency
- mental retardation

- migraine headaches
- neuroticism
- poor verbal ability
- poor spatial ability
- predisposition toward aggression
- psychosis

- reading disability
- schizophrenia
- school failure
- sleep difficulty
- slow physical development

Why is left-handedness associated with these ailments and complaints? We don't have to get melodramatic; left-handedness has not been singled out as a mark of major afflictions and infirmities. It simply fulfills certain conditions that make it an excellent candidate to serve as a signal that certain types of disorders may be present.

Rare Traits as Problem Signs

Animal breeders claim that, when they encounter an animal that appears different from others of its breed, there is a strong likelihood that the animal may have physical or other problems, even if the difference is apparently quite innocent, such as an unusual coat color, a difference in body shape, different fur characteristics, or even an atypical tail. Such characteristics are called *rare traits*, because they are seen only sporadically in a particular breed or species. Notice that such rare traits are not in themselves deformities, just differences. Since such visible characteristics are often signs or signals that there may be neurological, physical, or genetic abnormalities present in the animal, neuropsychologists and geneticists often call them *markers*.

It may seem ludicrous to suggest that *any* difference from the commonplace characteristics of the majority might be a sign of potential problems. Why should a characteristic, simply because it is uncommon, indicate that something may be wrong with the individual that shows it?

It is easy to demonstrate that apparently innocuous rare traits such as hair color do act as markers suggesting that various major physical, psychological, and neurological afflictions. Consider the "blue-marl" coloration found on some dogs, particularly collies; such silvery blue-grey markings occur in nature only infrequently. This rare coloration (now becoming less rare because it is being selected for by dog breeders who like its distinctive and elegant look) is often found to be associated with major abnormalities in the dog's vision or hearing. This same problem is found in many breeds of white dogs. White animals are also rare in the natural environment, except in snowy regions where the white

serves as a camouflage. When we study animals with this rare characteristic, we find that such animals show a higher risk of deafness and an
increased likelihood of developing emotional problems such as snappish-
ness, timidity, and a general appearance of being neurotic, if such a word
can be applied to animals such as dogs.

Much the same holds for human beings. Sticking with rare colors as
our example, there are problems found in rare-colored people. For instance, an albino person, whose skin appears to be bleached almost
white, often has major visual difficulties and a variety of other physical
problems such as a predisposition toward deafness and certain diseases
that appear to have no relationship to the missing skin pigment.

Differences in coloration are only one type of rare factor that can be
mentioned as a marker for various maladies and disorders. Many other
rare traits similarly suggest the presence of problems. For instance, in
relatively rare cases Siamese cats are born with a kink or a permanent
bend in the tail. This rare characteristic seems to be associated with
visual problems in the cats, such as a tendency to be cross-eyed and a
pronounced tendency for emotional instability and random aggressive-
ness.

It appears that rare physical characteristics in general, even though
they seem to have only cosmetic effects, often turn out to be associated
with various physical and psychological shortcomings or deficits. Consider the following list of relatively rare physical characteristics found in
human beings:

- Although everybody has one hair whorl where the hair tends to
  grow in a circular pattern on the head, two or more whorls in the
  hair is a rare trait.
- Ears seated low on the head.
- Two ears set at noticeably different heights on the head.
- Missing earlobes.
- Having a fifth finger (the "pinky") that appears curved (a slight C-
  shape bend) when the hand is placed flat on the table and viewed
  from the top.
- A third toe as long or longer than the second toe
- Webbing or partial attachment between the two middle toes.
- A particularly large gap between the first (big toe) and second toe.
- Tongue furrows or grooves that run front to back.
- The typical human palm has two large horizontal creases that run
  sideways across the hand (called by palm readers the *heart line* and

the *head line*); however, some rare individuals have only one such pronounced horizontal crease on the palm.

- On the palm, the lower horizontal crease (the *head line*) continuing all the way to the edge of the hand is another rare trait.
- Ultra-fine, virtually uncombable hair that some people call "electric," as it seems not to want to stay down flat.
- Certain fingerprint patterns are also quite rare, such as a hand with two or more *radial loops* (a simple loop pattern where the top of the loop points away from the thumb)

All these rare characteristics are referred to by researchers as *minor physical anomalties*. The first thing to notice about this list of rare features is that none of them seems to have any obvious connection to a person's psychological or neurological condition. Yet, like left-handedness, people with certain neuropsychological problems are more likely to have these traits than are people without obvious problems.[2] Let's take a quick look at some of the complaints associated with these rare traits. They include:

- attention deficits
- autism
- brain damage
- emotionality
- hyperactivity
- impulsivity
- juvenile delinquency
- learning disability
- low spatial ability
- low verbal ability
- mental retardation
- neuroticism
- predisposition toward aggression
- psychosis

A glance at this list and the one earlier in this chapter that catalogs the problems found more frequently in left-handers show a good deal of overlap. In fact, every item associated with our list of minor physical anomalies also appears on the left-handedness list! Is there something in common between left-handedness and a curved pinky finger, or an overly long third toe, or the existence of two hair whorls? The answer is "Yes." Don't look for a neurological, genetic, or physiological linkage, however; the common factor is a statistical one. The important fact is that left-handedness and all the other characteristics that we have just inventoried are statistically rare. This association between rare traits and pathological conditions is not magic, capricious, or unknowable in its nature, and it is not due to the operation of demons or a god that dislikes left-handers. Let me show how this association comes about.

Rare Traits and the Sign of the Left

With only about one out of every ten people being left-handed, it would certainly be classified as a relatively rare behavioral trait by most psychologists. This very rarity is the crucial quality that allows it to serve as a marker for certain problems. In order to see why this is the case, we don't have to talk about specific maladies, forms of brain injury, damage to the left hemisphere, or any other neurological factors. The theory that I will describe depends upon two simple requirements and a little bit of a numbers game. Actually, the theory is one that my frequent co-researcher Alan Searleman, of St. Lawrence University, and I called the *Rare Trait Marker Theory*. In our work on the theory we had to describe its operation and implications using some sophisticated mathematics; however, you won't have to worry about any mathematical operations in order to see how it works.[3] The basic concept behind this theory is really quite simple and is based upon some earlier suggestions by Paul Satz from UCLA, whom we have spoken about before.[4]

The Rare Trait Marker Theory does not single out left-handedness specifically, but actually could be used to describe an association between various pathological conditions and psychological problems and *any* rare trait. We could have chosen any of those minor physical abnormalities listed in the previous section or many other, similarly rare physiological or behavioral traits that we have not had the space to list here. Basically, three requirements must be met for the theory to work. The first is that we have a trait or characteristic that we can reliably say describes the majority of people in the population, like a genetically fixed characteristic (such as normal separation between the two middle toes). In addition there has to be some alternative characteristic that may occur in some individuals, instead of the common or dominant trait (such as webbing or partial attachment between the two middle toes). The second condition is that this alternative characteristic should be relatively rare. The third requirement is that there should be some form of pathology or abnormality that might prevent the common characteristic from occurring and allow the alternate rarer characteristic to develop (such as birth and pregnancy complications that may affect the normal development of the fetus).

While the rare trait marker theory allows us to make a set of predictions based upon any rare trait, our interests have to do with handedness. There are many reasons that left-handedness is a particularly good marker that may signal the presence of various pathological conditions and abnormalities, according to this theory. Let's see how this works.

To meet the first requirement of the theory we must accept the fact that the majority of people are genetically programmed to be right-handed, pretty much as a normal species characteristic. Let's also accept the fact that there may be an alternate genetic or developmental pattern that will make some people *naturally* left-handed. To meet our second requirement we need only observe that left-handedness is relatively rare. Let us assume, as an example, that 90 percent of the population, by following the main track laid out in their genes, will eventually arrive at a station along their course of development where they will be recognizable as right-handers. For the remaining 10 percent of the population, following their genetic main track means that they will develop into left-handers.

To meet our third requirement we must next suppose that there are some forms of pathology that can cause a person to deviate from his or her genetically programmed main-track handedness. Our last chapter showed that there are pathologies or injuries, possibly caused by a difficult birth or pregnancy complications, that might cause left-handedness. For this example, let's say that this set of complications switches the handedness of 10 percent of the population. (This 10 percent figure is chosen for the sake of argument and should not be taken as being a fixed, absolute value.) Because of some form of neural injury or damage, 10 percent of all right-handers will get switched off of their programmed main track and onto a *side track* that leads them to left-handedness. We can look at this process in a number of ways. For instance, we might say that the individuals are actually switched from right to left-handedness, but more likely what happens for these people is that normal consistent right-handedness (their main-track destination) doesn't develop because of neural or other damage. In other words, these people become non-right-handed, which means either left-handed, mixed-handed, or inconsistently-handed. A person who was genetically programmed to become right-handed but now is left-handed because of some form of birth related injury could be called *pathologically left-handed*. However, I will refer to such a person as a *side-track left-hander*, as the handedness came about by being switched off of his or her genetic main track. Although I have been concentrating on the side-track left-handers, it is important to remember that the same pathology that causes natural right-handers to deviate from their main track will also cause 10 percent of all main-track left-handers to switch their handedness. Thus, there will also be a set of *pathological right-handers*, or *side-track right-handers*.

If 10 percent of both left- and right-handers switch their handedness, why are we talking about a *sign of the left* in which left-handedness in particular is a signal that some form of pathology or problem might be present? Here is where the statistical factors, and the numerical magic, come in.

To understand what is going on, look at figure 9.1. Notice that it shows our starting population with its 90 percent main-track or natural right-handers and its 10 percent main-track left-handers. In the next part of the figure you see the effect of the pathology (which we assume is due to birth or pregnancy related complications). The pathological

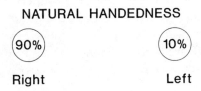

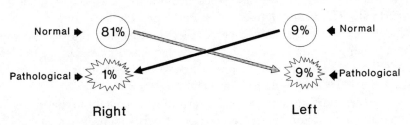

FIGURE 9.1: This diagram demonstrates how the Rare Trait Marker Model works. The circles represent the percentages of normal individuals while the squares represent percentages of pathologically affected individuals.

condition switches 10 percent of the right-handers, so that we end up with 9 percent (10 percent of 90 percent) as side-track or pathological left-handers. The same pathology also switches 10 percent of the left-handers, so that we end up with 1 percent (10 percent of 10 percent) as side-track or pathological right-handers. Notice what has happened. In our final population (after all of the pathological switching has occurred) we now have 18 percent left-handers, and half of these arrived at their left-handedness on the side track that they had been switched to by some injury or pathology. If we look at the group of left-handers and randomly select one of them, our chances of picking out a left-hander affected by pathology is 50 percent or 1 out of 2. Compare this to the group of right-handers. Of the 82 percent right-handers, only 1 percent arrived at their handedness by an injury or problem. The chance of picking out a side-track right-hander with pathology is only 1 out of 82. In other words, the likelihood that a left-hander has some form of neurological injury that switched his or her handedness is nearly 41 times greater than the likelihood that a right-hander had this sort of injury.

The fascinating thing about the rare trait marker theory is that it doesn't depend upon any specific physiological, injury, or disease mechanisms. It makes no assumptions about the vulnerability of various parts of the nervous system. In other words, we don't have to know why or how or even when a particular injury or damage occurred. All we need to know is that there are both a common and a rare trait and that some form of pathology (actually, *any* form of pathology) can produce the rare trait.

Certainly, under particular conditions the theory works better or worse. For instance, just how uncommon or infrequent the rare trait is in the population makes an important difference. The less common the rare trait is, the more likely it is that individuals who show it will have arrived at that trait by the side track provided by pathology. If we had started with 95 percent right-handers and 5 percent left-handers (instead of the 90 percent right- and 10 percent left-handedness that we assumed in our example), the likelihood that the left-hander arrived at his left-handedness though pathology jumps from 41 times higher than a right-hander to 117 times higher than a right-hander.

Another important feature that determines how well the theory works in any given situation is the percentage of people who are side-tracked by pathology or injury. Your first guess might be that the higher the rate of pathological switching, the better the system works. However, when we explored the matter mathematically, we found to our surprise that the smaller the percentage of people who are shifted pathologically, the greater the difference between left- and right-handers. If the percentage side tracked is only 1 percent (instead of the 10 percent in our example), then the likelihood that you will find a pathological left-hander goes from 41 times higher to 76 times higher. The usefulness of a rare trait as a potential sign of some abnormality is reduced if the rate of injury or pathology is too high! There is a trade-off here that is important for the researcher: As the rate of pathological shifting goes down, it becomes harder to find people with abnormalities, and it becomes more difficult to do the research. This situation reminds me of a comment made by the American science-fiction writer Paul Anderson, who said, "I have yet to see any problem, however complicated, which, when you looked at it in the right way, did not become more complicated." Completely by chance, it turns out that with the distribution of handedness at about 90 percent for the common trait and 10 percent for the rare trait and with a likely rate of pathological switched-handedness between 5 and 10 percent, we seem to have blundered upon the optimal combination of values to make the rare trait marker theory work most efficiently according to the mathematics. Apparently, fate even smiles upon neuropsychologists, sometimes.

Left-Handedness as a Marker

We have seen that left-handers are more likely to have some form of pathology than right-handers by the operation of the statistical processes that gave us the rare trait marker theory. We have also seen that the chance combination of numerical values are luckily (for the researcher) in a range that makes handedness a good sign of possible pathology. For another reason that left-handedness turns out to be a good marker for pathologies, we have to bring ourselves back to the physiology and leave the magic of numbers.

One reason that left-handedness is useful as a possible sign of damage is that the control of handedness is quite complex from the neurological point of view. Up to now I have spoken as if the only important aspect of hand control had to do with the relative dominance of the left or right cerebral hemispheres. When we are talking about handedness and hand control, however, as many as twenty-three brain centers and neural pathways may be involved. These include several different movement-control systems and position-sensing systems that originate in the cerebral cortex. Several other centers of control are located in the older sections of the brain (usually referred to as the midbrain), in addition to a set of pathways through the spinal cord and lower brain centers and some pathways between the two hemispheres.[5] The interesting fact is that injury or damage to *any* of these sites or systems may alter the natural development of handedness. In other words, side-track left-handedness may arise from damage to the cortex, midbrain, or lower brain centers. It can also occur if the damage affects movement-control systems, position-sensing systems, or any of a number of major neural pathways. Left-handedness is a particularly interesting feature because it is such a sensitive trait and may come about because of damage to a broad variety of different neural centers and systems.

The neuropsychological usefulness of left-handedness, as a possible sign for psychological and neurological problems and pathologies is really based upon chance and fortune, which brought together the three needed elements, namely, that: (1) Left-handedness is a relatively rare trait. (2) Handedness can be changed by pathological factors. (3) The pathologies that cause left-handedness are quite varied and may also cause or signal the presence of other problems, as we will see more clearly in the next chapter.

The combination of these features in exactly the right numerical relationships, all operating according to the rare trait marker theory, is what has made left-handedness such a good sign of neuropsychological problems in an individual. We could not have asked for a better indicator in some ways. As Shakespeare says in his play *Cymbeline*, "Fortune brings in some boats that are not steered."

When such rare opportunities are provided by nature, scientists are really duty-bound to snap them up and make the most of them, if knowledge is to advance. As the eminent French bacteriologist Charles Nicolle said, "Chance favours only those who know how to court her." There are many sorry instances where the history of science was delayed because people failed to recognize a chance occurrence that suggested an important relationship.

Left-handedness as a marker for problems is what clinical researchers call a *soft sign* for pathology, meaning that it is not something that you can directly cut out, weigh, or subject to direct chemical or physical analysis. Handedness is merely an observable behavior that indirectly suggests a problem, rather than a *hard sign*, which might be an observation of a damaged section of the nervous system. Hard signs almost always indicate pathology. Thus, a person who tests positively for HIV antibodies almost definitely has been exposed to the disease AIDS. Left-handedness is a soft sign in the sense that an individual who shows it is not definitely pathological, but rather is more likely to have some pathological condition than a person who does not show this behavioral sign.

There are some special groups who deviate from the normal and who suffer from certain clinical conditions that illustrate what we have been talking about. To understand what we mean by a soft sign, let's look at the relationship between handedness and two such conditions.

Mental Retardation. The psychologist Margaret-Ellen Pipe from the University of Otago in New Zealand recently reviewed the scientific evidence showing a relationship between handedness and mental retardation.[6] She looked at twenty-three different research reports covering a span of nearly eighty years, and found an amazing degree of agreement in their findings. She reports that left-handers are much more common in groups of retarded individuals, with some studies showing up to five times more left-handers than are found in groups of normal individuals. Notice, however, that all retardates are not left-handed, and certainly all left-handers are not retarded.

Schizophrenia. Another review of the scientific literature was conducted by Pierre Flor-Henry of the Department of Psychiatry at the University of Alberta.[7] He looked at the relationship between certain forms of psychopathology, particularly schizophrenia, and handedness. The pattern is very similar to that for retardation, with left-handers being two to five times more common in samples of schizophrenics than in samples of normal individuals. As before, remember that because individuals are left-handed does not mean that they will be schizophrenic. Instead, this finding suggests that if you are schizophrenic, you are more likely to be left-handed.

We have seen that left-handedness and mixed-handedness *may* be an indication that there is something neurologically awry in some individuals. Yet we know that the majority of left-handers seem to do quite well in the world, and are often successful, respected and appreciated members of society. Certainly, when I look at my left-handed son Ben, I do not feel as though I am looking at a damaged and pathological individual. He seems to be surviving his university courses and shows no psychological symptoms more terrible than a tendency to go to more live performances by the rock music group the Grateful Dead than some people might consider healthy. I do not live with a continual fear that because he is left-handed he will suddenly have a psychological breakdown, lapse into retardation, or lose his ability to function in society. As he is more typical of the majority of left-handers than groups of mentally deficient or psychopathological individuals, it is such people whom we should be concerned about. Is he different? Well, he is a left-hander, and does show some of the differences in his behavior and his life history that I have come to expect of normal, functional, left-handers. Next we'll consider some of the differences that make up the pattern typical of most southpaws.

10

Left-Hander Differences
and Deficiencies

B ased upon what we have learned so far, the blunt question that has
to be asked is whether left-handers are damaged or different in some
way? Even if we believe the evidence of the last two chapters, it is still
possible to argue that although a person may become left-handed because of some neural damage, the only residual left by this injury might
be left-handedness. That handedness has gone "awry" doesn't mean
that we have to predict other problems as well. Many scientists believe,
however, that left-handers are susceptible to a variety of problems to
a much greater degree than their right-handed friends and neigh-
bors. More important, these researchers suspect that these problems
are related, at least in part, to the neural injury that produced the left-
handedness in the first place. Their suspicions come about because of
what I call the *secondhand piano scenario*.

Suppose that you wanted to buy a used piano and happened to notice
one at some flea market or secondhand furniture store. One has to be
careful in buying an older piano, as they sometimes have problems and
don't work very well. The source of the problems is that most of the
moving parts are made of wood. If the piano has been heated and cooled
a lot or subjected to uneven temperatures (such as being placed between
a cold outside wall on one side and a heated room on the other), the
wood can warp. The warping may affect the keyboard and related struc-

tures so that the piano keys no longer are properly seated, making it difficult or even impossible to push some of the keys down. In addition to warping, there may be other forms of hidden damage. Because most of the older pianos used leather strips to help fling the hammers against the strings, it is possible that the strips have dried out or broken through exposure to warm dry air, lack of upkeep, or simply age. Even if the secondhand piano appears to be in reasonably good shape on the outside, the wise shopper should carefully check it out to make sure that it is in good working order.

Let's suppose that you walk over to the used piano that has caught your interest and press one of the black keys. Although everything looked fine, you now discover that this black key doesn't move. It appears to be stuck, as if it had been glued into place. Obviously something is wrong with this key. Given this bit of evidence, would you be willing to bet that at least one other key from the remaining 87 on this piano keyboard doesn't work right? My guess is that most people would be willing to take a modest bet that there is another key that doesn't work, since the whole piano must have been subjected to the same heating, cooling, dampness, or other conditions that caused the one key that you touched not to work.

You are probably thinking, "What does this scenario have to do with handedness?" Well, let's suppose that each of the black keys on the piano represents some brain center or pathway that is involved in determining or controlling handedness. If all of the black keys are working right, you are right-handed; however, if any one black key (actually some neural process that it represents here) doesn't work the way it should, you will be left-handed. In terms of this piano analogy, as one black key doesn't work, we can assume that you are left-handed. Now, let's suppose that the white keys represent other neurally controlled behaviors. These may be abilities or predispositions or any of a number of normal processes. If you have already found a black key that doesn't work, doesn't it seem likely that there might also be a white key on that same piano keyboard that doesn't function properly? Perhaps a white key which is near the nonfunctioning black key. The same conditions that caused the black key to malfunction are likely to affect the whole keyboard and to cause difficulties with white keys as well.

The kind of reasoning that we have just gone through is behind the search for problems in left-handers. The argument goes that, if left-handedness is caused by some type of damage or injury, then that same damage or injury might have caused other problems that could affect the physical or psychological status of the left-hander. If left-handedness is a sign of some form of damage (a black key doesn't work), then it is likely that there is other damage that has nothing to do with handedness directly (a white key won't work). The greater the original extent of the problem (that's the abuse to the piano), the more likely that we will find left-handedness (at least one black key that doesn't function) and also the greater the likelihood that we will find other problems (more white keys that don't work).

This kind of reasoning has led to some interesting research and some startling findings. Scientists have found a number of ways in which left-handers differ from right-handers, and the vast majority of these differences support the notion that left-handers have more problems. This is consistent with the damage theory of left-handedness, as it would be reasonable to presume that the same mechanism that caused the injury that resulted in left-handedness has also resulted in other problems and difficulties.

The Alinormal Left-Hander

Let me make one thing clear. I am not suggesting that left-handers shuffle and shamble through life, requiring custodial care because they are too damaged to survive on their own. For most left-handers, the problems that result from the injury or pathology that we believe is present are not very large. They tend to show up when we look carefully, with an eye toward certain types of difficulties that are often not apparent to the nonscientist observing an average left-hander. Getting this message across, however, has turned out to be more difficult than I originally expected.

Early in our work, when we first began to uncover evidence suggesting that neurological damage resulting from stressful births might account for a sizeable proportion of left-handedness, we found that there was a tendency for people (particularly people in the media) to overreact to these findings. The simple scientific data were presented in extremely dramatic and distorted ways to the public. Clearly the journalists were out to arouse interest and controversy, but what seemed to result from their efforts was mostly anxiety and annoyance on the part of left-handed readers. Of course, one really couldn't blame a left-hander who read headlines such as "Brain Damaged Lefties," or "Wrecked Nervous System Makes Southpaws," or "Left Hand—Spoiled Brain" for being upset.

It soon became clear to me that part of the problem lay in the words that I was using. I tended to use the term "pathological left-handedness" to refer to any left-handedness that came about from some form of injury or physical damage. This term is technically correct and has been used by a large number of neuropsychologists over the last twenty years. Unfortunately, the term "pathological" seems to have extremely negative implications that go beyond the common scientific definition, which is only "something that differs from normal because of some form of injury." In the mind of the general public, the label seems to expand so that it also is taken to imply that the pathologically affected individual could be described generally as "weak," "broken," "sick," "helpless," "ravaged," or "debilitated." The message that people seemed to be taking home with them was that left-handers, as a group, were infirm and incapacitated in some major ways. Understandably, this state of affairs was making some left-handers very unhappy. Evidence for this came from the stream of hostile letters that began to make their way to my office. People would write things like:

> How dare you imply that left-handers are brain damaged? My father was left-handed and was an extremely respected surgeon. He also finished very high in his class in medical school. If you knew what you were talking about you would stop making such empty accusations about people who merely use a different hand when they are doing things.

or:

> You have some nerve calling left-handers pathological. Both of my sons are left-handed. One of them is a Phi Beta Kappa graduate of Yale and the other has just finished his law degree at Chicago. I intend to consult with my lawyer son to see if some sort of legal action can be taken to stop this form of slander that you are putting out through the media.

or:

> My daughter is very upset about an article that you wrote in the *Los Angeles Times*. Her friend at school showed it to her, and now they are all laughing at her and calling her brain damaged and retarded. A university professor like yourself should know better than to go around picking on people because they are left-handed and ruining their lives. You ought to be ashamed of yourself and you should publicly retract your article.

Of course, I did not write any of the newspaper articles referred to.

When an article is about a person's work, people tend to assume that the person being discussed has written the newspaper report as well. If I had written these columns, I certainly would not have tried to sensationalize the results as the journalists did. When we have published our research in scientific journals, our intentions were not to imply that, because a person was a left-hander, that person was automatically supposed to be classified as impaired.

To try to avoid the implications that the public was drawing from the word "pathological," our research group began to look for a different label that might not trigger these emotional responses from readers and this sensationalism from journalists. Rather than referring to left-handers as being *abnormal*, we have come to refer to them as being *alinormal*. The *ali* in "alinormal" is the same as the *ali* in "alibi", and it means "elsewhere" or "otherwise", while *normal* has its usual meaning. Thus we could say that although left-handedness itself may arise from pathological influences, we begin with the presumption that any given left-hander is otherwise normal. Any problems which the typical left-hander might have are usually presumed not to be incapacitating for the individual. On the other hand, we do expect that there would be noticeable differences between alinormal left-handers and typical right-handers and that some of these differences would be consistent with the notion that left-handedness is associated with some forms of neuropathology. Evidence supporting such a viewpoint seems to be scattered all through the research literature. Left- and right-handers seem to differ in many aspects of their behavior and physical development.

The Slow-Growing Southpaw

Researchers have often suggested that we grow into our pattern of handedness. Infants and very young children often show mixed patterns of handedness. Sometimes, for instance, the young child may pick up food with his or her right hand, and then the next time might do it with the left hand, suggesting that handedness has not yet completely "set." At some point, between about three and six years of age, handedness comes to be quite well established. Some scientists have suggested that this trend reflects growth patterns that are going on in the brain and nervous system.[1] The two hemispheres of the brain grow at different rates, and one (usually the left) gradually establishes its dominance. It is this dominant hemisphere that determines your handedness.

Suppose that something (say some form of birth stress, or some other form of injury) damages the newborn child. One consequence of such damage might be to slow the normal growth process. The theory offered in such instances is that, as the normal process of growth and development causes an individual to become right-handed, the group of individuals with the slower growth pattern might be less likely to develop the expected pattern of strong and consistent right-handedness. In other words, they are more likely to be left-handed. Turning this argument on its head, the neuropsychologist would expect that, as a group, it should be possible to predict that left-handers would mature more slowly than right-handers. In other words, for the neuropsychologist, left-handedness (a broken black key in our piano scenario) might serve as a sign or a signal that the normal growth and developmental processes are delayed (a broken white key).

In our laboratory, we decided to pursue this question, to see if, indeed, left-handers were slower in their physical development than right-handers.[2] Trying to determine the answer is harder than it seems. Clear indications of the level of a person's physical development are needed. What would be preferred is some sort of a clear-cut marker or abrupt change that occurs during the course of development of each individual, so that we could determine when left- and right-handers reach that stage of development. This would allow us to see if people with different handedness mature at different rates. The most obvious set of changes that human beings undergo during their process of growing up occur during puberty. At puberty, individuals begin to develop most of their adult physical characteristics, and their bodies undergo rapid and dramatic changes. These changes affect the individual's height, weight, voice, body shape, skin characteristics, and the functioning of the sex organs. Different individuals reach puberty at different ages. Generally speaking, the better an individual's health status is, the earlier he or she reaches puberty. Looking for the timing of physical signs of puberty and sexual maturity might be a good way to see if left- and right-handers mature at the same rate.

For women there are some very obvious signals that they have reached sexual maturity. The signs that an observer is most likely to notice include the change in the size of the maturing girl's breasts, the width of her hips relative to her shoulders, and the change in skin texture from that of a child to the soft elastic skin pattern of the adult human female. The single event associated with her changing body that is most likely to be remembered by a woman is the occurrence of her first menstrual period. Most women remember this event clearly and can recall the age at which this occurred with reasonably good accuracy. For many it is remembered as a traumatic event, and hence this event is usually clearly stamped into memory. Although, on average, in North America the age that the first menstrual period occurs at about twelve and a half years of age, some girls may begin menstruating as early as ten and a half years, while others may reach eighteen years of age before menarche.

We decided that the age at which the first menstrual period began would be a good indication of how quickly a woman was developing. Quickly maturing women would reach this developmental stage at a younger age. Therefore, we asked 713 college-aged women to recall the age at which they had their first period. As the average age of this group of women was only a bit older than 18 years, we expected that the memory of this event would still be quite vivid and easily recalled. Naturally, we also determined if each woman was left- or right-handed as well. The average North American woman begins to menstruate at about twelve and a half years of age, and the data show that 75 percent of all women have their first period before they are fourteen. We decided to call anyone who does not have a period until fourteen or older a slow-maturing female. When we analyzed our data, we found that left-handed women were 59 percent more likely than right-handed women to have their first menstrual period after they were fourteen years old. This result can be interpreted as meaning that left-handed women are developing physically at a slower rate than their right-handed counterparts.

To conduct a similar investigation for males is a bit more difficult, as a readily visible marker of when a man reaches sexual maturity is not as clear. We certainly have no striking physical event to be easily described and remembered. We do know that males tend to mature more slowly than females. The average male reaches puberty at about fourteen and a half years of age, although some may be two or three years ahead of or behind this age. Although the technical definition of puberty involves the age at which the first live sperm are produced, this is not an event that men are apt to remember or even recognize. Other signs of sexual maturity include the lowering of the voice and the growth of the shoulders relative to the waist. These changes are visible, but occur over an extended time and are not usually noticeable to the growing adolescent. Perhaps the most memorable change for the male during the path to puberty is the change in his pattern of bodily hair. Most males can recall, somewhat vaguely, the age at which they first noticed hair on their chest or around their genitals. A much more memorable event for most men, however, is the age at which they began to shave. This event is memorable because it usually involves getting together the equipment and eventually placing the steel blade against the face. For the adolescent male, the first shave maybe as traumatic as first period for a woman, and may cause almost as much blood to be shed.

We decided to use the age of appearance of adult-pattern body hair as an indication of the rate at which males were maturing. We asked 467 male university students to remember the age at which they began to shave and also the age at which they first remember seeing the adult pattern of bodily hair over various parts of their body. The average age of puberty is fourteen and a half years in North American males; as 75 percent of all males show adult-pattern body hair before the age of sixteen, we considered any male who took longer to be a slow-maturing individual. Our results were very similar to the results for the women. Left-handed males were 57 percent more likely to fall into the delayed growth group than were the right-handed males. Remember, this pattern is what you would predict if left-handers are delayed in their growth relative to right-handers. The left-handers thus show the characteristics associated with sexual maturity at a later age than do the right-handers.

There is another feature of puberty that might also serve as an indicator of how rapidly individuals are developing, and that is an individual's height. A sudden surge in growth occurs around puberty for human beings. This tends to be most obvious around sixth or seventh grade. Unfortunately, most people don't have a clue to how tall they were in sixth and seventh grade as far as measured height in inches or centimeters. On the other hand, virtually everybody can recall their size in relative terms. In other words, you can probably tell me whether you were taller or shorter than most of your classmates around the end of your primary school days.

When we asked both the men and women whom we had tested before to recall their height relative to their classmates at around sixth grade, we found strong evidence that left-handers were maturing more slowly. Left-handed women were 78 percent more likely to report that they were shorter than their classmates in grade school than were right-handed women. For men, left-handers were 52 percent more likely than right-handers to remember that they were shorter than their friends toward the end of primary school. All of this evidence seems to support the notion that left-handers may have delayed growth and development.

If we accept the fact that southpaws develop more slowly, there are still two possibilities to consider. The first is that left-handers mature more slowly, but eventually catch up to their right-handed companions. The other possibility is that once the major period of growth is past, development stops. This would mean that, once having fallen behind in their rate of maturing, left-handers never catch up. We decided to check these two alternatives out experimentally.

Obviously, if left-handers do not make up the lost ground in their growth, they should have a smaller body size. Body size is measured quite easily by the height and weight of the individuals involved. I knew, before I even started this study, that the size differences that I would be looking for would not be very large because, in my previous studies of attitudes toward left-handers and the labels used for them, I had never run into "left-handed" being used to convey the idea of "short" or "slim" or "little" or "runt" in any of the slang phrases that I had studied. If the differences were small, then I would need to measure the height and weight of a lot of people to get a good estimate of whether there was a difference between the size of left- and right-handers.

As my research funds have never been lavish, I looked for some way of getting information about body size and handedness that would not require the expense of bringing hundreds of people into my laboratory to take their measurements. Fortunately, there was a way to get the data that I needed without directly measuring anybody in the lab. This took advantage of the fact that baseball is a sport that is in love with statistics. Periodically, baseball records are put out in the form of "encyclopedias" that list vital data on every player who ever played in the major leagues. While the nature of the data available on any one player varies a bit, depending upon how long ago the player was active, it usually includes the height and weight of each player. It also usually includes the hand that the player threw a ball with and the side that the player batted from.

I dug up a copy of such a baseball encyclopedia,[3] and had one of my very patient research assistants enter the data from every one of the 3,707 pitchers who had played major league baseball up to 1975. I restricted myself to pitchers, as it became obvious from the data that there were systematic differences in the size of players depending upon the position that they normally played. For instance, catchers tend to be somewhat heavier, and often a bit shorter, than most other players, and shortstops tend to be a bit lighter weight. Furthermore, I reasoned that there were enough pitchers to make a reasonable estimate. Finally, the throwing hand of a pitcher is apt to be a good estimate of his natural handedness. Although there are many "switch hitters," players who bat from either side, I can't ever remember hearing of a "switch pitcher" (although I know that writing this is bound to cause a wave of correspondence from afficinados of the sport, who doubtless will provide the names of one or more such individuals).

Now if left-handers mature more slowly (as we have seen) and if they then stop their growth at about the same age that right-handers do, lefties should be a bit smaller than their right-handed colleagues. This is exactly what I found.[4] The difference in height was small but reliable. Left-handed pitchers averaged about a half-inch shorter (1.23 cm) over-all than right-handed pitchers. There was also a systematic weight differ-ence, with left-handed pitchers running about 3 pounds lighter (1.35 kg) than their right-handed teammates.

The importance of these results is not in the size of the difference but rather in the fact that this pattern of difference between left- and right-handers is exactly what would have been predicted from the notion that left-handers grow and develop more slowly than do right-handers. Such data suggest that not just the rate but also the final level of development that the individual reaches differ as a function of handedness. Left-handers simply don't seem to reach their full growth potential. This might be the case for the nervous system as well. If left-handers have a nervous system that has not matured to the extent that a right-hander's has, this might predict differences in behaviors and abilities for people, depending upon their handedness.

Learning and the Left-Hander

Suggestions that left-handedness might be associated with learning diffi-culties probably started with the observation that left-handedness is more common in groups of retarded individuals, a fact we mentioned earlier. This observation eventually led researchers to ask if there was a relationship between left-handedness and some of the milder forms of learning problems. In some respects this sort of a question comes right out of the issue of how quickly and completely individuals mature. It has been suggested that people with learning difficulties are people whose development has been delayed, so that they never achieve the level of maturity of their nervous system that would allow the most efficient processing of information.[5] You now only have to go one step further in terms of speculation. As left-handedness is associated with slow devel-opment and learning disabilities are associated with slow development, then it should be possible to suggest that left-handedness should be more common in groups of individuals with learning problems.[6]

A variety of learning disabilities have been measured. One of the most common is *dyslexia*, which usually shows up as reading difficulty in which the dyslexic individual has trouble interpreting the strings of symbols that make up a word or a sentence. Thus a dyslexic might read the word "saw" for the printed word "was." Writing difficulties often appear in the form of letter reversals, and dyslexic individuals may write b for d, q for p, and so forth. Such problems can greatly impair a child's performance in school.

A good deal of evidence shows that the number of left-handers is greater in groups of learning disabled and dyslexic people. For instance, one study compared 500 consistent left-handers to 900 consistent right-handers. Approximately 12 percent of the left-handers reported learning difficulties such as dyslexia while only 1 percent of the right-handers did. In other words, left-handers were 12 times more likely to have this learning disability.[7]

Even in groups of individuals in whom there is no evidence of a learning disability, left- and right-handers perform differently, with most researchers finding a slight difference in favor of right-handers in certain intellectual abilities or academic skills. For example, in our laboratory we have tested university students. This means that we can be sure that we were not dealing with any severely learning disabled individuals, but even in this group we found that the left-handers didn't do quite as well as the right-handers in vocabulary tests, in tests of arithmetic ability, and in certain types of problem-solving tasks. The differences were quite reliable, but not very large, which is consistent with our notion that left-handers are alinormal rather than abnormal.[8] Similar results were found in a study of records of academic achievement in a high school in Somerset, England. There it was found that right-handers did better in virtually every school subject tested. Again, the differences were reliable but small, with an average difference between left- and right-handers of only about three percentage points in their grades.[9]

Differences in learning and thinking ability between left- and right-handers, however, are not always consistent. Some researchers have found no differences at all in some areas of ability. Others have found that the pattern depends upon the sex of the individual, with left-handed males often showing the poorest overall performance. Part of the reason for the inconsistency has to do with the fact that systematic differences in the abilities of left- and right-handers don't seem to show up until after puberty. In young school children, handedness is seldom found to be related to learning or to problem-solving ability. In adults the results are much clearer. The differences don't reliably make themselves visible until high school or, at the earliest, junior high school, when the children are around thirteen or older.[8]

Some Left-Hander Talents

The picture is not all gloom and intellectual dullness for left-handers, however. In our laboratory we did find certain tests, involving the ability to visualize objects and to mentally manipulate their images, that produced the reverse pattern. A typical example is the *Mental Rotation Test*. A sample item from this test is shown in figure 10.1. Notice that we start with a "test" item, which looks like an object made up of ten blocks glued together. The person's task is to look at the three items next to the example that are marked "target items." One of these figures is exactly the same object as the test item, only it is rotated so that you are looking at it from a different angle. The other two items are different in their shape, and no matter how you rotate them, they will never look like the example. The person being tested has to pick out the object that is the same shape as the test object. In this task, which requires the ability to create an image of an object in your mind and to maneuver it around, twisting and turning the image mentally, we find that left-handers are better than right-handers.[8]

A test like the mental rotation test is useful because this kind of mental imaging skill is an important part of certain scientific applications of mathematics. It is particularly useful in subjects such as in physics, chemistry and engineering, which require a certain degree of geometrical imaging and reasoning. A study conducted at Oxford University looked at the handedness of university faculty members and found that left-handers were much more common in these applied mathematical subject areas than in theoretical mathematics, which does not require these visualization skills.[10]

TEST ITEM   **ROTATED TARGET ITEMS**

FIGURE 10.1: A sample item from the Mental Rotation Test, where the task is to determine which of the three test items is the same as the test item, rotated into a different orientation.

This same set of skills probably explains why there are so many left-handed chess players, since the game of chess requires the ability to visualize geometric patterns and how they would change for each given move.[11] Similarly these visualization skills may also explain the over-abundance of left-handed architects and artists that we discussed in chapter 7.[12]

There is also some evidence that suggests that left-handers tend to be more *extreme* in their overall abilities. By extreme we mean that the intellectual abilities of southpaws are often a case of feast or famine. To illustrate the famine part, we have already seen that there are more left-handers in learning disabled groups and in more extremely intellectually disadvantaged groups such as mental retardates. There is, however, a feast part as well. This is shown by the fact that there is an unexpectedly high number of left-handers in certain groups of extremely bright individuals. For example, the psychologist Camilla Benbow and her research associates from Iowa State University have been studying exceptionally bright and intellectually precocious young (high school age) individuals. To give you some idea of the degree of talent that she is dealing with, she has singled out students whose *Scholastic Aptitude Test* scores (a college admission criterion) are extremely high. The cut-off scores that Benbow used would place a student as being the top one in 10,000 students. When Benbow looked at the handedness of this extremely bright group of students, she found that they are more than twice as likely to be left-handed than are the general run of students taking this exam.[13] The implication is that left-handers are apt to be extremely dull or extremely bright.

Criminality and Delinquency

In 1903 a Professor Cesare Lombroso noted that, in his studies of criminals, he tended to find a disproportionate number of left-handers. Male criminals were three times more likely to be left-handed, and female criminals five times more likely to be left-handers. This caused him to conclude, "I do not dream at all of saying that all left-handed people are wicked, but that left-handedness, united to many other traits, may contribute to form one of the worst characters among the human species."[14]

Lombroso's damning association of left-handedness with wickedness and criminality seems to have been part of a general pattern of negative feelings about left-handedness. For instance, popular journalists often make it a point to call it to public attention when a particularly villain-ous individual is left-handed. Thus, among criminals, some of the more spectacular and disturbing criminal left-handers include:

• *Billy the Kid*: The infamous William H. Bonney has become, in many people's minds, the model of the western badman. Bonney was born in New York City in 1859. His family moved from there, first to Kansas and then to New Mexico. Before Bonney had reached the age of sixteen he had killed several men in arguments in saloons and gam-bling halls. Billy the Kid, as he came to be called, is believed to have started the practice of carving a notch in the handle of his pistol for each victim. It is reported that this left-hander had carved twenty-one notches in his gun, representing as many dead men, by the time he reached the age twenty-one. Bonney led a brutal gang of cattle rustlers and killers during the Lincoln County cattle wars. He was eventually captured and sentenced to hang. After a spectacular escape, he was hun-ted down and shot to death by the right-handed Sheriff Pat Garrett.

• *Jack the Ripper*: Perhaps the first and the most spectacular of the urban serial sex murderers was Jack the Ripper. His killing spree is thought by some to have begun on the Bank Holiday of 6 August 1888. The victim that day was named Martha Turner, and she was a prostitute living in London's rundown Whitechapel district, in the East End. Turner was killed at around 3 A.M. by someone who stabbed her thirty-nine times with a sharp knife or bayonet-like weapon. Dr. Timothy Kel-eene examined the body and concluded that the wounds seemed to have been made by a left-handed man. On Friday, 31 August 1888, Mary Ann Nichols was killed by having her throat cut. Afterwards she was disembowelled. Bruises on the side of her face and the fact that her throat was slashed from left to right led the examiner, Dr. Ralph Llewel-lyn, to conclude that the killer was likely left-handed. This very same left-to-right throat slash was found on all of the subsequent victims of the Ripper's wrath, namely, Annie Chapman, Elizabeth Stride, Cather-ine Eddows, and Mary Kelly. Because of the evidence that the killer may have been left-handed, some writers have suggested that the Ripper might have been the left-handed Duke of Clarence, who was grandson of Queen Victoria, and who may have gone mad as a side effect of infection from syphilis.

• *John Dillinger*: Born in Indianapolis, Indiana, John Dillinger became one of the most noted bank robbers and murderers of the Prohibition era. When he was paroled from prison after an attempted robbery, Dil-linger formed a gang, which proceeded to terrorize the American midwest during 1933. He was flamboyant and arrogant. He played to the press, and journalists were eager to write up his exploits. In a bit of grandstanding, he once wrote a letter to Henry Ford, to tell him that he always drove Ford Motor Cars because they made the best escape vehicles. Dillinger's reputation grew, fed in part by two well-publicized escapes from jail. Because he was responsible for at least sixteen killings, the FBI labelled this southpaw the very first Public Enemy Number One. He was eventually shot down outside a Chicago theater by a contingent of federal agents under the direction of the right-handed FBI agent Melvin Purvis.

• *The Boston Strangler*: To shift to a more recent case, we have Albert Henry DeSalvo, who reduced the city of Boston to near panic in the early 1960s as the "Boston Strangler." The police believe that the left-handed DeSalvo was responsible for over 300 rapes and sexual assaults prior to and during his killing spree. According to DeSalvo's confession, he also committed thirteen murders between 14 June 1962 and 4 January 1964. Most of these murders involved rape and strangulation, with the bodies left in obscene postures with a bow knotted around their neck. It is interesting that DeSalvo was not identified by the police "Strangler Bureau," which was set up to respond to the brutal string of murders and to calm the rising wave of fear that gripped Boston. Instead, his confession was obtained and taped by his lawyer, the brilliant attorney F. Lee Bailey, who was just beginning his rapid rise to national prominence. This is particularly interesting because F. Lee Bailey is also a left-hander!

Now, of course, a few major criminals who are left-handed should not be sufficient to stigmatize all left-handers as potentially criminal or delinquent. However, a steady stream of research since Lombroso's original pronouncements seems to suggest that an unusually large number of left-handers get into trouble with the law. Several studies have shown that the number of left-handed inmates in reform schools is unexpectedly large.[15] Furthermore, a study in a reform school in Alabama found that the more strongly left-handed the individuals were, the more likely it was that the reform school dormitory staff would rate them as showing high levels of conduct disorders.[16]

The psychologist Cyril Burt felt that left-handers have an anti-authority attitude and uncooperative natures, which would produce just the sort of behaviors that would get a child into difficulty with the law or other officials. He observed:

Again and again in my case summaries the left-handed child is described by those who know him as stubborn and wilful. At times he is visibly of an assertive type, domineering, overbearing, and openly rebellious against all of the dictates of authority.[17]

The evidence linking left-handedness with criminality and delinquency has been slowly accumulating. For instance, one study began by looking at all 9,125 children born between 1959 and 1961 at one particular hospital in Copenhagen. At about twelve years of age a group of these children were carefully tested for their handedness. Some six years later, when the children were about eighteen, researchers checked the Danish police register to see if any had any problems with the law. Although there weren't enough delinquent girls in the group to allow the researchers to draw any conclusions, the data from the boys was quite clear. Strongly left-handed boys were more than twice as likely to have been arrested at least once than were the right-handed boys.[18]

My own laboratory has recently collected some data that relate to the criminality and delinquency issue as well. During the course of our research we have been testing the personalities of left- and right-handers using a variety of specialized psychological scales. One of these is the *Social Nonconformity* scale, which is a part of the *Psychological Screening Inventory.*[19] This scale was designed to measure how similar the person being tested is to a group of convicted prisoners whose antisocial behaviors led to their being jailed for offenses ranging from minor infractions up through violent crimes. The rationale behind using such a scale is that, if a person gets a high score on this measure, he or she has many of the same behavior characteristics as this criminal group has. Such individuals are apt to agree with statements such as, "I break more laws than many people" or "My school teachers had some problems with me." They would also tend to disagree with statements like, "I have never broken a major law" or "I like to obey the law." In our research, we tested 494 university students on the Social Nonconformity scale and found that left-handers had consistently higher scores than right-handers, meaning that the attitudes of the left-handers were more similar to those of known and convicted lawbreakers.

Personality Differences

Several researchers have suggested personality differences between left- and right-handers. One of the most vigorous, and negative, in his description of the personality of left-handers was Abraham Blau, former

Chief Psychiatrist at the New York University Clinic, whom we mentioned in chapter 4. Blau's theory was that left-handedness was a sign of emotional negativism. He believed that the left-hander was a basically hostile and negative person, which was proven by his very unwillingness to learn to be right-handed. In his view, left-handedness is adopted as an act of protest, anger, and aggression by a young child who has few other ways to express his hostility. Blau is quite strident in his expression of his ideas, writing:

My theory of negativistic sinistrality is that it springs from a contrary emotional attitude to the learning of right-handedness. Sinistrality is thus nothing more than an expression of infantile negativism and falls into the same category as other well-known reactions of a similar nature, such as contrariety in feeding and elimination, retardation in speech and general perverseness insofar as the infant with meager outlets can express it.[20]

Dr. Blau eventually reaches the damning conclusion that left-handedness should be used by psychiatrists as a definite sign that the person showing it has personality difficulties. Fortunately for the left-hander, few other scientists have reached such a negative conclusion about the personality of left-handers.

There are a number of studies that suggest that there are real personality differences between left- and right-handers. One common finding is that left-handers appear to be more anxious than right-handers. For example, one investigation involving 266 San Jose State University students confirmed that left-handers score high on psychological tests that measure how anxious a person is and how likely they are to become anxious in various situations.[21]

Another illustration of the relationship between left-handedness and anxiety comes from a study conducted among medical students. Specifically, the participants were 141 general surgery residents participating in the Loyola University training program over a six year period. When tested for psychological characteristics, the left-handed surgical residents were found to be much more responsive to stress and, in addition, they were notably more cautious in their behaviors than were the right-handed surgical residents.[22]

Left-handers seem to be more anxious about nearly everything. Things that particularly seem to worry left-handed students more than right-handers include how they are doing in school, their relationships with others, their health and appearance, their career development, money concerns, and time pressures.[23] It is possible that all of this worrying may also explain why left-handers seem to be a bit less emotionally stable than right-handers.[24]

My own laboratory has recently began to look at the personality traits of left-handers. We analyzed some data from an ongoing project and found some systematic differences between left- and right-handed personalities, particularly in the way individuals respond to other people socially. Using a group of 523 young adults, we presented them with the *Interpersonal Adjective Scale*, a list of 64 words that describe personality characteristics. Each person had to rate how well each word described himself or herself. The data revealed that left-handers were more likely to describe themselves as being *introverted*. They tended to feel that they were "bashful" and "shy" rather than "outgoing," "talkative," and "cheerful." Left-handers were also more *aloof* in their characteristics. They tended to describe themselves as being more "distant," "antisocial," and "unneighborly" and less "friendly" and "approachable" than right-handers did when describing themselves. Along the same lines, left-handers have a personality that may be considered to be *cold*. They admit to being a bit "ruthless" and "unsympathetic," as opposed to right-handers, who claim to be more "tenderhearted" and "kind." Finally, left-handers seem to be a bit more *quarrelsome*. They are more likely to describe their behaviors as "impolite" and "discourteous" and are less likely to describe their behaviors as "cordial" and "courteous." The resulting picture of the personality of the left-hander is of an individual who keeps to himself and tends to be a bit unresponsive and abrasive in his or her social interactions as compared to right-handers.

And in Passing . . .

A series of other differences between left-and right-handers are difficult to categorize but probably ought to mentioned because you might find them interesting or amusing, such as:

- *Hair color.* While it is unclear whether blondes have more fun, a survey of 1,117 individuals in the Boston metropolitan area did indicate that blondes are twice as likely to be left- or mixed-handed than are people with darker hair colors.[25]
- *Eating habits.* A study published in South Africa suggests that people who are vegetarians are more likely to be left-handed.[26]
- *Right-left confusion.* A survey of 607 people in Texas questioned how well people could tell their right from their left side. Some of the

questions asked whether the individual had difficulty when he or she had to quickly judge his or her left or right, or whether they had problems in quickly deciding which way to turn when someone giving them directions tells them to go left or right. Left-handers were about one and a half times more likely to report that they "always" or "frequently" had such confusions in telling their left from the right sides.[27]

- *Tongue-rolling ability.* One recent study of 948 individuals enrolled in the Faculty of Education of Ohio State University looked at tongue-rolling ability and handedness. Tongue rollers are individuals who can turn up one or both sides of their tongue, an ability that is important if you wish to be able to whistle musically. They report that many fewer left-handers have this ability than right-handers.[28]

- *Sex of children.* Perhaps one of the most puzzling recent findings about handedness comes from the University College in London, where a researcher gathered published data on 27,420 individuals and then looked at their handedness and the handedness of their parents. He reports that, if both parents are right-handed, their chance of having a male child is greater. If at least one parent is left-handed, the chance that their offspring will be female goes up by 17 percent.[29]

We have now listed a number of differences between left- and right-handers, which suggest that the psychology, development, personality and the behavior of left-handers may differ from those of right-handers. While some of these comparisons reflect on matters that affect the individual's life-style in major ways, another set of characteristics may place the left-hander's life in actual jeopardy. Let us now look at the health implications of being left-handed.

11

Health and the Left-Hander

It was the writer and newspaper columnist John Mortimer who said, "There is no human activity, eating, sleeping, drinking or sex, which some doctor, some where, won't discover leads directly to cardiac arrest."[1] In some respects I am fulfilling Mortimer's prophesy when I am forced to inform you that certain health implications are associated with being left-handed, although the good news is that, at least to the best of my knowledge, left-handedness does not lead to cardiac arrest.

One might suspect that left-handers could be subject to physical difficulties that might affect fitness and vigor, simply from the reasoning that we used in the last chapter in the secondhand piano scenario. If left-handedness is due to some form of birth-related or pregnancy-related neural damage, it is likely that other neural control centers and perhaps certain organs may have been damaged as well. If these damaged organs or neural pathways are important for the maintenance of normal health and normal bodily functioning, this might cause left-handers to have a somewhat poorer health status.

We became interested in the relationship between handedness and health because one of the themes of my neuropsychological research has to do with what a person's behaviors can tell us about that person's physiology and health. This research area is often called *behavioral medicine*. Several scientific journals deal exclusively with research on this topic, and an international organization meets annually to discuss the newest research findings on this subject. In the area of behavioral medicine three different approaches are used. The first looks at how the individual's behaviors can affect his or her health status directly. From this approach one might ask how smoking, drinking, or exercise (all behaviors under a person's direct control) affect health and what can be done to alter these behaviors. The second looks at how physiological conditions can affect behavior. Here questions might deal with how a certain genetic makeup might predict criminality or psychological disturbance. The third approach looks at how particular behaviors can be used to predict the existence or likelihood that certain physical conditions exist or may eventually develop in a person. My own interests are with the second and third approaches. With reference to handedness, this means looking at physiological factors that can cause a person to develop into a left-or a right-hander and looking at which physical conditions might be predicted by a person's being left- or right-handed. My research on the direct health implications of handedness came about indirectly. Our lab was looking at another set of problems when the issue of handedness came up.

Sleep and the Left-Hander

I have always had some interest in the problem of sleep, because it is a behavior that takes up one-third of our life and is very sensitive to many psychological and physiological factors. For example, one of the major symptoms of *depressive neurosis* is a change in a person's sleep pattern. The most common complaint associated with depression deals with a particular form of insomnia in which the person goes to sleep without much difficulty, but then awakens very early, well before daybreak, and can't fall back to sleep again. In some other forms of neurotic disorders we may find *hypersomnia*, where the person sleeps for prolonged periods, often for twelve hours or more a day.

In my laboratory an intermittent research program has been looking at sleep patterns and their relationship to other problems. I was interested in the effects of minor birth stressors or pregnancy difficulties on sleep patterns, having been attracted to this problem when research began to be published indicating that children who have experienced birth stressors or a difficult pregnancy are apt to have problems with sleep, mostly difficulty in falling asleep or frequently waking during the night. The types of birth-related problems that seemed to produce sleep disorders included premature birth, low weight at birth, and breathing difficulties.[2]

With the help of Alan Searleman of St. Lawrence University in New

York State, I decided to test the relationship between birth difficulties and sleep disorders. Specifically, we wanted to extend the previous research to see if the insomnia experienced by birth-stressed children was simply a childhood problem or whether the effects persisted through to adulthood. To answer this question we asked over a thousand college students if they suffered from any sleep problems.[3] We next contacted their mothers and determined whether any difficulties had been associated with the birth of these children. We were interested in any birth stressors from the following list:

- premature birth
- an overly long period of labor
- breech birth
- breathing difficulty at birth
- low birth weight
- Caesarian delivery
- multiple birth
- Rh incompatibility

We also asked the mothers to tell us how well their children slept when they were infants, particularly when at around six months of age.

The results were quite clear. When children had had a difficult birth, their mothers were much more likely to report these infants also suffered from sleep difficulties. Furthermore, these sleep difficulties were likely to continue through to adulthood. We found that in about 75 percent of the cases, if mothers reported that their infants had sleep problems, eighteen years later, as young adults, these individuals were still reporting sleep problems.

Alan Searleman and I had worked together on a number of other earlier projects, and several of these had involved the relationship between handedness and birth stressors. It was probably unsurprising that we noticed that the list of birth stressors that produced sleep disruptions were very similar to the list of birth stressors described in Chapter 8 as associated with increased levels of left-handedness. This immediately suggested to us that left-handers as a group might also suffer from insomnia more than right-handers. It certainly seemed worth looking into.

To see if there was any relationship between sleep disorders and left-handedness, we began another study that ultimately involved 1,274 participants.[4] We first measured the handedness of each person in the study and then determined if they suffered from either of the two most common sleep problems: namely, trouble falling asleep and frequent awakening during the night. The results were really quite striking. Left-handers were nearly twice as likely to have disrupted sleep because they woke frequently during the night than were right-handers. In addition, left-handers were two and a half times more likely to have trouble falling asleep than were their right-handed contemporaries. These findings confirmed our suspicions that there was a link between left-handedness and insomnia. We concluded that to be a left-hander means that one may suffer many sleepless nights.

Sensory Disorders

Insomnia is not the only problem that left-handers seem to be more susceptible to. Some research has provided evidence for an unexpected connection between left-handedness and various visual and hearing problems. Although the mechanism that links handedness to the sensory systems is not fully clear, it may merely be another example of the process that I have mentioned several times already: If there was some form of injury or neural damage sufficient to cause the left-handedness, it seems likely that other systems may have been damaged also. The likelihood that any other system may be damaged will probably be related to just how complex and widespread the neural control mechanisms are for that system. Certainly the functioning of the eye and the ear involves a lot of neural processing and many different brain pathways and analysis centers. This would make these systems vulnerable targets for any random damage due to the kind of birth stressors that may result in the failure to develop right-handedness.

A Harvard Medical School ophthalmologist followed up the suggestion made by some earlier scientists that there might be an association between handedness and *squint*.[5] Squint is the technical term for the condition of being cross-eyed. There are several types of cross-eyedness. The most common type is *esotropia*, which means that the eyes are turned too far inward (toward the nose) as opposed to *exotropia*, where the eyes are turned outward (referred to as "wall-eyed"). This researcher tested people at the University Hospital in Boston and the Boston City Hospital and also patients showing up for ophthalmological treatment in several private medical practices. He found that, compared to non-cross-eyed patients, the group of esotropically cross-eyed patients contained more than twice as many individuals who were not right-handed (that is, were left- or mixed-handed). Thus, at least for this form of visual problem, left-handers seem to be at greater risk.

Hearing also seems to be related to handedness. One group of researchers looked at the handedness of deaf students enrolled in the Virginia School for the Deaf and Blind in Staunton, Virginia (a high school for the visually and hearing impaired) and also at Gallaudet College in Washington, D.C. (a university with a special program for the deaf).[6] To qualify for the study, individuals had to be deaf. In addition, all participants must have had some form of deafness that had started at a very early age, before the person had had time to develop language skills. Finally, the subjects of this study had to be free of any detectable brain malfunctions other than that which might be causing the deafness. The handedness of these students was compared to that of normally hearing students enrolled at the University of Virginia. The resulting data showed that, of the hearing students, 11 percent were non-right-handed; of the deaf students, 28 percent were. In other words, deaf students were two and a half times more likely to be non-right-handed than were hearing students.

Studies such as these suggest that left-handers are more likely to be suffering from visual or hearing impairments than are right-handers.

The Testosterone Connection

Over the past ten or so years, researchers have uncovered an entire set of health-related problems that affect left-handers more than right-handers. This particular set of problems is linked together by a hormonal factor. While many of the resulting health problems are minor and fairly common ailments, a few are more serious difficulties.

The story of the discovery of this set of handedness-related health problems started with a pair of observations. The first observation was not very new. It was the well-known fact that men are more likely to be left-handed than women. The second observation came to light during a conversation that the late Norman Geschwind of Harvard Medical School had with one of his associates, a medical doctor. He noted that it seemed to him that certain diseases seemed to be more common in left-handers. These two ideas somehow fused together in Geschwind's mind and resulted in a series of neuropsychological speculations and a large number of experimental studies, which have been carried on since his death by his colleague and research collaborator Albert Galaburda, also at Harvard Medical School.[7] For Geschwind and Galaburda the story of left-handedness begins in the womb. They agree that left-handedness comes about through abnormal conditions during pregnancy and delivery, and the culprit is not one of the birth stressors that we have discussed before but rather the common sex hormone *testosterone.*

Testosterone is the hormone that is responsible for giving male characteristics to an individual. It is the release of massive doses of testosterone at and after puberty that is responsible for the voice change in males, the development of facial hair, and even the onset of the normal male pattern of balding. For the developing fetus, the presence of high levels of testosterone is responsible for the development of masculine genitalia. A developing male child is bathed before birth in testosterone secreted into the amniotic fluid in which the fetus floats. Much of the testosterone is produced by his own testes as soon as they are formed; however, some testosterone is produced by the mother. Small amounts are secreted into the womb from her ovaries and placenta; therefore under certain conditions, even developing female children can be exposed to sizeable amounts of this hormone.

According to Geschwind and Galaburda, testosterone also affects the brain of the developing infant. Specifically, it slows the rate of development of the left hemisphere of the brain, which is normally responsible for the control of the right hand and also houses the language control centers. This abnormal pattern of brain growth may result in the left hemisphere's not achieving its full growth potential, allowing the right hemisphere (controlling the left hand) to be more dominant, at least relatively speaking. This shift in brain dominance may then cause an individual who otherwise would have developed into a right-hander to become left-handed, because the left side of the brain did not mature properly and cannot enforce a leadership role.

These speculations about the effects of testosterone explain some research findings very well. For instance, males are exposed to more testosterone in the uterus, because their own organs generate this hormone. This means that the chances that a male will be left-handed should be greater than the chances that a female will be left-handed, which of course, was one of the observations that led Geschwind to start looking at testosterone in the first place. The fact is that males are about one and a half times more likely to be left-handed than females.

Testosterone also affects the development of other organs besides the brain. For instance, it tends to suppress growth of the thymus gland. The thymus gland is a double-lobed organ located in the lower neck region, behind the breastbone. It is particularly important for the development of the body's immune system, which is designed to protect us from infection. If the thymus gland is not functioning properly a person

can develop various problems ranging from allergies to increased susceptibility to diseases or even greater risk of tumor growth.

In human beings, immune-system disorders make themselves known
in several ways. Normally the immune system rallies to defend the body
from specific *antigens*. An antigen is usually a virus or a bacteria, which
is recognized as being a foreign substance in the body. *Lymphocytes*,
which are white blood cells, are formed in several places in the body,
with one of the most important locations being the thymus gland. Part
of the job of a lymphocyte is to recognize that the proteins that make
up viruses and bacteria are not the usual body-related substances but
rather foreign or alien matter that might be dangerous to the individual.
If the normal development of the thymus gland and other related sites
is retarded, the ability of certain lymphocytes to distinguish a dangerous
invading foreign substance from a harmless substance is sometimes affected. This can result in the body's mounting a defensive reaction to
something as harmless as grass pollens or household dust. Such reactions result in the symptom patterns that we usually refer to as *allergy*
or *hypersensitivity*. Common allergic symptoms come about because of
the formation of specific antibodies, which then cause certain cells (the
mast cells) to release substances including *histamine*. Histamine and some
of the other compounds related to it produce the familiar allergic symptoms that include skin rashes, itching, sneezing, runny nose, watery
eyes, swelling, breathing difficulties, and muscle contractions that result
in stiffness and pain.

Medical researchers generally identify particular allergies on the basis
of the specific immune response triggered and the type of antibodies
released. One particular allergic pattern is quite common. It involves
the release of the antibody *immunoglobin E*. When immunoglobin E interacts with the lymphocytes produced in the thymus gland, it produces
fairly immediate allergy symptoms. People whose allergic reaction involves this antibody are usually called *atopic* individuals. This atopic
pattern is actually the basis of a number of the allergic reactions, including some which are very common and familiar to most people. For instance:

• *Hay fever.* This allergic response is quite common in the spring in
many geographical regions. It involves symptoms which are mostly in
the nose. Sneezing, runny nose and so forth are often triggered by sea-
sonally produced pollens from grass, trees and weeds (such as the ever-
present ragweed). The secondary effects sometimes include watery or
itchy eyes.

• *Allergic rhinitis.* For some people allergic symptoms similar to those of hay fever persist throughout the year, rather than having seasonal peaks. These allergic responses are triggered by household dust. To be more precise, it is not the dust itself but a particular mite found in house dust. Other substances that might cause these symptoms are animal fur or feathers or the skin dander produced by some animals. When the allergic symptoms go on all year, doctors tend to refer to the problem as allergic rhinitis, rather than hay fever, although the immune system reaction is virtually identical.

• *Conjunctivitis.* Atopic allergic reactions may also show up as an inflammation of the skin covering the eye and inner eyelids known as conjunctivitis. Symptoms may include redness, occasional itching or tenderness, and usually some form of sticky or watery discharges from the eye.

• *Asthma.* A more serious atopic allergic reaction pattern is asthma. Its symptoms include wheezing, coughing, and severe breathing difficulty, the results of an allergy-like response to certain substances inhaled in the air such as pollen, animal dander, fur, certain spores, or dust. An attack can also be generated by certain foods (eggs, shellfish, and chocolate are common causes) and some drugs (aspirin is a frequent culprit). The allergic response involves swelling and the accumulation of thick layers of mucous on the passageways leading to the lungs, which in turn leads to the breathing difficulties. Major attacks may require the use of oxygen to relieve the symptoms. Serious, sudden-onset attacks are also treated with adrenaline and certain steroid compounds. Many asthma sufferers carry inhalers that provide aerosol versions of such drugs for emergency use.

• *Skin Problems.* Difficulties with the immune system not only affect the respiratory system and the eyes but also can produce a variety of skin symptoms, particularly *eczema*. Eczema is not a disease but more a description of a particular set of symptoms, which include a red scaly skin rash, sometimes with crusts or scabs. The rash may be dry or have a watery discharge and is often accompanied by various degrees of itching or burning. Certain forms of eczema, such as some types of *urticaria* (a reddened and swollen form of skin rash) also seem to be the result of a malfunctioning immune system. These seem to follow the pattern associated with some of the other atopic forms of allergic responses.

• *Other Allergic Responses.* A variety of other allergies, particularly many common food allergies and insect sting allergies, follow the atopic pattern of response. It has been suggested that a number of these may actually involve the immune system in some ways, particularly as many allergic symptoms seem to involve an overreaction of the immune system to substances that are not intrinsically dangerous to the body.

We have spent this much time describing the atopic group of allergic responses because they involve the lymphocytes produced by the thymus gland. Such problems are much more common in people whose thymus gland is not operating at full capacity. This is important to our discussion of handedness because, according to Geschwind and Galaburda, exposure to raised levels of the hormone testosterone while the individual is still developing in the womb is responsible for retarding the growth of the thymus gland. Also, according to the theory, the same intrauterine exposure to high levels of testosterone is believed to be responsible for delaying or interrupting the development of the left hemisphere, thus pushing the individual toward left-handedness.

Putting all of these theoretical speculations together leads us to a clear prediction about health and handedness. As a testosterone imbalance can cause some forms of immune system difficulties and also may cause left-handedness in some individuals, we ought to find higher rates of immune diseases in left-handers. We can even be more specific and predict that the kinds of immune problems that ought to plague the left-hander more than the right-hander should include the atopic problems such as hay fever, asthma, allergic rhinitis, conjunctivitis, eczema, urticaria, and a variety of food and other allergies.

The relationship between atopic diseases and left-handedness was first explored in a study in Glasgow, Scotland.[8] It involved 1,092 individuals who were asked whether they were susceptible to any of three problems typical of immune system malfunctioning, namely, hay fever, asthma, and eczema. The results demonstrated an unexpectedly high degree of association between handedness and these maladies. In fact, the data showed that left-handers were eleven and a half times more likely to report these atopic symptoms than were right-handers. Since that first study, several other tests of the same hypothesis have been conducted. Most find similar results, with left-handers seemingly more susceptible to atopic diseases. In so doing, these studies seem also to be confirming the predicted association between left-handedness and deficiencies in the immune system.

As an example of these subsequent studies of handedness and allergic symptoms, we might consider an investigation conducted in London, England. This study measured the handedness of 313 patients who were attending an allergy clinic at St. Mary's Hospital.[9] Obviously, such individuals had noticeable allergic symptoms severe enough to cause them to seek medical assistance. The patients that the researchers were most interested in were suffering from asthma, allergic rhinitis, eczema, or urticaria-type skin rashes. The handedness of these people was then compared to 350 individuals selected at random from people who happened to be at Paddington and King's Cross railway stations when the researchers were there. These "random people" are probably quite representative of the general population of England. Overall, the patients in the allergy clinic were 70 percent more likely to be left-handed than were the people who were not allergy patients.

To further test the theory, the allergy patients were also tested for the precise nature of their allergic reaction using a skin test procedure that looks for the specific antibodies associated with the atopic disease pattern. Remember, it is the atopic pattern of allergic responses that are most strongly associated with problems with the immune system. As predicted, the people who showed the atopic type of antibodies (namely, *immunoglobin E*) in their response were much more likely to be left-handed than the nonpatient group. In fact they were nearly 80 percent more likely to be left-handed.

Another study conducted in Michigan looked at people who were patients of an allergist and those who were attending a health screening clinic.[10] These results, based upon 853 participants, were almost identical to the results of the London study. People who reported allergies were 80 percent more likely to be left-handed. This study also unearthed an intriguing bit of additional data. These researchers looked at the handedness of the children of asthmatic patients. They found that these children are 62 percent more likely to be left-handed, perhaps suggesting that the testosterone imbalance that the parent may have been exposed to is passed on to the children, perhaps through some genetic mechanism. In any event, both the London study and the Michigan study reach the same conclusions, namely, that left-handers are more common in groups of allergy suffers, particularly those with atopic allergies. This is what we would expect if there was some relationship between immune deficiencies and left-handedness.

A particularly interesting extension of the kind of research that we have been discussing includes susceptibility to *migraine headaches*. Migraines are particularly severe headaches that differ in their symptoms from the common types of tension headaches that most people are familiar with. One difference is that migraine headaches will often only involve one side of the head. The pain is often quite stabbing in its nature and usually is felt more to the front and side of the head than tension headaches are. Another difference is that the migraine headache may be accompanied by visual disturbances such as flashes, points, streaks, or zigzags of light. The person may even be bothered by double vision during the headache. Other symptoms may include sweating, which may be a bit bizarre, as such migraine-associated sweating often occurs on only one side of the body. For some people there may stomach problems that result in vomiting as well.

Some researchers have suggested that migraine headaches may be another symptom associated with immune system disorders. If so, we ought to find that migraines are also related to handedness. Some earlier reports seemed to show that left-handers were more likely to have migraine headaches than were right-handers, which supports this theoretical notion.[7] The occurrence of headaches in general was looked at in 374 students enrolled in a public high school in a rural community in Michigan.[11] Researchers determined the number of students who had been forced to miss classes during the previous year because of headaches. They found that the percentage of left-handers suffering such severe headaches was double the percentage of right-handers.

The Autoimmune Connection

The problems with allergies, headaches, sleep disruption, and allergies might all fit into the *alinormal* description of left-handers that we spoke about in the last chapter. These problems, while annoying or uncomfortable, do not incapacitate the person in such a way as to force us to classify the sufferer as being damaged, diseased, or pathologically nonfunctional. Unfortunately, the testosterone exposure that leads to immune system malfunctioning does suggest that left-handers may have a higher risk of having some fairly severe difficulties and disease states as well.

The more severe problems are the result of *autoimmune difficulties*. We have already seen that, if the immune system is not functioning properly, some harmless substances that are inhaled or eaten may be treated as foreign and potentially harmful. It is the body's defensive reaction to such substances that leads to the usual allergic symptoms. One curious variation of immune system malfunctioning comes about when certain proteins that the body normally produces are not recognized. Some secretions or cells associated with the body's internal organs are seen as foreign substances and are reacted to as an invading bacteria or virus would be. When this happens we are faced with an autoimmunity problem or an *autoallergy*. Autoimmune responses are allergic reactions to your own body products. The key to understanding the concept is the word root *auto*, which means "self." Autoimmunity means that the immune system allows the lymphocytes to mount an attack on the person's own body cells and organs.

It is believed that autoimmunity problems are more extreme variations of the immune system malfunctioning just discussed and they are apparently caused by the very same mechanisms. Specifically, when the fetus is subjected to hormonal imbalances (such as high levels of testosterone), growth of the thymus gland and related structures is affected. This places the individual at risk for developing both immune diseases and autoimmune diseases. The same mechanism makes it more likely that a person will be left-handed. We would expect higher rates of autoimmune diseases in left-handers, and this prediction has been confirmed for a number of autoimmune problems.[12]

Let's consider some of the autoimmune diseases which seem to be more common in left-handers:

• *Hashimoto's thyroiditis*. One of the more important problems involves the thyroid gland, a two-lobed organ that lies in front of the trachea in the neck. The thyroid secretes certain hormones that play a crucial role in regulating the rate at which the cells can use or *oxidize* nutrients. Because of this, the thyroid is vital to regulating a person's rate of growth and energy level. A common, but quite significant, thyroid problem called *Hashimoto's thyroiditis* is associated with autoimmune system problems. It is also called *lymphocytic thyroiditis*, since the lymphocytes are found acting as antibodies against the hormones produced by the person's own thyroid gland. In some instances these lymphocytes may attack the thyroid gland itself. The symptoms usually include goiter (a swelling in the base of the neck), pain, and fever. They also include the usual symptoms associated with an underactive thyroid gland, namely: reduced energy, mental dullness, and cool, dry, puffy skin. The usual treatment involves lifelong replacement therapy, with continued doses of thyroid hormone.

• *Myasthenia gravis*. Another autoimmune disease found more commonly in left-handers is myasthenia gravis, a disease of the junctions between the nervous system and the muscles. It leads to fatigue and weakness of the muscles in general. When affecting the eye, it can lead to double vision and drooping eyelids. It can also affect the muscles controlling breathing, swallowing, and coughing, which in turn, in severe cases, may lead to respiratory failure. Sometimes, in order to stop the flow of attacking lymphocytes that cause the problem, the thymus gland must be removed.

• *Stomach and gastrointestinal diseases.* A series of inflammatory diseases of the stomach and gastrointestinal tracts seem to have autoimmune connections. *Crohn's disease* is the most important of these. It is sometimes called *regional ileitis*, as the most common site of the damage is in the lower three-fifths of the small intestines, called the ileum. This section runs about 24 feet (7.5 meters) in length in the average adult male. In some instances, other parts of the gastrointestinal tract can be involved as well. This disease may extend over many years, displaying symptoms that include abdominal pain, weight loss, anemia, dehydration, and possible blockage of the intestinal passageway. A closely related disease is *ulcerative colitis*, which produces similar symptoms with the addition of some rectal bleeding. These digestive-system problems appear to be associated with autoimmune difficulties. The specific mechanism of inflammatory bowel disease symptoms is a reaction produced by the immune system in which lymphocytes actually attack the inner surfaces of the person's own gastrointestinal system causing inflammation, bleeding, ulcers, and weakening of the walls of the digestive tract.

• *Diabetes.* In Greek the word *diabetes* means "passing through." It has come to designate a set a diseases in which excessive urination is one of the visible symptoms. *Diabetes mellitus* is a disease in which there is an inadequate secretion of the hormone insulin, which controls the blood sugar level. Too high a blood sugar level can lead to a variety of complications such as kidney disease, arteriosclerosis, disorders of the nervous system that affect feeling and muscle control, increased susceptibility to infections, and many other problems which can have the effect of shortening an individual's life span. There are two common types of diabetes mellitus. The first is *juvenile onset* or *insulin-dependent* diabetes (usually called Type I), which begins to show its symptoms between childhood and early adulthood. The second type is *late onset* or *non–insulin dependent* diabetes (Type II), which shows up in middle age or later. The nature of these two types of diabetes is quite different. Late onset diabetes often results from factors associated with pancreas failure such as obesity, environmental factors, sometimes viral infections, and most certainly a genetic predisposition. Although enough insulin is produced to avoid some of the most severe diabetic symptoms, not enough is produced to meet the body's needs. Juvenile onset diabetes, however, is quite different. It appears to be due to autoimmune problems. What seems to happen is that the body does not recognize the *islet cells* (the cells in the pancreas that make and secrete insulin) and react to these cells or their secretions as if they were a foreign invader such as an infectious virus. Antibodies are created, which then attack the islet cells and damage or eliminate their ability to make insulin. Often, virtually no insulin is found in the blood of such patients. In this form of diabetes the individual's condition fluctuates considerably, and it is often difficult to maintain a stable condition. Insulin administration is usually needed in order to keep the individual alive.

Several studies[13] have shown that all of the autoimmune problems described above are more common in left-handers. For instance, there are reports that left-handers may be twice as likely as right-handers to suffer from juvenile onset diabetes. The number of left-handers is particularly high among male diabetics. The relationship between diabetes and handedness is not as clear in females. When we look at patients with Hashimoto's thyroiditis, we also find an overabundance of left-handers. Left-handed women appear to be three times more likely to have Crohn's disease and ulcerative colitis than their right-handed counterparts. In other words, the gloomy news is that left-handers seem to be particularly susceptible to autoimmune diseases and problems.

Alcoholism

Some other problems, although behavioral in nature, do have health implications and also seem to be related to handedness. One of these behavioral problems is *alcoholism*. Alcoholism, defined as a form of compulsive drinking, is one of the most serious public health concerns in contemporary society. This disease is generally progressive and often results in both physical and psychological dependence. Alcohol dependency, when prolonged or severe, almost always leads to physical problems. Alcoholics often suffer from malnutrition, mental disturbances, neural damage, loss of certain aspects of visual function, and damage to the liver. Ultimately, the cumulative effect of alcohol dependency and its negative effects on various organs of the body may lead to death.

Although I was quite surprised when I first learned of it, there seems to be an association between alcoholism and left-handedness. I found that a number of researchers had looked at patients hospitalized for alcohol abuse in order to determine their handedness. In general, all had reported that there were more left- or mixed-handed individuals in these patient groups. The effects were most noticeable among men where, in some cases, the number of left-handers was nearly four times the percentage found in the general nonalcoholic population.[13] One puzzling finding with respect to alcoholism and handedness is the fact that individuals with an alcoholic father are also much more likely not only to be alcoholic, but to be left-handed as well.

For left-handers the trouble doesn't stop with the development of the alcoholic symptoms, but affects the success of their treatment, too. Specifically, left-handed alcoholics seem to be less likely to respond well to therapeutic programs designed to treat their alcoholism. In one study that looked at 64 alcoholics receiving therapy for their problem, the researchers determined how many relapses into drinking each individual had during the treatment regime. The goal was to have six months of total abstinence from alcohol. Patients who were left-handed had nearly three times as many relapses, hence they required a considerably longer time in therapy. Among the patients who had the most trouble avoiding alcohol for six months, 86 percent were left-handed. Compare this to the fact that, among the group that had the least trouble avoiding alcohol, only 12 percent were left-handed.[14]

Another study monitored a sample of alcoholic men during a full year of treatment for compulsive drinking. At the end of the year of hospitalization for alcoholism, 56 percent of the right-handers were listed as being "improved" while only 29 percent of the left-handers made it to the "improved" category. In other words, compared to right-handed alcoholics, left-handers were only half as likely to improve under direct treatment.[15]

Left-handers seem not only more likely to be drinkers, but also more prone to be smokers. One research project studied a community in Michigan and surveyed about 1,100 people. In this group, left-handers were more likely to be smokers and more likely to report that they smoked more than ten cigarettes a day; they were more likely to be both drinkers and smokers as well.[16]

Why do we find more left-handed smokers and drinkers? A particularly suggestive piece of data suggests that left-handers have different brain responses to psychologically active chemicals than do right-handers. One researcher from the Department of Psychiatry at the University of New York at Stony Brook looked at the data from fourteen studies that measured changes in the electrical activity of the brain after individuals had been given one of a variety of different drugs. These studies all used electroencephalograph recordings, commonly know as EEGs, to measure the activity of the brain in response to these chemicals. Left-

and right-handers did differ in terms of their EEG recordings. In general, the brains of left-handers showed greater changes in response to these drugs than did the brains of the right-handers. There were quite a variety of drugs that left-handers were more responsive to, including an antihistamine, several sedatives, an antidepressant, an antipsychotic, and several experimental drug compounds and even the common painkiller aspirin. The clear conclusion is that the brains of left-handers react more vigorously to a variety of substances.[17] Perhaps this increased reactivity makes it easier for left-handers to become dependent upon or addicted to substances such as alcohol or nicotine.

Homosexuality

Homosexuality refers to individuals who are sexually attracted predominantly to others of the same gender. The root *homo* comes from the Greek word for "same." Homosexuality has been called many things at various times, including a sin, an illness, a behavior disturbance, a way of life, a perversion, a normal variant of sexual behavior, and a crime. For many years the mental health profession officially championed the belief that homosexuality was a psychological disorder. In 1973 this position was officially modified. Under the revised view, only those homosexuals who feel personally troubled by their own behavior and who want their sexual orientation to be changed to the heterosexual pattern are now considered candidates for psychological treatment. This change in attitude seems to have come about because of evidence that many (some say most) homosexuals are well adapted to their alternate life style. They usually are productive, working members of the community, who don't show any evidence of being psychologically disturbed and seem to be quite happy with their sexual orientation.

Many theories have been offered to try to explain homosexuality. Biologically based theories originally suggested that homosexuality might be due to some hormonal imbalance. For example, it has been suggested that male homosexuals might be suffering from a deficiency in testosterone or a surplus of *estrogen* (the major female hormone). Female homosexuals (lesbians) are then said to be suffering from the reverse hormonal imbalance, either a deficiency in estrogen or an excess of (or the effects of early exposure to) testosterone. Research, however, has provided mixed evidence for this viewpoint, with some research suggesting that hormonal factors are important[18] while other research has suggested that hormonal factors are not crucial in determining homosexual behaviors.[19]

If an imbalance of the sex hormones, particularly of testosterone, does play a role in homosexuality, and if there is a link between testosterone levels and left-handedness, then we ought to find that homosexuals have different patterns of handedness than heterosexuals do. Specifically, lesbians, who might be women with higher than normal levels of testosterone or testosterone exposure during their early development, ought to be more likely to be left-handed. Male homosexuals, if they have lower levels of testosterone, should be less likely to be left-handed than the general heterosexual population.

An alternate to the hormone theory of homosexuality has to do with the rare trait marker theory discussed in chapter 9. If we suggest that heterosexual behavior is what has been genetically programmed into human beings, then homosexuality might be viewed as a rare trait. This rare trait might come about due to some kind of damage or stress (perhaps during pregnancy or birth) that interferes with the normal genetic programming. Homosexuality might appear as an alternate form of behavior as the result of such early physiological difficulties. If homosexuality is caused by the pathological results of such birth stressors, then we might expect to see an association between this variant of sexual behavior and left-handedness. Remember that we have already seen evidence that left-handedness is due to such early problems and the resulting neurological damage that they may leave behind. If this speculation is true, then both male and female homosexuals should be more likely to be left-handed.

Several studies have looked at handedness and homosexuality. One of the first was conducted at the clinic for the treatment of venereal diseases at Guy's Hospital in London.[20] This study involved 100 heterosexual and 94 homosexual males. The handedness measures classified the participants as consistently or strongly right-handed or not consistently right-handed. In other words, the non-right-handed group consisted of both left- and mixed-handed individuals. When the handedness of the heterosexual group of men was compared to the handedness of the homosexual men, it was found that the homosexual group contained nearly twice as many mixed and left-handed individuals. In fact, over half of the homosexuals were not consistently right-handed. Remember, that if male homosexuality was caused by reduced testosterone we would have expected *fewer* left-handed male homosexuals. As this research indicates that there are more left-handed homosexual males, it probably was not a hormonal imbalance that caused the homosexuality in the first place. The finding or more left-handed male homosexuals is what we would have expected if homosexuality was caused by some form of neural damage or other pathology. The argument is that, as left-handedness is likely to be caused by some form of damage probably due to birth or pregnancy stress, other signs of damage might also be expected. Homosexuality might then simply be another soft sign or another "rare trait" that serves as a sign of stress or damage along with left-handedness. Since the investigation I described was published, other research has confirmed the finding that there is an overabundance of left-handers among male homosexuals.[21]

The relationship between handedness and female homosexuality was demonstrated in a Canadian study conducted in Hamilton, Ontario.[22] The participants were recruited from the membership of a local homosexual organization. In this study it was found that there was a very high percentage of non-right-handers in the group of female homosexuals. In fact, the rate of lesbians who turned out to be left-or mixed-handed amounted to 69 percent of the group, which is more than four times that found among heterosexual females. For women, both the hormonal imbalance theory and the neuropathology explanations of homosexuality predict increased left-handedness among lesbians, and these predictions are clearly confirmed by the research data.

Please note that the finding that the majority of homosexuals are left- or mixed-handed does not mean that the majority of left- or mixed-handers are homosexual. If we look at the data for female homosexuals that we outlined a moment ago we can see this more clearly. To begin with, only about 2 percent of the female population is estimated to be homosexual in any of their behaviors. From this fact and from a knowledge of the number of left- and right-handers in the general population, we can compute that about 1 percent of all consistently right-handed women will be homosexual while about 4 percent of all left- and mixed-handed women will be homosexual. Although this means that left- and mixed-handed women are four times more likely to be homosexual than are consistently right-handed women, it still means that 96 percent of all left- and mixed-handed women are heterosexual. Similar values could be computed for male homosexuals. We would say that the risk of homosexuality is higher for left- or mixed-handed people, but the vast majority of non-right-handers is not affected by this sexual orientation.

My laboratory recently has recently become involved in the issue of sexual orientation and handedness. Diane Watson, a psychiatrist and the head of the Sexual Dysphoria Clinic at the Vancouver General Hospital, has been collaborating with me in a research project involving *transsexuals*, individuals who wish to be a member of the opposite sex. For instance, a transsexual man wants to become—indeed feels that he really is—a woman. He wants to replace his penis with a vagina. Such individuals often apply for sex change operations, which involve extended and continuing hormonal treatment, several bouts of surgery, and psychological counselling to allow full adjustment as a member of the opposite sex. Males wishing to become females are about five times more common than females wishing to become males.

One of the better-known examples of transsexualism is the English journalist who covered the British expedition that climbed Mount Everest. As a member of the team he was James Morris. Some years later, after surgery to effect a sex change, he became Jan Morris. In her autobiographical book, *Conundrum*, she outlines what goes on in the mind of a transsexual. Such an individual wants a relationship with someone of the same (genetic) sex, but not a homosexual one. The transsexual pictures the desired relationship as heterosexual. The frustration felt by transsexuals is that they feel such a relationship is prevented by a genetic accident that has placed them in a body of the wrong sex. This motivation spurs them to seek some drastic remedy such as a sex-change operation.

Our study looked at a small group of male transsexuals who had applied for sex-change operations and were now attending the clinic, in various stages of hormonal treatment prior to surgery. We measured their sidedness and then compared it to a larger sample of randomly selected males of the same age. In a nontranssexual group of individuals of the same age as the patients we found about 12 percent left-handedness. Among the transsexuals, however, 36 percent were left-handed. Transsexuals were nearly three times more likely to be left-handed than were people with a heterosexual orientation.

It is interesting to note that the transsexuals were also more likely to be left-sided in things other than handedness. Transsexuals turned out to be one-third more likely to be left-footed, twice as likely to be left-eyed, and two-thirds more likely to be left-eared.

It thus appears that differences in sexual behaviors, particularly homosexuality and transsexuality, appear to be directly related to handedness. Left-handers (and mixed-handers) appear to be more common in certain groups of individuals who engage in variations of sexual behavior different from what is generally perceived as "standard" or "usual" among the majority of the population.

Depression and Suicide

One last set of depressing findings deals with handedness and suicide. Establishing a link between these two items is not as speculative as one might think at first. The first stage starts with the observation that, in groups of adolescents who commit suicide, an unusually large percentage of individuals have a history of birth stressors and pregnancy complications. Such suicide victims are often found to have had breathing difficulties at birth, premature births, problems during delivery or a mother who suffered from infection or disease while pregnant with them.[23] Notice that some of these birth and pregnancy problems are the same as those that we have suggested might be the cause of left-handedness in a large number of individuals.

The second set of observations has to do with depression. One of the most common psychological symptoms associated with suicide is depression. Usually, fairly long and deep bouts of depression have been noticed well in advance of any suicide attempt. When suicide is relatively unexpected, it often involves people who have a tendency toward depression. Sometimes unexpected suicides occur in a person with *bipolar affective problems*, such as a *manic-depressive* disturbance. Such a manic-depressive person will tend to have mood swings that alternate between extreme "highs" and very marked "lows." Psychologists refer to the "high" period as the manic phase, where the person is happy, talkative, and outgoing. The "low" periods are referred to as the depressive phase, where the person is depressed, anxious, overly sensitive, unhappy, and unresponsive to other people and tends to withdraw from others. During such a depressive phase, people often refer to themselves as "worthless" and suggest that their lives are "hopeless" and "not worth living." A person with this type of problem can go from a manic to a depressive condition in a matter of seconds. When suicide is attempted by such people it is almost always found to have occurred during the depressive phase of their condition. Suicide and depression are so closely linked that psychologists often consider thoughts about suicide to be a *symptom* of depression, and questions such as "Do you ever think about ending your own life?" appear on many questionnaires designed to measure depression.

There seems to be a good deal of evidence suggesting a relationship between handedness and depression. Although it is not always the case, the most common finding is that individuals diagnosed as suffering from depression and anxiety symptoms are more likely to be left-handed.[24] In one investigation it was found that depressive patients were about three times more likely to be left-handed than were normal individuals.[25] In addition, there is the puzzling finding that children of depressive individuals were six times more likely to be left-handed as well.

The manic-depressive condition also seems to be associated with handedness. Several studies have shown that people with this form of psychological disturbance are more likely to be left-handed.[26] Perhaps one of the most striking and bizarre illustrations of the linkage between depression and left-handedness comes from the case history of a manic-depressive patient. This case was described by Lewis C. Bruce and published in the scientific journal *Brain* in a paper entitled "Notes of a case of dual brain action."[27] This extraordinary and exceptional case involved a 47-year-old Welsh sailor who suffered from a manic-depressive illness. Welsh was this man's first language, although he later learned to speak English quite well. When the sailor was in his manic phase, where he was excited and "talkative and mischievous," all of the evidence showed that he was clearly right-handed. During this phase he also understood both Welsh and English. When he was under the influence of the depressive phase of his illness, where he became melancholic, morose, and relatively unresponsive, he was then completely left-handed. During this phase he no longer could understand speech in his second language, English. During the transitions between his depression and his mania, he was ambidextrous. This case is particularly interesting because it summarizes the general findings of researchers all in one individual. Notice that it is during depression that this individual shows his left-handedness, as might be expected if there was an association between left-sideness and depression.

We can now combine the two lines of evidence that we have discussed in this section, namely: (1) suicidal individuals show a high probability of having suffered from the same pattern of birth stressors that we know causes left-handedness, and (2) left-handers are more likely to be subject to depression, a psychological condition known to be associated with suicide. This clearly leads to the prediction that left-handers may be more likely to attempt suicide than their right-handed contemporaries.

There is an interesting study that seems to confirm this prediction. It looked at people enlisted in the U.S. Navy, who had been sent to the Naval Regional Medical Center in Great Lakes, Illinois. Each of the seamen tested had been referred to this medical facility after he had attempted to commit suicide at least once. The most common suicidal techniques involved slashing the wrists or trying to poison themselves with an overdose of sleeping pills or some other such substance. When handedness was measured in these people, the percentage of left-handers was extremely large in this group of attempted suicides. In fact, the percentage of left-handers was three times higher than in the general, non-suicidal population.[28]

Musings

This has been a fairly dark set of findings. Left-handers seem to be subject to a variety of problems that may have strongly negative health implications. As I slowly became aware of this data, each new bit of information seemed to hit home a bit harder and to demand more of my attention. There seemed to be some sort of link between the findings that left-handers had more health-related problems and the earlier research puzzle that I had never fully resolved about why left-handers are so rare among older groups of individuals. I knew that it was time to turn the energy of my laboratory toward testing a hypothesis which, if proven true, was going to make many people unhappy.

12

Do Left-Hands Die Younger?

I t was the fall of 1987, and I was going through one of those periods where a particular research problem was becoming an irritant because of my own inability to understand fully what was going on. It had been seven or eight years since Clare Porac and I had collected the data that indicated that there were very few older left-handers. When we first discussed this puzzling problem in this book, we showed our results as a graph (figure 4.1).

The data showed that when we measured the handedness of 20-year-olds, about 13 percent of the group were left-handers, but this percentage dropped off very quickly among older groups of people. When we looked at the handedness of 50-year-olds, we found that only around 5 percent of them were left-handed. We had lost over half of the left-handers by this time. At age 80 and above, it was hard to locate any left-handers at all. We found that left-handers made up less than one-half of one percent of this oldest age group. If we start off with 13 percent left-handers at age 20 and end up with less than 1 percent at age 80, over this period of time 96 percent of our original set of left-handers have disappeared. This pattern of results had been reproduced by other researchers in other laboratories around the world since our original finding.[1] All had reported fewer left-handers in groups of older individuals, so our findings had been confirmed. Neither we nor these other researchers had a convincing answer to the question, "Where have all the older left-handers gone?"

As with most unanswered questions I have encountered, the "Case of the Disappearing Southpaws," as I had come to call it, occasionally popped into my thoughts as though to check and see if I had come up with a solution since we last met. It had forced its way into my thoughts on this morning, and I was beginning to empathize with the Greek physiologist and philosopher Alcmaeon who grumpily noted that "Men perish because they cannot join the beginning to the end." I have certainly felt, many times, that the absence of a particular answer to some research question that I was working on was bound to do me in. It would be a clear case of death by frustration. Absence of the answer to this particular problem left me out of sorts and in a grouchy and irritable mood, which matched the weather outside.

I don't like feeling sullen, so I thought that I might make this rainy autumn day in Vancouver a bit brighter for me by dropping into the office of Diane Halpern. Diane Halpern is a psychologist from California State University at San Bernardino. She had just finished a stint as the acting Dean of Graduate Studies there and was now on a research sabbatical. She had come to the University of British Columbia to work with me for a few months. Diane is one of those special people whom I have been lucky to work with during my career. She, like Clare Porac of the University of Victoria, who has been a co-investigator with me for many years, is an experimental psychologist with a broad range of interests. Modern scientists tend to specialize in very narrow subject areas, which focuses their interests and makes it easier to keep abreast of new findings in their field. A few, however, have maintained wider and more general interests, covering a much broader range of problems in their field. Such individuals always seemed to me to be a bit brighter, more productive, and certainly more enthusiastic about research.

I leaned on the edge of the desk in Diane's office and we began to chat about various and sundry matters when Diane looked at me and, with a tone that we train clinical psychologists to use with their patients, asked, "You seem to be a bit distracted today. Is something wrong?"

"No, I've just been stuck on a problem which I find interesting but a bit frustrating." Since the floodgates were already opened, I promptly proceeded to tell her about the data showing the disappearance of left-handers in older groups.

As soon as I stopped talking Diane began to consider the issue, initially wending her way down pathways that I had been over many times in the past. "Maybe it's just that the older people were trained in schools or in households that forced them to use their right hand. You know there was a good deal of pressure on lefties back then. Another possibility is that left-handers simply learn to do more things with their right hand because so much of the world is set up for right-handers. In other words, it could be that a lot of the older people that your measurements say are right-handers are really converted left-handers."

"That's Clare Porac's favorite hypothesis," I said. "I call it the *modification theory*. It's based on the idea that left-handers disappear from the population because they are gradually changed into right-handers."

I next found myself summarizing some of the data introduced in chapter 4 of this book. "The problem with the modification theory is that it doesn't work. We've already been able to show that the number of left-handed adults hasn't changed since the turn of the century, which I take this as evidence that social pressure to change handedness doesn't work. The other point is that it is really difficult to change the handedness of a person. It only works in one out of every three or four cases, then only if you catch the person very young, and then only for the specific actions that you train. No—simple learning factors can't account for the slow and gradual disappearance of left-handers that we observe."

Diane looked at me for a moment or two. She was holding a pen in her hand exactly the way that a dart player might hold a dart to throw at a target. She pointed it at me and prompted, "You have another idea?"

Oh yes, I had another idea, but to spell it out was to risk being labeled a bit of a crank and a crackpot. Diane, however, was a friend as well as a colleague. One can say some silly and speculative things to friends and expect to be forgiven if they turn out to be wrong.

"Let me propose a hypothesis different from the modification theory. Let me offer what I might call the *elimination theory*. According to this notion, the reason we don't find many older left-handers is that they are not there to find."

"Are you saying that they die off at a younger age?" Diane asked.

"Yes."

Diane stared across the room and then said, "Convince me that your idea makes sense."

Here it was, the time to lay it all out. What Diane needed was the pattern of research results that had led me to this point. So I gave her a quick précis of the data that I thought were relevant.

"Look," I said, "we already know that a lot of left-handers become left-handed because they have been exposed to some sort of birth stress.

Since you know that I feel that right-handed is what we are all programmed to be, we can presume that the left-handedness came about because of some form of neural damage which kept some people from reaching the right-handedness that everybody was designed for. Now suppose that the left-handedness is the most benign and innocent of the changes that this birth stress brought about. Suppose that some other organs or other aspects of the nervous system have also been damaged. We already know that left-handers have a lot more problems. They grow more slowly, have sleep problems, have a lot of both immune system and autoimmunity problems, more headaches, and a whole flock of other problems.

"Look, I know that left-handedness is not a disease. I'm not suggesting that southpaws should all be immediately put on life support equipment as soon as their handedness becomes set, just so that we might be spared the embarrassment of having them all die in the streets at age ten. All that I am proposing is that if left-handers have sustained some form of neural or organ damage, due to the end results of birth stress, or if their immune systems are not up to par, then this could affect a left-hander's health status. They might not be as resilient as right-handers if there is a disease or some injury. This means that their survival rate might be a bit lower than that of right-handers. We don't need much of a difference, a percentage or two, in terms of survival rate per year, to end up with left-handers disappearing more rapidly than right-handers, and perhaps, being virtually extinct by the time we look at 80-year-olds and older."

I had hurried through my arguments in the hopes of finishing before the storm of disbelief broke. Diane, however, seemed to be listening intently and thinking about the lines of research that I had outlined. She now spoke again.

"That's a fascinating theory," she said. "I wouldn't like to hear it if I were a left-hander, and I would probably need some strong evidence to make me even consider that it might be true. Have you done anything to test it yet?"

"No. I've thought about some possible ways of testing the theory, but I always run into the same problem. You see, what you need to test this hypothesis is a group of people whose handedness you know. They also have to be dead so that we can determine their lifespan. This is a bit of a problem, since it is hard to determine a person's handedness after they have died. These records are not part of the death certificate, most doctors don't record it, and, of course, after the individual has died it's a bit late to give them a questionnaire to fill out."

Diane put down her pen and leaned back in her chair. "This is really a challenge," she said. "I'm sure that there has to be some way to get this kind of data. I mean, suppose that we were looking at someone who was a baseball pitcher. Certainly people would notice which hand he threw a ball with. There would also be records on when he died if he were famous. Aren't there books listing this sort of thing?"

The answer was like most other insights that I have encountered. Once stated, it seemed simple and obvious. When faced by such an insight you invariably start muttering to yourself various phrases like, "It's so simple, I should have thought of it." The problem is, that such solutions are only simple looking backwards, *after* the answer has already been spelled out.

"Yes, there certainly are records for baseball," I said.

"Well," said Diane, "why don't we look them up and test your hypothesis? If you're right, then when we look at how long baseball players live, the left-handed ones should die younger." Then she added, with the practicality of a researcher who has had to struggle for research funds all of her professional life, as we both had, "Besides, if the records are already published somewhere, this should be a really inexpensive project to do. If it works out we can always do the study in a more formal way—if we can figure out how to get the handedness data from everyday, nonfamous dead people."

It all seemed so straightforward. A trip to the library, and then we would have the answer to my recurring and nagging question. Little did Diane or I know that we were kicking open a door that would lead to much more than a low-cost solution to a question raised by some earlier data. We were soon to learn that Robert Hertz, the anthropologist, might have been warning us, or making a prediction about our results when he observed:

> It is a notion current among the Maori that the right is the "side of life" (and of strength) while the left is the "side of death" (and of weakness). Fortunate and life-giving influences enter us from the right and through our right side; and, inversely, death and misery penetrate to the core of our being from the left.[2]

The Baseball Study

The more I thought about the published data on baseball players, the more that I liked the idea. There were many advantages to using such a group of people. To begin with, if we are looking at life span, we know that sex of the individual is an important factor. In general, men die younger than women. This difference in life span may be due to specific behaviors that men engage in. Men are more often engaged in occupations where they can be injured or killed. For instance, men are more likely to be killed while engaged in military, rescue, criminal, or police activities than are women. There are also differences in the rate of smoking and drinking of men and women, which probably contribute to sex-related differences in life span. Biological differences between men and women may affect health risks. There is, for instance, the suggestion that men may have a less efficient immune system than women.[3] All this indicated that it would be more efficient to conduct our first investigation using only one sex. Men would be preferred for our purposes because there are more left-handed men than women, and we can get more useful data entries more easily.

Two other features made this endeavor sound good. First of all, it seemed important that handedness measures be taken while the individual is still young, but not too young. Certainly, by the age of 18 or 20 years, when the player enters major league play, we can assume that handedness is well established and unlikely to suffer from further pressures to switch left-handers to right-handedness. Further, it seemed desirable to eliminate any extraneous influences that might affect the results. Therefore, it seemed important that the people we considered should be healthy, at least at the start of the study. Professional baseball players certainly fit these requirements. They are clearly healthy to begin with, and, as the active playing years tend to be in the early twenties, measures of handedness would have been taken before many left-handers would have disappeared from the population.

A trip to the library revealed that there was a book called *The Baseball Encyclopedia*.[4] This is a fat book, which is updated periodically. It contains information not only about famous ball players but also about every person who ever played baseball in the major leagues, whether he was a "star" or not. In most instances the information is concisely presented. All entries do include the date of birth—and the date of death, if the individual is deceased. They also include the hand that the person threw with and the side the person batted from. The edition we used had statistics completed up to 1975.

We hired a young undergraduate whose unenviable task was to type into a computer the relevant data about every major league player who had passed away before 1975. Several weeks later, when she had finished this task, we began the data analysis.

Our first task was to decide on some way of scoring the handedness of each person. Obviously we didn't have questionnaire or interview data from these players, but we wanted to make sure that we would only be looking at strong right-handers and comparing them to strong left-handers. For this reason we decided that a person would be scored as right-handed only if he used his right hand for both throwing and batting. If there was any indication that players had ever changed handedness or that they threw with both hands or were "switch hitters," they were not scored as strong right-handers. The same type of decision went into selecting our strong left-handers. We were going to exclude from our analysis anybody who was weakly right- or left-handed, mixed-handed, or ambidextrous. We felt that looking at clearly right- or left-handers would give us the best indication of any relationship between handedness and life span. In the end, this method of classification left us with 2,271 individuals whose handedness and whose life span we knew.

For data like this, there are many ways that we can conduct the analyses. One way is to pick an age and to see how many people survive up to that age. Suppose that we pick a really advanced age, such as 90 years, as our value. We found that two and a half percent of our starting group of right-handed ball players made it to that ripe old age, while less than one half of one percent of left-handers made it to age 90. This means that a right-hander has a chance of reaching 90 years of age which is five times greater than that of a left-hander!

In our estimation, the clearest and most sensible way to look at the results of this study involved the use of the notion of risk. We would ask the question, "Does being left-handed say anything about a person's risk of dying in any given year or at any given age?" To answer this question we decided to look at each age of death separately. For the purposes of our analysis we decided that if the risk at any give age of a left- or a right-hander dying differed by less than half a percent we could ignore it as being too small to matter. We looked at each age of death separately from age 20 (the age when the first death occurs in our set of ball players) on through the full age range (to 109). What we found is that there was no real difference in the risk of death for left- and right-handed baseball players up to age 33. From that age onward, the percentage of right-handers who survived was higher. In 52 of 58 instances in which the difference in survival between the left and right-handers was large enough to be meaningful, we found that the right-handers had a lower risk of dying. In effect, the data showed us that, for any given age, the percentage of left-handers who will die will run around 2 percent higher than the rate for right-handers.

While this figure might not sound tremendously large, we can get a feel for the nature of this difference by asking whether you would knowingly select an airline for your next trip if you knew that the chance of your dying on it was 2 percent higher than for other airlines? If we were looking at the proportion of left-handers in the population, this difference in the relative survival would cause a gradual decrease in the percentage of southpaws. Over a period of many years, with this higher risk of death in each year, the full population of left-handers would disappear well before the last right-hander had passed away, which is, of course, what we found.[5] The oldest left-hander made it to age 91, and the oldest right-hander made it to age 109, an 18-year difference!

Once we had the data analyzed, we published it as a short article in the scientific journal *Nature*[6] so that others would know that we had a possible explanation for the observation that the percentage of left-handers in the general population dwindles as the population grows older. For an article that was less than a thousand words long, the amount of controversy and attention it drew was remarkable, and well beyond anything that Diane and I had ever expected. We are scientists with few aspirations toward being celebrities. We both have a strong desire for the quiet and privacy that research and scholarly writing require. For a period of several months, however, this privacy was shattered.

The story was immediately picked up by the major news wire services and sent out worldwide. The major radio and TV networks picked up the item, and I even got a phone call from my mother, who said that she nearly drowned because she inhaled her coffee when she heard my voice talking about the life span of left-handers on the radio during the morning network news. A long string of media interviews seemed to fill my working days for weeks afterward. There were some bizarre highlights to this attention, as when a TV team was sent all the way from Australia to interview us on the left-handedness findings. Others had to do with the nature of the magazines that picked up the story. In addition to the more traditional news outlets (such as *U.S. News and World Report*) or the science magazines (such as *Omni* or *New Scientist*), reports appeared in unexpected places. My daughter Rebecca, who was clearly taking some delight in all of this, even sent me a clipping on this work from *Weight Watchers Magazine*, which caused me some mirth when I wondered if the item ever would have appeared if the editors had ever seen my portly middle-aged silhouette.

Not only the sources, but the tone of the media coverage varied quite a bit. Some simply reported the material as a new and interesting scientific finding that suggested left-handers might have a shorter life span.

Others showed some disbelief. The media reports that bothered Diane and me the most were the articles and broadcast pieces that adopted a snide and derogatory attitude, treating the finding that some 10 percent of the population might have a shorter life span as if it were a joke. For example, an article on our research published in *Psychology Today* had the insensitive title, "So Long, Southpaw." The effect of these negative and derisive headlines was perhaps predictable, but shocking nonetheless. Apparently people took this jesting tone as coming from us, rather than from the journalists reviewing and reporting our work. I began to receive abusive and threatening phone calls, such as one that went, "You right-handers think that you'll live longer than us left-handers but you won't if we kill you first." I immediately instituted a policy of having all calls go through my answering machine so that I would not have to deal with this kind of abuse directly. It also caused me to wonder what sort of can of worms we had opened up in our research.

Although Diane and I had not expected the intense public reaction that resulted from our study, we certainly had expected some reaction from the scientific community. Because our idea that left-handers had a shorter life span was relatively novel, we had predicted that response to this theory would follow the usual pattern for most scientific discoveries that have eventually proved themselves to be valid and have had broad implications. First it would be ignored, then it would be attacked, and finally it would be taken for granted. Since the stage of being ignored had been skipped, it seemed likely that we would immediately encounter the attack stage, and we did not have long to wait.

Perhaps it was predictable that the two major comments on our findings were either authored or directed by left-handers and that none of the attacks was initiated by psychologists or neuropsychologists who knew the data that had led us to conduct the study in the first place. The initial comment came from E.K. Wood,[7] who is described in one article as being "neither left-handed nor a scientist"[8] but whose analyses were directed by E. Sterl Phinney, a left-handed professor of theoretical astrophysics from the California Institute of Technology. Another broadside came from Max Anderson, a left-handed free-lance statistician, working out of his home in Vancouver.[9] Both comments pointed out some of the problems associated with working with *archival data*. Archival data is any set of records available through published sources, data banks, historical records, and the like. Newspaper archives, libraries, census data, traffic accident reports, or sports records are often used as sources for data. The researcher comes along at some later time and tries to use this existing data to answer a current research question, as we did with the baseball records. Inevitably the data is not as complete as the investigator would like, and it is frequently in a form that is not very convenient or amenable to easy processing. This means that the researcher has to use very clear definitions as to what constitutes valid data, and the scientist may have to engage in some complex statistical procedures to extract a meaningful answer to the research question. All of this means that, when using archival data, the strength and reliability of results that the researcher gets depends not only upon the specific set of records used but, as in our case, upon the definition of handedness and the specific statistical tests used to determine the significance of the findings. We had known all this in advance and already had plans to go beyond the archival material in our research.

Even before people had responded to our first study, Diane and I had recognized that we were now committed to further research. As the initial data had suggested that there might be a relationship between left-handedness and reduced longevity, we knew that we would eventually have to go out and collect data from the "real world" to confirm this finding. We could not rely on data solely from published reports on an elite group of very healthy athletes, all of whom were male and all of whom were quite special in some ways. This kind of data was all right for a quick inexpensive look at the issue, but what we really needed was new data, drawn from the general population, collected under scientifically controlled conditions. This would be a much more expensive and time-consuming research project, of course. Hopefully, if we were correct in our original conclusions, this type of data would provide us with an answer sufficiently clear so that complex statistical analyses would not be needed to prove the point. This new study was already through the design stage before the baseball-player study had even been published.

The California Study

Our first plan was quite a simple one in concept, but turned out to be more difficult than we anticipated in practice. The plan was to consult death certificates to obtain the names of recently deceased individuals. There were some problems here. Handedness is not listed on death records, nor is it usually part of a person's medical records. Because the deceased person can no longer supply us with the information, his or her handedness would have to be obtained from some other source. A next of kin or a close friend is almost always listed on the death certificates; thus the most direct way to determine the handedness of the deceased seemed to involve contacting this person to see if they recalled this information.

Even from the start, it became clear that conducting this kind of study was going to involve problems. We first approached the government agency that keeps vital statistics for the Province of British Columbia, in Canada. They made it quite clear that they were not going to cooperate with any project that involved contacting the next of kin. I pointed out the safeguards that we had considered so that we would not offend anybody or intrude on their privacy. They responded by noting that they could not stop me from examining these documents, as death certificates are public records, but they also indicated that they would make it as difficult and expensive as they possible could. When I pressed them about their reluctance, they told me that whenever the next of kin had been contacted by researchers in the past it had always led to a public outcry and to pressure on the ministry staff. They were simply not going to go through it again. I was sure that I was just dealing with a group of civil servants who were afraid of any publicity and were overreacting to our proposed project. Still, I couldn't think of any way to get around them. Since it seemed that the data would be very difficult for me to get locally, I contacted Diane, who was by then back in California, and told her that we would have to find another source of death records.

"No problem," she said. "We'll just do it here. I'm sure that Americans are not as sensitive as Canadians and that we won't have any difficulties at this end." We didn't know just how wrong her prediction would turn out to be.

Two inland counties in Southern California were selected as the source of the death certificates.[10] Before we started, however, we had to lay out some ground rules. We did not want to appear to be ghouls or to be insensitive to people's feelings when they were grieving over the death of a loved one. For these reasons, Diane consulted a bereavement counsellor whose specialty is to help people deal with their grief and loss after the death of a friend or family member. The counsellor suggested that we should not contact anyone until at least nine months had passed since the death. In addition, we should make the contact fairly gentle and not follow up or press people to respond to our queries. For ethical and humane reasons we did not contact the next of kin when the deceased was a child of six or younger or if the death had come about because of murder or suicide. These cases are too sensitive to deal with, and we did not want to inflict any unnecessary discomfort on families who had lost people through such tragedies. Once having established these guidelines and cleared the research with the University Research

Ethics Committee, we felt that we could conduct this investigation with a minimum of problems.

Diane organized a team of seven research assistants to help in gathering the data. First they had to go through the vital records, starting with deaths that had occurred at least nine months before, working backwards through the files. A total of 2,875 death certificates were examined, and a very brief questionnaire was sent to the next of kin listed on the record. An enclosed letter explained that the results might prove to be "useful for scientific and medical purposes," which we sincerely feel is true. In order to eliminate any possibility that we might contaminate the responses, we did not tell people that our hope was to look at handedness and life span nor did we give them any information about the research question or the major focus of the investigation. We did, however, assure individuals that all of their responses were completely anonymous.

To make the situation as quick and painless as possible, we simply asked each individual to fill out a postage-paid card, which asked about a half-dozen questions. To determine the handedness of the person, we asked which hand the deceased used for writing, for drawing, and for throwing a ball. A small number on the address side of each card provided coded data taken from the death certificate, giving the age at death, the sex of the individual, and the cause of death but no indication of the name of the deceased. In other words, we kept our pledge of anonymity by making sure that we could not identify the specific person from whom each card came or the name of the deceased. We also made no attempt to follow up the questionnaire in any way. We hoped that many of the next of kin would help us out with this project and reasoned that if the questionnaire was returned and filled out it meant that that person felt that this task was not too difficult or painful. If the person chose to not fill it out, we would abide by their choice with no pressure or reminder notes.

We were very pleased and touched by the number of people who responded to our questionnaire. Some even included personal notes and additional information. On the other hand, the warnings from the people in the Vital Statistics Department in Canada also turned out to be true. Even with the most gentle of approaches, some people became quite upset about any questions about their deceased loved ones. Diane received several nasty responses from some of the next of kin. We knew that these represented only a tiny minority of people who were overreacting, but, rather than cause discomfort to anyone, we decided to end the data collection as soon as we had the minimum number of cases to allow us to analyze the data properly. When we finished the study, 1033 people had replied, better than one-third of the total contacted. After eliminating returns where the deceased did not have full use of both hands or where the next of kin did not recall which hand the person used, we ended up with 987 usable responses.

Based on the reports from the next of kin, we classified an individual as right-handed if he or she performed all three activities that we surveyed (writing, drawing, and throwing a ball) with the right hand. We were insisting that the person be strongly right-handed to be counted as a right-hander, much as we did with the baseball player data. Of course, this means that our left-handed group contains both left-handed and mixed-handed individuals.

When we analyzed the data in terms of life span, the first thing that we noticed was that it confirmed the already well-known finding that there is an advantage in being a woman, regardless of handedness. In our study the average life span of a woman was 77 years and 5 months while the life span of a man averaged only 71 years and 4 months. According to our data, women live 6 years and 1 month longer on average, roughly the same results obtained by other researchers. Our major interest, of course, was in handedness, rather than the effect of sex, but the fact that we were confirming well-known relationships gave us some assurance that there was nothing unusual about our test group of people.

On the basis of our baseball-player data, we had, of course, expected that the left-handers would have a somewhat shorter life span. We had also expected that we would have to use some sophisticated statistical-analysis techniques to confirm this effect, perhaps another analysis of annual risk of dying or the like, as we had done in the first study. We had no expectation that the size of the difference would be anywhere near the size we actually obtained. The difference in life span between left- and right-handers was sufficiently large that all we needed to do to show it was to look at the average life spans of the two handedness groups. The average age of death for the right-handers was 75 years, while the average age of death for the left-handers was 66 years. In other words, according to this data, left-handers have a life span that is 9 years shorter! Notice that this means that handedness actually has a larger effect on life span than does a person's sex.

Why are the effects so large in this group, compared to our baseball-player sample? It probably has to do with some of the factors that we had worried about in the first place. After all, professional baseball players are much more healthy than the average person; otherwise, they wouldn't have made it to the level of playing on a major league team. People who were sickly to begin with would not make it into the baseball records and thus would have been excluded from our data. Perhaps most of the left-handers who are at higher risk of early death did not reach the levels of performance needed to get into the elite sample of individuals that we were looking at in the baseball study. Probably, as we are now looking at more typical people, the effects are larger because we have a broader range of health status to look at.

There are some interesting features about this data. For instance, sex and handedness combine to produce slightly different effects of handedness on the life spans of men and women. This can be seen in figure 12.1. While right-handed women live to an average of 77 years and 8 months, left-handed women have an average life span of 72 years and 10 months, meaning that right-handed women live 4 years and 10 months longer. For men, however, the effects of handedness are twice as strong. Right-handed men live an average of 72 years and 4 months as compared to left-handed men, who have an average life span of only 62 years and 3 months. Left-handedness can cost a man 10 years and 1 month in terms of life expectancy. Left-handedness is thus a much more

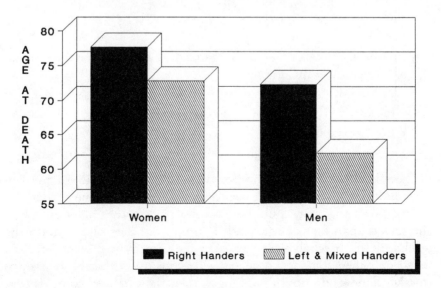

FIGURE 12.1: The relative life span of left- and right-handers.

dangerous attribute for men than for women, although it is costly to both sexes in terms of life span.

We had predicted that left-handedness would be associated with a shorter life span; that seemed to be the only sensible explanation remaining to explain why the percentage of left-handers in the population grew smaller when we looked at groups of older individuals. If we eliminate historical pressures toward right-handed use earlier this century and also eliminate the effectiveness of learning effects that might gradually make left-handers into right-handers, then a difference in life span seems to be the most likely explanation for our "disappearing southpaws." We already knew that left-handedness was linked to a number of factors that might be associated with reduced survival ability. These included:

- a history of birth or pregnancy complications
- a slower pattern of growth
- sleep problems
- immune system difficulties
- possible neurological damage
- autoimmune problems
- higher susceptibility to a number of diseases including:
  - some forms of diabetes
  - epilepsy
  - various thyroid problems
  - myasthenia gravis
- a tendency to certain behavior patterns that may place the individual in jeopardy including:
  - alcoholism
  - increased criminality or antisocial behaviors
  - homosexuality
  - certain psychopathological conditions, such as schizophrenia.

These health difficulties and behavioral tendencies, more typical of left-handers, all have negative health implications. Any one of them, or several taken together, could be part of a pattern that may result in a shorter life span for the left-handed group. Our data also confirm the results of the baseball-player study, using directly collected data and much-simplified statistical analyses. The conclusion that both reach is that left-handers do not live as long as their right-handed counterparts.

Another Reason

It is true that medical and behavioral factors we have reviewed could explain a difference in the life span of left-and right-handers such as the one we observed. There is, however, another factor that seems to have a great effect upon the life expectancy of the left-hander. Some additional analyses of the data from the California study suggested that our technological, industrialized, and highly mechanized environment might actually be "eating" left-handers. Not only do left-handers have higher levels of health risk from all the sources we have discussed in the previous chapters, but our California data showed that left-handers may be at risk from an environment that has been specifically set up for the safety and the convenience of right-handers. In the next chapter we will see how a world engineered for right-handers can be deadly to left-handers.

13

A World for Right-Handers

The preceding two chapters were probably a bit gloomy, with their dire statements about the health and the expected life span of left-handers. Those chapters focused mostly on the physical status and vigor of the southpaw. Let's shift our focus to deal with the world the left-hander lives in. As you will soon see, the way the world is set up will also affect the physical and psychological well-being of the left-hander.

If you are left-handed, what I am going say here will be "old hat" and obvious. If you are right-handed, what I will tell you will probably be a revelation, as it will point out some features of the environment that you may never have thought of. The issue begins with the fact that nine out of ten people are right-handed, which means that nine out of ten people responsible for designing tools, implements, machines, work spaces, homes, and the general technical environment will also be right-handed. If I am an engineer designing a product so that it will be safe and comfortable to use, I will tend to assume that everyone is just like me. What is convenient for me should be convenient for everyone else. The notion that the designer uses is that all human beings are pretty much the same. As there is a 90 percent chance that I will be right-handed, unless there is some reason why I should think about handedness as a factor, I will design the product to be comfortable for a right-hander.

To understand ways in which the environment is set up against the interests of left-handers, you might want to look at the bimonthly *Left-hander Magazine*. It regularly publishes a column called *Perspective*, based upon submissions from left-handed readers. Each edition of this column usually presents an anecdote about the difficulties associated with being a left-hander in a right-hander's world. Most of these complaints have to do with tools, implements, machines, and architectural design. It is startling, at least for the right-hander, to see how many such complaints there are.

One of the tools that causes a lot of gripes from left-handers is the common scissors. Scissors provide a good introduction into the right-handed bias to the world. Most scissors have handles shaped so that one hole is angled correctly for the right thumb and the other hole correctly shaped to fit three or four fingers of the right hand. Inserting the left thumb into the thumbhole requires bending this digit backward, which, to put it simply, hurts. Inserting the fingers of the left hand into the larger hole in the handle causes the tapered edges (tapered the wrong way for a left-hander) to dig into the user's skin. Left-handers complain about the torment of twisting their hands to manipulate scissors and then being criticized by parents or teachers when their craft work and paper cutouts were not as neatly executed as those of their right-handed friends or classmates.

Scissors are one of the few items of right-handed technology that have evolved to the point where left-handed versions of the tool may be found here and there. Unfortunately, this seems to be the case only for paper and sewing scissors. In the industrial realm we find that metal shears, leather shears, hedge shears, pruning scissors, tailor's pinking scissors, and even barber's hair-cutting scissors are still available only in the right-handed design from the usual retail outlets. Electric scissors and the barber's or hairdresser's electric clippers are virtually always right-handed in their design, with the start button placed so that it can be operated only by the thumb of the right hand. On electric hair clippers, the guide that directs the hair into the cutter is often beveled to accommodate the natural movements of the right hand and is consequently awkward for left-handed operators.

The Right-Handed Kitchen

Many common articles frequently trouble left-handers. From the kitchen, one of the most common complaints concerns the can opener. This simple instrument is designed to be held with the left hand while the cutting gear is operated by rotating a handle with the right hand. As figure 13.1 shows, this design forces the left-hander into a set of

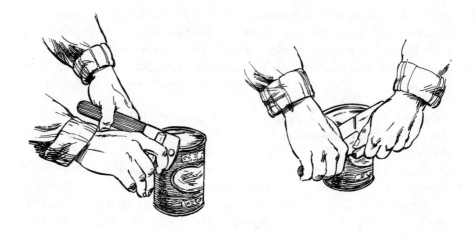

Right-hander   **Left-hander**

FIGURE 13.1: A left-hander has a much more difficult time in using the standard manual can opener.

ungainly contortions. Even these acrobatics do not provide a comfortable solution for the left-hander, as the gearing on most openers is designed so that the turning knob rotates away from the body, a more powerful, comfortable, and controlled movement than rotating the hand toward the body. Left-handers must reverse this pattern to use the more awkward inward turn or must cross the body with the arm to rotate the hand outward. The hands and lower arms of the southpaw in this bizarre position rest close to the jagged edges of the open lid inviting cuts and nicks. Using a wall-mounted can opener is not much easier. Often the left-hander gives up and adopts a right-handed pattern of use, with additional fatigue and frustration. I have always wondered whether the inventor of "boil in the bag" frozen food products might not have been a left-hander looking for a way to get prepared foods to the table without a can opener.

The kitchen is actually a microcosm of the world designed for the right-hander. Let's consider the simple soup ladle. Typically it has a lip or spout nicked into the side so that the soup can be conveniently poured out with little spilling or dripping. The left-hander has to do without this aid, as the pouring lip is on the wrong side. Pouring from the smooth, rounded side is bound to cause left-handed servers to splash the liquid. Many items used for pouring or draining have a similar problem. Some espresso and turkish coffee pots have the spout on the left and a handle on the side, as do some cooking pans, gravy boats, and beverage servers—quite convenient for the right-hander but an awkward bother for the left-hander. Examples of utensils partial to right-handers may be seen in figure 13.2.

Many electric coffee makers have the water reservoir on the left, forcing the user to reach for the carafe from the right as is shown in figure 13.3. Clearly this right-handed design either forces the left-hander to operate with his or her weaker and less agile right-hand or invites spills and splatters as the carafe is pulled out by the left-hand, "sneaking around" the upright portion of the appliance that blocks access to the carafe of coffee. Filling the reservoir demonstrates more design considerations. In this particular unit, the lid opens to the left, allowing easy right-handed access for pouring water into the machine but making use of the left hand quite difficult. The southpaw must either go around or over the obstructing lid or hope that his or her right hand is strong and agile enough to accomplish the task without sloshing water all over.

Many measuring cups are also right-handed. Although they can be held in either hand and the spout is symmetrically placed, the measuring

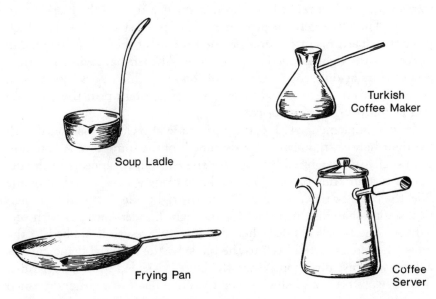

FIGURE 13.2: Typical kitchen items designed to aid the right-hander in pouring or serving hot liquids, but which are inappropriately designed for the left-hander.

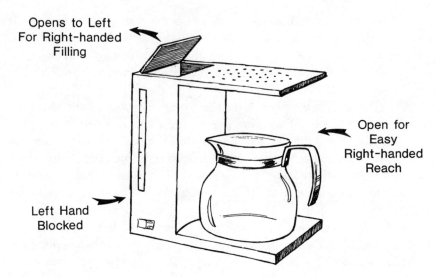

Opens to Left
For Right-handed
Filling

Open for
Easy
Right-handed
Reach

Left Hand
Blocked

FIGURE 13.3: An automatic coffee maker which is clearly designed for the right-hander.

lines or markings often appear on one side only, naturally, the left side. The left-hander must either put the cup down and then turn it around to read the liquid level or look through the cup to read the markings in reverse. The same general problem holds for most coffee mugs which place their patterns or pictures on the left side of the cup, where it can be seen by the right-handed coffee drinker. The left-handed person then gets to stare at only the blank side of the mug which does little to add an aesthetic touch to the grim prospect of getting up in the morning and facing your first cup of coffee.

Kitchen implements with cutting edges are also clearly fashioned with the right-hander in mind, to the detriment of the southpaw. A common but usually unrecognized bias against the left-hander appears in the design of certain knife blades. When a knife blade is bevelled on only one side, the bevel or taper is invariably on the right side. Such an asymmetrical wedge shape is functional for the right-hander because, with one flat and one bevelled side, when downward pressure is applied to the knife, the force exerted back to the blade by the material being cut has a slight sideways direction. When the knife is wielded by a right-hander, this sideways pressure helps to keep the knife blade upright and pushed against the food, as figure 13.4 shows. For the left-hander, however, a one-sided bevel is a disaster: If the southpaw tries to hold the knife straight up and down, the force pushing back on the knife will tend to

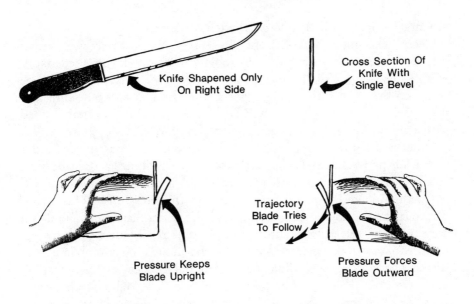

Knife Shapened Only
On Right Side

Cross Section Of
Knife With
Single Bevel

Trajectory
Blade Tries
To Follow

Pressure Keeps
Blade Upright

Pressure Forces
Blade Outward

Right-handed Slice   **Left-handed Slice**

FIGURE 13.4: A typical knife, bevelled on the right side, assists the right-hander by producing a force which holds the blade upright, while for the left-hander it causes the blade to tend to curve outward toward the slice.

push it away from the large piece and out into the slice, producing half a slice because the knife wants to travel in an curve. A left-hander tends to compensate for the tendency of the blade to slip by angling the entire knife so that it points more sharply inward and applying a counter-twist to the blade. This complex movement means that the knife is under somewhat more tenuous control. In addition, the sharpened edge ends up aimed directly toward the left-hander's right hand, which is holding the thing being sliced, a clear invitation to accidentally cutting a chunk out of the supporting right hand as well as the food.

As if cutting problems were not enough disadvantage, this design also makes knife sharpening unmanageable for the left-hander. This bevel requires that the sharpener be held in the right hand and the blade stationary in the left or that the blade be held in the right hand and rubbed against a stationary sharpening wand held in the left hand. Either of these patterns of movements sharpens the knife by scraping away metal on the right side where the bevel is. A left-hander whose active movements are made with the left hand is naturally oriented to attempt to sharpen the knife on the left, unbevelled side.

Electric carving knives offer the same problems as the single-bevelled kitchen knife, with an additional problem to compound the left-hander's slicing woes. Usually, the on-off control switch is designed to be operated by the thumb of the right hand assumed to be holding the instrument. In addition, the handle of the appliance is often shaped specifically to fit the fingers of the right hand.

Other power-driven appliances in the kitchen are generally no kinder to the left-hander. A typical electric food slicer is about as right-handed as you can get. The one shown in figure 13.5 is designed to be operated by holding down the power-on switch with the left thumb. This layout was to make the appliance safe to use, as the switch has to be held down continuously; releasing it automatically stops the blade from turning. Unfortunately it also means that the left hand must be immobile during slicing operations. According to the original conception of the appliance, the food should be held and moved by the right hand. Notice that, for the right-hander, the right arm pushing the food flares out and safely away from the blade while the left hand drapes easily over the back of the machine with the fingers far from the rotating blade. For the left-hander, however, this design is a disaster. The southpaw must cross arms, with the right hand on the switch and the left crossed over to push the food forward. Both arms and hands are actually in jeopardy with this action. The left arm clearly crosses over the platform and in

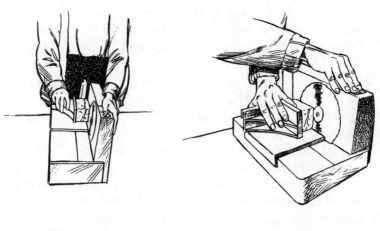

Right-hander   **Left-hander**

FIGURE 13.5: An electric food slicer designed for right-handed use, and the posture that a left-hander might take to operate it.

front of the blade. Leaning too far forward or slipping may cause a nasty cut. The right hand is also in some jeopardy since it drapes out into the working area and rests over the blade. Fatigue or inattention, which might cause the hand to droop slightly, will bring it into direct contact with the moving blade.

Numerous other examples of the right-handed bias to our world can be found in the kitchen and its immediate surrounds. Salad and pastry forks often have one tine made somewhat thicker than the others, so that the diner can use the fork to cut through lettuce or pie crust without a knife. When only one of the outside tines is thicker, it is always on the left, because the fork is designed for the right-handed user who will naturally turn the left side downwards, tines toward the person, which is the right-hander's most natural cutting motion.

Right-handed design features show up in a number of other implements. In my own kitchen utensil drawer, I find a pastry server serrated on the left side for right-handed cutting action. A similar asymmetrical pattern of serrations are incorporated in my grapefruit sectioning knife. My cheese server is angled and sloped so that only the right hand can use it properly. My utility drawer also contains an ice cream scoop, which has a moveable loop to help ease the ice cream out. The clearing loop is activated by pushing a lever with the thumb. As the expectation is that the scoop is held in the right hand, the lever is designed to be operated by the right thumb. If left-hander holds the scoop with his left thumb on the lever, the scoop is backward and unusable. My utility drawer also contains a single-blade potato peeler with the handle to the right, making it a comfortable gadget for the right hander but also impossible for the left-hander to use with the normal whittling motion, away from the body, for which it was designed.

For larger appliances the prejudice in favor of the right-hander continues. Have you noticed that the microwave oven is right-handed? Most microwaves have a door that opens from right to left, providing easy access for the right hand but an awkward and partially blocked reaching angle for the left hand. This pattern of favoring the right-hander in door opening appears in other appliances such as clothes dryers. Further, controls for the microwave (as for many other appliances) are almost always on the far right where they will be most convenient for a right-hander standing directly in front of the device.

Even the kitchen sink in most homes is designed for a right-hander, with the drain board on the left. The expectation is that the dominant right hand will be the active hand engaged in the washing actions, while the less-used left hand will be consigned to placing the washed item on the drain board.

Right-Handed Favoritism in School

School is not any kinder to the left-hander than the kitchen. Our left-to-right writing pattern is set up for a right-handed writer. The most comfortable and controlled hand movement is a pull across the body. For the right-hander it is a left-to-right movement, and for the left-hander it is reversed. In the majority of written languages, letters are written in this left-to-right sequence. Even in those languages that use a right-to-left script (such as Hebrew), the curve of the letters favors the right hand.

For the left-hander, writing is far from simple. First, the southpaw is forced to move in a direction that is uncomfortable for the left hand. Next, the left-hander is forced to make curves that are the reverse of what the left hand would most naturally and correctly draw. Finally, the left hand, when held in the normal writing posture, drags over the line that was just written. I still have a very clear image of a former mathematics professor of mine who was left-handed. As most mathematics instructors tend to do, he spent a lot of his lecture time writing equations and examples on the chalkboard. One had to be very fast and alert to copy the equations properly when he was at work, because he would scribble the beginning of an equation and then, as he progressed through it, inadvertently smear the chalk marks with the sleeve of his left hand as he formed the next set of symbols. At the end of each exercise the blackboard had a series of complex equations and also a set of random smudge marks dribbling across the chalked lines of mathematics. These smudges often obscured or obliterated valuable information such as subscripts and other technical notations. The professor, of course, displayed white chalk streaks on his tweed sports jacket as further evidence of the right-sided bias to written matter. It is possible that it is to avoid such smearing that many left-handers adopt the hooked writing style in which their hand is held above the line they are writing on.

The right-handed bias to written language shows up in some of the implements commonly used in schools. For example, the simple spiral-bound notebook used by many students shows clear partiality for the right-hander. Students are often expected to write notes on one side of the page, because the ink tends to bleed through to the other side, and they are usually instructed to write on the right-hand page. This expectation is confirmed by the fact that the pages are often three-hole punched (on the left side of the right-hand leaf) so that individual pages can be torn out and entered into a loose-leaf binder. While right-handers notice nothing special about this arrangement, left-handers are left with a very uncomfortable writing arrangement. Their arms are forced to rest on and to drag across the metal spiral coil, as can be seen in figure 13.6.

Even such commonplace items as rulers have a bias. The natural sequence of movements for drawing a straight line of a predetermined length involves positioning the ruler, holding the writing implement against the straight edge, and then pulling the pen along the ruler, in a direction across the body, as can be seen in the upper part of figure 13.7. For the ease of the right-handed user, the numbers are lower on the left and increase as you move to the right. This makes sense for the right-hander because the motion of drawing the line usually begins at the "zero inch" location on the far left and continues along the ruler until it reaches the mark indicating the desired length, somewhere to the right. The number corresponding to the current length of the line is always visible. For the left-hander, however, this process is not so efficient, requiring the left-hander to cover the numbers while drawing the line with a pulling motion across the body from right to left. The left-hander also covers the end of the ruler, as can be seen in the lower part of figure 13.7, causing is a tendency for the pen to suddenly drop off the end of the ruler if the line is drawn too quickly and the unseen "zero inch" point is reached before the pen can be stopped. The alternative, starting at the low-numbered left side and pushing the pen or pencil, is not practical, as such pushing may cause the point of the drawing instrument to dig into and tear the paper. Even if this is not the case, the southpaw's hand will ride over the line just drawn and, if ink is used,

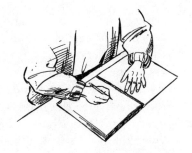 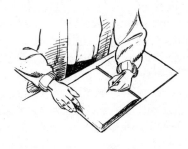

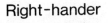

Right-hander　　　　　**Left-hander**

FIGURE 13.6: Left-handers must uncomfortably drag their arms over the metal spiral of a notebook when taking notes.

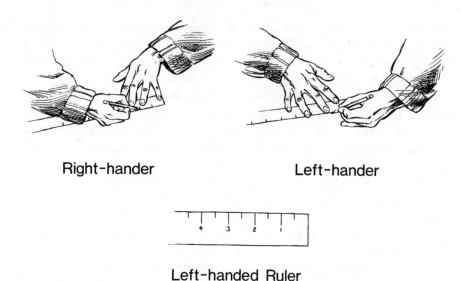

Right-hander   **Left-hander**

Left-handed Ruler

FIGURE 13.7: Typical left-handed line drawing posture covers the numbers and obscures the end of the ruler. Also shown is a reversed ruler which would simplify the process for left-handers.

may smear the end product. To be practical a left-hander should use a reversed ruler with numbering starting on the right (see figure 13.7). Although I am told that such devices now exist in some specialty stores, I have no recollection of ever seeing such a reversed ruler used by any of my fellow students. I certainly can remember many left-handers struggling through art and geometry classes with smudged lines or lines that end with a kinked "tail" caused by the pencil's inadvertent plunge over the end of the ruler. The left-hander's drawing problems are compounded in more complex drafting and drawing equipment. T-squares, drafting machines, and technically scaled rulers are not available in left-handed designs from the usual art and drafting suppliers.

There are other impediments to the success of the left-handed pupil. One common complaint is the relative scarcity of desks with left-handed writing tablets. Theoretically, if society were responsive to the needs of the left-hander, approximately one out of every ten desks (that is the ones with the side mounted writing surfaces) would have the fixed tablet mounted on the left side. One morning I looked at the auditorium in which I teach an introductory psychology course. The room contains approximately 250 seats with fixed arms for writing. Not one was left-handed. I mentioned this to one of the right-handed administrators of our university's physical plant division, the administrative unit responsible for such things. He attempted to reassure me that "There are enough left-handed desks in the university. You can probably find some of them in other lecture halls." I'm sure that is cold comfort to the twenty-five or so left-handers in my lecture section who end up twisted to the side as they attempt to take their notes. The possibility that there may be left-handed desks in other lecture theaters does not help them in this lecture hall where there are none. Furthermore, I doubt that one out of every ten desks in any of our lecture halls or classrooms is rigged for the ease and comfort of the left-hander.

The Right-Handed Office

In the modern office, left-handers still have a few strikes against them in terms of design, although they fare a bit better in the office than in other areas of the environment. One of the most common items in the modern office is the typewriter or computer keyboard. Strangely enough, the standard keyboard layout favors the left-hander.

The standard keyboard design is called the "QWERTY" layout because in the American version the top row of letters begins with the letters "QWERTY," as can be seen in figure 13.8. In this design 57 percent of the work is done by the left hand, which probably explains why so many championship speed typists have been left-handers. This outcome favoring the southpaw accidentally came about because of an attempt to overcome a mechanical design problem. With the older manual typewriters each keystroke caused a metal bar to swing down or forward to hit the paper. If the typist worked too quickly, the metal typebars would collide and jam the mechanism. The design solution was to relocate the keys so that letters often are typed immediately after one another, such as "i" and "e," would be placed on opposite sides of the machine. This placement made it less likely that the bars corresponding to these rapidly struck letters would collide. The fact that more work would be done by the left hand was a minor flaw in the design that apparently went unnoticed.

Since the QWERTY keyboard was introduced, some attempts to improve the layout involved changing the physical presentation of the keys to accommodate the mirror-image symmetry of the hands or to conform to the spacing and agility of individual fingers. Others try to rearrange the letters on the keyboard. The most elaborately developed keyboard arrangement was the result of the careful work of A.N. Dvorak in the 1940s. Dvorak, a founder of the field of *human engineering*, specialized

STANDARD QWERTY KEYBOARD

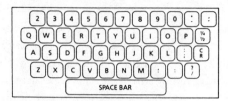

DVORAK KEYBOARD

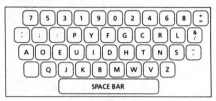

COMPUTER KEYBOARD

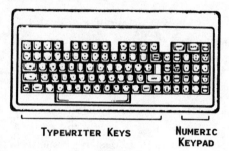

TYPEWRITER KEYS   NUMERIC KEYPAD

FIGURE 13.8: The standard QWERTY keyboard with it's left hand bias, the "improved" DVORAK keyboard with a right hand bias and a standard computer terminal keyboard with the numeric keypad set up for the convenience of the right-hander.

in developing equipment that better fit the bodies and movement patterns of workers. Such considerations are especially important in situations where the workers have to make many repetitive movements. He was able to show that with an alternate typewriter keyboard (now called the Dvorak keyboard in his honor) groups of mostly right-handed individuals actually typed about 10 percent faster, with noticeably fewer errors. He accomplished this by rearranging the keyboard so that it had a more "natural" layout—natural, of course, for the right-handed majority, thus taking away the southpaw's advantage in typing. In Dvorak's keyboard arrangement, 56 percent of the workload is on the right hand.

The Dvorak keyboard, although often discussed, has never been very successful, not because the right-handed world would not like to see it introduced but because it would be too disruptive to attempt to change people's habits at this stage. Millions of people would have to learn a new style of typewriting, and millions of typewriters and keyboards would have to be changed. Since the QWERTY layout works well enough, there is little motivation to change, meaning that left-handed typists continue to have a bit of an edge.

This is not to say that the right-hander has not managed to enforce his habits on the design of the contemporary keyboard. For instance, with the introduction of computers into the work place, a new design of keyboard has developed. This contains the usual QWERTY typewriter layout, but also contains a numeric keypad, designed to facilitate the entry of numerical data. This keypad is, of course, placed to the right of the keyboard (see figure 13.8) so that it is easy and natural for the right-hander to use but requires the left-hander to cross his body or shift his position completely to use it.

There are other subtle handedness biases in the office. Adding machines and desk calculators usually have their adding, subtraction, totalling, and other mathematical function keys on the right side. I remember some of the older manual adding machines, which had to be cranked after each entry. Of course, the crank was on the right side. Computer printers have a right-handed bias, as the controls such as the on-off switch, the patten pressure lever, and most of the function switches are most often on the right side. On the computer itself, floppy disk drives are usually located on the right side of the computer chassis. Even the common copying machine favors the right-hander, as the paper feed end is usually located on the right so that the sheets to be copied can be manipulated by the right hand.

Telephones seem to be an exception to the usual right-handed rule of equipment design. The cord of the receiver is usually attached to the left side of the phone base. If the cradle that holds the receiver is asymmetrical, it is usually placed to the left where it would be more naturally picked up by the left hand and then placed against the left ear. While this arrangement seems to favor the left-hander, it was actually created for the right-hander's comfort. If you hold the phone receiver in your left hand, your right hand is free to dial the number, make notes, or jot down messages. If you are using a pay phone, the right hand is available to insert coins into the slot, which is, of course, placed on the right side of the phone. For the left-hander to be able to perform these tasks, he or she must shift the phone to the right hand, which causes the cord to drape itself across the dial and in front of the body in an annoying and interfering manner. At the pay phone, left-handers must cross their body with the left hand to dial or insert coins.

Leaving the office for a moment and stepping out into the hall to get a cup of coffee will show the continuing right-hand tendency in the world. If you look at a coin-operated coffee-dispensing machine you will see that it is, like most machines, a right-hander's device. For instance, the coin slot is on the right. The buttons to select your beverage choice are on the right. Even the door to the compartment holding the hot coffee is right-handed, swinging open to the left so that the right hand can slip in and take the beverage. The metal bracket that keeps the cup upright is open to the right, and if left-handers try to use their dominant left hand to remove the coffee, the positioning is so awkward that they are almost guaranteed to spill the liquid on themselves during the extraction process.

The Right-Handed Workplace

In industrial settings such as factories, mills, machine shops, or any other place where heavy tools or equipment are used, we find an environment quite badly designed for the left-hander. Most power tools and machines are very strongly right-handed. Let's just consider a few items. The familiar drill press is usually designed so that the handle that lowers the drill downward is on the right side, for ease of use by a right-hander. The left hand is presumed to be holding the material down on the drill stand table. If the left-hander attempts to use his left hand to lower the bit he will effectively block his view of the item that he is trying to drill, as can be seen in figure 13.9. It is hard to place a hole accurately if your view is partially obstructed by your own arm.

Saws are especially bad for the left-hander. One of the more commonly used saws in many metal and wood shops is the band saw, clearly designed with the right-hander's needs in mind. The band saw opens to the right for maximal freedom of movement for the right-hander's dominant hand. In figure 13.10, you will notice that the movements on the left side are actually blocked by the upright. This machine is clearly based upon a conception that the work, that is, the material to be cut, will be held by the right hand. When the right hand is used, the arm and elbow flare out to the side, safely away from the saw blade. If a left-hander wants to use this equipment he must either use his right hand to hold the work (which will be weaker and more awkward) or cross his

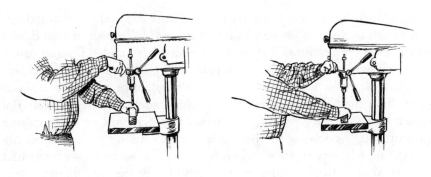

Right-hander   **Left-hander**

FIGURE 13.9: When a left-hander uses a drill press his arm crosses in front of his body and blocks his view of the work.

body with his left hand, which places his arm directly in line with the saw blade and seems to invite a bad cut.

Portable power tools are no better in terms of their design. A portable power saw is indisputably engineered so that it will be held with the right hand. Held in the right hand, the motor serves as an effective shield between the operator and the rotating saw blade. The left-hander does not have this added protection, because holding the tool in the left

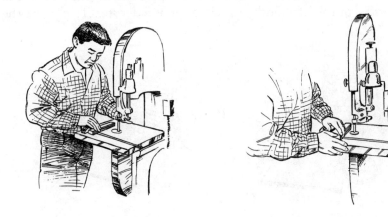

Right-hander   **Left-hander**

FIGURE 13.10: A right-hander safely uses the band saw; for the left-hander, the arm crossed in front of the blade invites danger.

hand places the saw blade nearly flush against the body, inviting disaster, as can be seen in figure 13.11. I discussed this aspect of tool design when I was on a radio talk show once, and a left-handed listener called in to tell me a story. He said he was pleased that I had mentioned this problem as people had always doubted him when he told a story about what happened to him when he was using such a saw. The material which he was cutting was difficult to get through, and he was applying pressure on the saw, with the blade next to his hip, when suddenly something felt very strange. When he stopped the saw to see what had happened he noticed that his pants were in the process of slipping down; he had sawed through his own belt.

Many of the portable power tools, such as drills or the electric saw that we were just speaking about, have safety switches that must be depressed before the trigger will activate the machine. This switch is usually in a position where it can easily be depressed by the right thumb (see figure 13.11). Because of this, and the specific shape of the handles, guards and trigger grips, these tools are often difficult, unwieldy, awkward and fatiguing for a left-hander to use. For example, the electric chain saw is clearly designed to be operated by a right-hander, with only passive support provided by the left-hand. A trigger activates the saw, and, for added protection of the user, the safety switch mentioned above must be depressed before the trigger will allow the saw to operate. This design is meant to prevent inadvertent trigger contacts from starting the blades. The safety switch is conveniently placed for the thumb of the right hand. For the left-hander the situation is a disaster. To operate the

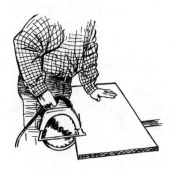
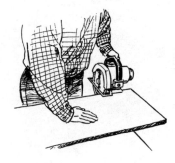

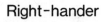

Right-hander   **Left-hander**

FIGURE 13.11: A portable power saw is more safely used by a left-hander places the blade very close to his body.

saw left-handed, the operator has to cross his arms, placing the body
somewhat off balance and reducing the degree of fine control that the
operator has over the machine. Furthermore, in this crossed-arm position with the left hand on the trigger handle, the safety switch is now
permanently depressed by the closed hand, which is wrapped around it
in the "wrong" direction. Not only does the safety switch now not do
what it was supposed to, but, by digging into the palm of the left-handed
operator, it acts as a source of discomfort and a possible contributor to
accidental loss of control of the machine. The gasoline-powered chain
saw adds an additional difficulty, as the saw is meant to be started by
holding it in the left hand and pulling the start cord with the right.
Reversing the hands places the saw bar dangerously close to the operator.

Around a machine shop or a mill, you will find more right-handed
bias the more closely you analyze the situation. On-off switches and
safety switches seem to be set up for the convenience of the right-hander.
Assembly lines make the presumption that everyone is right-handed in
the placement of parts, the direction that the belt moves, and the positioning of the workers. Heavy earth-moving equipment, such as cranes,
scrapers, and spreaders, usually place the most important and frequently
used controls at the right side, for comfortable use by the right-hander.
For instance, the lever that raises, lowers, and alters the angle of the
blade of a bulldozer is found placed conveniently for the right-hander
at the right side. Also, many hand tools with cutting edges bear evidence of a right-handed design. Scythes are curved for right-handed use,
adjustable cutting blades are advanced by the right thumb, trowels are
edge-grooved for right-handed use, and the list goes on.

Left-handed doctors, dentists, and scientists do not fare much better.
Surgical instruments are almost always right-handed in their design, and
left-handed medical cutting instruments must often be specially made,
if they are obtainable at all. In surgical theaters the usual setup for the
anesthetist places most of the controls under the right hand. The most
common dentistry station is right-handed. Left-handed dental students
are often forced to switch to right-handed operation to accommodate
to these restrictions, although convertible dentistry units are becoming
somewhat more common.

Chemical and pharmaceutical equipment, much like kitchen equipment, often shows the same right-sided design considerations. For example, the common chemical beaker, like the kitchen measuring cup, often
has markings on only one side, the left side, where it will be visible to
a person holding this piece of glassware in his right hand; and pouring

lips on crucibles are often placed so that they can be used only when held in the right hand.

Other pieces of laboratory equipment suffer from the same right-handed design bias. The standard microscope has the focus and light adjustment knobs on the right side, which is where you will also find the on-off switches for the chemical centrifuge, spectroanalysis units, and other analytical equipment. The exposure controls on most x-ray and other high-tech diagnostic units are also on the right, placing left-handers at a disadvantage as they are forced to use some inelegant contortions while reaching for vital switches and knobs.

Perhaps the greatest industrial disservice to the left-hander has to do with instruments that require twisting or turning. For example, adjustment knobs or even threaded screws and bolts show a clear preference for the right-hander. *Ergonomics* or *human engineering* is the scientific discipline that focuses on the study of human movements and behavior patterns with the goal of best designing jobs and machines to fit the worker. One fact that has clearly emerged from ergonomic studies has to do with the way in which hands habitually turn. For the right hand, the most powerful, most natural, and best-controlled movements involve clockwise rotation, while for the left hand, counterclockwise rotation is best. This has implications for many aspects of machine control. For instance, it is when increasing the speed or power of a machine that the most control and care is required. This is why the custom is to have a clockwise turn associated with "more" or "faster."

This turning bias also determined the direction in which screws or bolts are threaded. Screws are invariably threaded so that a clockwise motion is associated with driving the screw forward. The forward driving of the screw usually requires maximum strength and continuous pressure and control to keep the screwdriver from slipping out of the slot in the screw head. Notice that this clockwise turning pattern places the left-hander at a clear disadvantage. The left-hander's natural turning tendency is counterclockwise, which means that he will suffer from a reduction in strength and control when using a screwdriver to advance a screw for insertion.

Numerous variations on this right-handed, clockwise theme may be found. One example, which caused some amusement to a friend of mine, dealt with the common corkscrew. Corkscrews, just like threaded machinery components, must be turned clockwise to advance the spiral prong into the cork. A short while ago, I had a little party at my home. We had set up some bottles of wine on a counter so that people could serve themselves. One of my colleagues was looking around for the corkscrew to open one of the bottles. On impulse I reached into our utensil drawer and pulled out a wing-type corkscrew that one of my students had given to me as a gag gift. Although it appeared to be quite a normal corkscrew, it was designed for a left-hander. This means that to advance the prong you had to turn the handle counterclockwise. My friend took this utensil and tried to open the bottle of wine. He placed the corkscrew over the bottle and turned clockwise. Nothing happened, of course, since the point was being dragged backwards across the cork instead of being advanced. He checked the point of the corkscrew and then tried again, pushing hard and sputtering, "There's something wrong with this thing!" It never occurred to him to reverse his hand movements and to turn the handle counterclockwise. When I finally showed him what was happening and explained the nature of the device, he was able to open the bottle. He thought that this was amusing enough so that he stayed by the bar most of the night. When people came by he would announce that they couldn't have anything to drink unless they passed a "sobriety test," which consisted of opening a bottle of wine with the corkscrew he gave them. The only one who passed without any hints from him was a left-handed graduate student of mine who started clockwise (showing much experience with a right-handed world) but immediately reversed her direction of turning after one or two turns.

Right-Handers at Play

Even at leisure or while engaging in sports, the left-hander is assailed by restrictions on activities and design flaws. The common camera is notoriously right-handed. The shutter release button is on the right side, the film advance is designed to be activated with the right thumb, and so forth. In loading the film, the camera is usually designed to open to the left, so that there is a large open area for the right hand to operate, while left-handed action is partially obstructed by the open camera back between the southpaw's hand and the film. The same right-sided bias is shown in many motion picture and video cameras, which have moulded pistol grips with trigger-type camera activation switches. Of course, the pistol grip is specifically formed for the right hand. In some instances the video camera will virtually force exclusive right-handed use. One such video camera that I saw recently had the eyepiece of the viewfinder mounted on the left side of the camera body in such a way that, when holding the camera with the right hand, the right side of the face rested against the camera body and the right eye was perfectly aligned with the eyepiece. If a left-hander attempted to use this camera holding the trigger grip with his left hand and resting the camera against the left side of his face, he would find that there was no way that he could sight the camera, since the eyepiece would be on the other side of the camera and completely unavailable for use (except, perhaps, by a person standing next to him).

To be a successful hunter or fisherman one must also be right-handed. Rifles are clearly instruments designed for the right-hander. Bolt action rifles have the operating lever on the right side. With this arrangement the operations needed for the insertion and ejection of cartridges with the left hand become possible only for circus contortionists. The chamber that holds the cartridge opens to the right for easy loading with the right hand. This right-sided chamber entrance makes use of automatic and semiautomatic weapons extremely difficult and dangerous for the left-hander. The expended cartridges are ejected from the chamber after each shot. If their trajectory is slightly downward the hot casings will tend to hit the left-hander's arm, which is extended along the stock to brace the weapon. If the rifle is held against the left shoulder and the cartridges eject high and backwards, the shooter's head, eye, or nose may be in the direct line of their flight. The only solution to this problem seems to be to hold the weapon against the right shoulder, which virtually forces right-handed trigger operation.

Fishing rods are also right-handed. Typical fly-casting rods or deep-sea fishing rods tend to be designed for right-handed use. Specifically, the winding lever used to take in the line after the fish is hooked is placed at the right side. For the left-hander the reel handle is on the wrong side. In the usual position the reel is optimally placed for right-handed action using the most comfortable form of whole-hand rotary motion. Ergonomists and human engineers have shown that the optimal winding movement involves the hand moving away from the body at the top of the motion and toward the body as it returns in the lower part of the movement. The simplest solution attempted by left-handers usually involves turning the fishing rod upside down, which places the take-up handle on the left side. Unfortunately this doesn't work very well, as in that orientation the line is more likely to foul and the rod tends to rotate in the hand, as the weight of the reel is on top causing fatigue and some loss of control. Mounting the reel "backwards" so that the take-up handle is on the left runs into problems with the actual pattern of movements. Now the rotary hand motions involve pulling into the body at the top of the motion and pushing away at the low point, which most people find to be less comfortable and more tiring actions. It is the difficulty with this reversed winding motion that makes the use of manual eggbeaters and manual twist drills so unwieldy and fatiguing for the left-hander as well.

Several team sports also provide equipment and playing problems for the southpaw. Field hockey, for example, is difficult for the left-hander because field hockey sticks are not made in a left-handed version. The stick is usually made so that the flat striking surface is on the left side while the right side is rounded. According to the All England Women's Hockey Association: "Any player using a left-handed stick would find it almost impossible to keep to the rules. They would find it difficult to receive the ball, or to get the ball away from other players. A 'bully' [which is a procedure to get the ball into play where players face each other, alternating between striking the ground and each other's stick; after three repetitions of this pattern of movements, the ball is played] would also be impossible with a left-handed stick, and so would the avoidance of obstructing . . . ".[1] Fortunately, there is always ice hockey, where left-handers are permitted and left-handed sticks do exist.

In polo the left-hander has difficulties as well, not with equipment but rather with the pattern of play. Because collisions are very dangerous for both the horse and rider, there are very strict rules controlling a player's right of way. These specify the circumstances where the player can go for the ball or must give way to another player. These right-of-way rules are so strongly oriented toward the right-handed player that the left-hander would often find himself forced into awkward hitting positions and sharper direction changes than the right-handed player in order to play "legally." This is important, as serious penalties are inflicted on players who do not follow the expected pattern of play. The Hurlingham Polo Club, which controls polo in Britain and many parts of the Commonwealth and serves as the model for most other polo clubs in the world, decided that it was safer for the sport simply to prohibit left-handed playing of the game. Even Prince Charles, heir to the throne of England, who is a natural left-hander, has been forced to play polo right-handed if he wishes to play at all.

For the left-hander who is banned from polo and field hockey, who finds hunting and fishing too awkward because of the equipment, it might seem that it would better to stay at home and watch TV or listen to the stereo or read a book. Even in this passive set of activities the left-hander will still find evidence for the right-handed bent to the world. For example, a record player has its tone arm and controls on the right side for easier right-handed access. Most TVs have their controls on the right, as do most stereo tuners, compact disk players, and tape recorders.

Even books are right-handed. Books are designed so that the leaf on the right side is turned as you advance through the pages. This is very comfortable for the right-hander whose right hand is more agile, but may cause a certain degree of fumbling for the left-hander, who must use his nondominant hand to lift a thin sheet of paper so that the page may be turned. This fact was recognized by the publishers of *Lefthander Magazine*, who have reversed the usual page order on their publication. As the magazine is designed for left-handers, it is published with the usual page sequence reversed. Page 1 is at the rightmost leaf (usually the back cover of a magazine) and the pages are turned from left to right for the comfort of the left-hander.

The examples I have given (only a small sample of the large number available) demonstrate that the world, our technology, and our constructed environment have been clearly engineered with a distinct right-handed bias. Many of these items might seem fairly trivial and might seem to have only nuisance value. For example, the right-handed design bias to clothing is clear but seems to have no earthshaking consequences. What difference does it make if a man's dress shirt has only one pocket, placed on the left side where it can be most easily reached by the right hand reaching across the body? Does it really matter that the fly in men's trousers, shorts, and underwear is designed with a flap that makes it more convenient to reach in with the right hand? What are the far-reaching effects of the fact that zippers are made so that the part that requires the most accurate manipulation is placed on the right side?

While such items may seem inconsequential, they affect the comfort of the left-hander and the level of daily hassles and frustrations. Clearly, if such design features were totally trivial, there would be no set convention associated with them and no bias would be evident. Controls would be set on either side of machines, pouring lips would sometimes be on the right and other times on the left, and pockets would appear randomly on either side of shirtfronts. However, the fact that so many items are oriented toward right-handed convenience suggests that these design features do affect the ease of use of many appliances and tools and must affect the comfort of the users. If the matter were simply one of comfort, however, we might be able to dismiss it without much more discussion. However, in some instances these right-handed design features can have a major impact on the safety of the left-hander. The lives of southpaws may be lost because of such design features, the problem that we will turn to in the next chapter.

14

The Hazardous Life
of the Southpaw

A long tradition labels left-handers "clumsy," "awkward," and accident prone. For example, the British psychologist Sir Cyril Burt painted such an extreme and unflattering picture of southpaws when he wrote:

> Not infrequently the left-handed child shows widespread difficulties in almost every form of finer muscular coordination . . . they shuffle and shamble, they flounder about like seals out of water. Awkward in the house, and clumsy in their games, they are fumblers and bunglers at whatever they do.[1]

Burt concluded that it was in the nature of the left-hander to be clumsy and uncoordinated. Some forms of clumsiness might be seen as consistent with our suggestions that left-handers may have suffered from birth-stress-related injuries. If the left-handedness was the result of some sort of neurological damage, left-handed individuals might not have as fine control over their limbs as undamaged right-handers might have. However this conclusion is hard to defend. How can one brand all left-handers as being stumbling, gawky klutzes and then in the next breath speak about the many great athletes who have been left-handed? Certainly, no one would call people like baseball's Babe Ruth, Lou Gehrig, Ted Williams, Sandy Koufax, Lefty Grove, or Reggie Jackson clumsy. I doubt that tennis stars like Jimmy Connors, Rod Laver, and John McEnroe or golf heroes Arnold Palmer and Ben Hogan would be accused of being "fumblers and bunglers." Yet all these individuals are left-handed. The reputation for ungainliness on the part of left-handers is not due to anything inherent in the left-hander but may have to do with other factors.

The Left-Hander in a Right-Handed World

One of the major reasons that left-handers appear to be clumsy and poorly coordinated comes from the fact that the world was primarily designed by right-handers for the comfort and convenience of right-handers. In the last chapter we saw many of the ways in which our man-made environment is constructed in favor of the right-hander.

Consider the poor left-handed child struggling with a can opener designed for right-handed use. As the child contorts and struggles to use this tool, which is ill-designed for left-handedness, it is virtually inevitable that some of the contents of the can will end up on the kitchen counter or the child's shirtfront. Right-handed parents and others are not apt to consider tool or utensil design when they find the resultant mess. Their other (right-handed) children have probably had no trouble with this simple task; therefore the obvious conclusion is that this child must be inept, poorly coordinated, and lacking in dexterity.

The same thing happens in the school. The southpaw child struggles with implements designed for the right-hander, and most teachers pay little attention to handedness. For example, most schools have only right-handed scissors. As a consequence, the left-handed child ends up with arts and craft projects that look like San Francisco after the Great Earthquake of 1906. The child doesn't even seem to be able to draw a straight line without smudging or falling off of the end of the ruler. Furthermore, the child's handwriting is streaked, wanders off the line, slants backwards, and suffers from poorly formed letters. The right-handed teacher often does not stop to consider that he or she is dealing with a left-handed child struggling with right-handed implements and a right-handed handwriting system. It is much easier to label the child uncoordinated and not very skillful.

Even in games and dances, the left-hander sometimes appears to be awkward and ungainly, not because of physical coordination but rather because left- and right-handers have different ways of moving their bodies. These differences have to do with turning preferences or what are sometimes called "veering biases." People who design museum exhibits, supermarket layouts, or department store displays take advantage of these veering biases. As is mentioned in some ergonomic textbooks, the majority of people have a distinct right—turn preference. After passing through an entrance, people have a tendency to turn to the right or to rotate their body in a clockwise direction. This turning bias is strong enough so that one self-help book, which was trying to show people how to get faster service and to avoid crowds and lines, was entitled *Always Turn Left*, suggesting that in this way you would go where the crowd was not.

In speaking about turning tendencies, however, it is important to note that the predilection to turn right is much stronger in the right-hander than in the left-hander. One year, as part of a laboratory project conducted by one of my experimental psychology classes, we demonstrated this fact. Each student had to bring in several friends (one at a time) to serve as test subjects. Each person to be tested was asked to step into a room and to fill out a questionnaire. The room contained two desks, one on the right side of the entrance and the other on the left. Identical desks were set at an equal distance from the door so there were no obvious factors that might influence which one was selected. In general, people tended to step into the room carrying the questionnaire and to take whichever desk they turned toward. The questionnaire was to determine handedness, and the experimenters simply noted the direction that each person turned when he or she entered the room. The results indicated that, just as the ergonomic textbooks suggest, the vast majority of the people tested did turn right. When the data was analyzed on the basis of the handedness of the people, it was found that the majority of right-handers turned to the right while the majority of left-handers turned to the left. In fact, left-handers were two and a half times more likely to turn left than were right-handers. Other more formal studies have confirmed the fact that left- and right-handers have different turning tendencies. For example, when asked to turn around on the spot, right-handers have a natural tendency to rotate their bodies to the right, resulting in a clockwise pirouette, while left-handers rotate more naturally to the left resulting in a counterclockwise turn.[2]

The effect of the different turning biases of right- and left-handers varies with the nature of the activity involved. Ballroom dancing is designed to have a right-handed man dance with a right-handed woman. This is confirmed by the fact that the flow of the dancers around the room, as well as the expected direction of most turns and twirls in the dance, involves a clockwise motion for both partners. In marching bands, the standard direction of parade turns is clockwise, toward the right. The standard military turn, the *about face*, involves clockwise rotations. It is not surprising that left-handers, always forced in the direction away from their natural counterclockwise turning tendencies, are more apt to make mistakes or to be slower or less graceful in their body movements, which merely adds to their reputation for being clumsy.

The tendency for the left-hander to turn in the direction opposite to that habitually used by the right-hander seems to have been a major factor in forcing one president of the United States out of office. Gerald Ford became the laughingstock of the nation because of his many mishaps. He was always bumping into his honor guard, colliding with members of his entourage, and tangling arms or legs with honored visitors during photo sessions. One very famous photo showed the results of President Ford turning unexpectedly to the left, only to knock into an aide. This collision, which then caused Ford nearly to tumble down the stairs of an airplane, was published in virtually every newspaper across the country. In reality, Ford was not clumsy. In his youth he had been an athlete, and he had kept himself in very good physical condition. He was a large man, as spry and agile as one might expect for a person of his size. His problem was that he was left-handed. All of the protocol associated with the president is based upon the assumption that he is right-handed. People are placed so that they will be in the appropriate positions when the usually right-handed president makes the common right turn or clockwise rotation. For the left-handed president, everything is on the wrong side, which makes collisions and tangles much more likely. The press played Ford's apparent awkward ungainliness for all that it was worth. Pictures of the president blundering around seemed to be an endless source of humor. The humor was, of course, the same kind of humor associated with the old movie slapstick gags, in which it is supposedly much funnier if a cream pie hits someone of high status (for example, an appropriately dressed queen, countess, mayor, or banker). Here, instead of cream pie in the face of the king, it is a fit of gawkiness that hits the president. The problem for Ford was that "clumsy" also carries to its observer connotations of "stupid." In no time at all, "dumb Gerald Ford," walking into walls and muttering nonsense, became the staple of every stand-up comedian in the United States. When election year came around, the White House staff attempted to minimize the effect that these stories and pictures were having on the president's public image. To do this they put an embargo on official press releases and photos of such awkward events. Unfortunately, the damage had already been done, and the public simply did not want to elect a "bumbling" president. Yet, Ford really only suffered from being a southpaw in a right-hander's world.[3]

A few years ago I found myself at one of those cocktail parties to which "important people" are invited so that they can be displayed to the more common folk, such as me. I was introduced to a man who had some position on President Ronald Reagan's White House staff. Since we both had drinks in our hands, I thought that I could get away with asking a question that had bothered me for a while.

"I remember that Ford ran into trouble because of his left-handedness," I started. "You know, banging into everyone and tripping around. How does Reagan avoid that sort of embarrassment, such as turning in the wrong direction and all of that, since he's left-handed too?" I asked.

"Well," came the somewhat hesitant answer, "he did have a long term as governor of the State of California which gave him an opportunity to work some of those problems out. The trick that we use is to let the president stand out about a half a step in front of us, or, if that's not possible, then to give him a full step of distance on either side. In that way, no matter which way he turns, he doesn't tangle with anyone else."

He looked at me and then added, with a bit of a malevolent grin, "We also make sure that all of the members of the press know that if they publish photos of any 'events' that make the president look like a stumbler or an oaf that they will never get close enough to him to take another photo, and neither will anyone else from their paper or magazine."

The Left-Hander at Risk

The examples just described, of the left-hander running afoul of the world designed for the right-handed, may merely be amusing to the uninvolved right-hander or annoying to the left-hander who must confront these problems on a daily basis. However, amusement or annoyance are not the only outcomes of our right-handed technology. There are reasons to believe that the right-handed design of the world may actually constitute a danger for the left-hander.

Consider some of the power tools discussed in the previous chapter, such as the band saw shown in figure 13.10. The left-handed worker is forced to use this tool despite its right-handed design if he wants to work in an industry that utilizes this kind of machine. There are two ways in which the left-hander might accommodate to these design problems.

The first is to give in to the pressure of the right-handed world and begin to manipulate the work with the right hand. The more demanding task of holding and moving the material to be cut then has to be done with the left-hander's nondominant right hand. By definition this hand is less expert for the southpaw; it works with less efficiency, less agility, and is more subject to fatigue. The other way that the left-hander might accommodate is to insist on using his left hand. This requires adopting an extremely awkward body position, and, for the band saw, as we saw in figure 13.10, the arm must pass in front of the moving saw blade.

Neither solution is really acceptable. Both are set-ups for accidents. If the less-expert right hand is used, its clumsiness may result in a problem, as it simply lacks adequate control for some delicate or precise movements. If the contorted and twisted position body position is adopted so that the left hand can be used, any slip may produce a disaster.

If you think that I am overstating the point, let me describe a visit to a mill in Western Canada. This mill specialized in cutting cedar logs into roofing shingles and shakes (much larger shingle-like cuts used on roofs or as house siding). The mill contained the usual large number of saws and log-splitting devices, all of which had the usual right-handed design features. At the time of my visit twenty-one men were working on the mill floor, four of whom were left-handed. Every one of the four left-handers (100 percent) was missing at least part of one finger from mill-related accidents with the saws. Of the 17 right-handers, only two (12 percent) were missing parts of digits from such accidents. The left-handers were eight times more likely to suffer from an accident that resulted in their losing a finger or part of a finger in this mill.

Power saws are not the only devices that have a right-handed bias. As we found out in the previous chapter, most of the large electrically driven machines have this bias, including drill presses, metal cutting mills, metal spinners and shapers, sheet metal brakes, lathes, power punches, and die cutters. Large industrial machines, cranes, bulldozers, scrapers, and similar devices also have this problem. Controls are set up for the right-hander, safety switches are located for best use by the right hand, and on it goes.

What are the consequences of this right-handed design? It is easy to imagine situations where the results of this bias might be quite serious. Certainly, a second or so lost by a left-hander, groping for a safety switch conveniently placed for a right-hander but totally out of reach for the left-hander, may make the difference between a safe shutdown and an injured worker. Left-handers manipulating controls with the right hand will be slower, less precise, and more likely to fatigue. A tired worker, moving more slowly and with less accuracy, is often a danger to himself and to others.

Remember that power tools and big machines are not the only culprits. We also seen that hand tools, whether they be single bevelled knives, can openers, scissors, metal shears, carving tools, or even surgical instruments, have handles and blades shaped for right-handed use. The left-hander must either use them in the "wrong" hand or suffer discomfort, loss of precise control, and fatigue. The end result may be blades that slip while being used and workers who sustain injury from their own awkwardness because of being forced to use a tool ill designed for their dominant hand. In the kitchen, working with ladles and pouring spouts that are set up for the right-hander places the left-hander at risk of burns and scalds from splattering hot liquids caused by reduced control.

Even the turning bias of the left-hander places them at risk. Right-handers expect that everyone has their own clockwise and rightward turning tendencies. The left-hander who turns in the opposite direction makes it more likely that he or she will suffer from collisions with other individuals. Such collisions can result in falls, spills, or even serious injuries. As left-handers are more likely to make the unexpected movement, they are more likely to be involved in such misadventures.

The Accident-Prone Left-Hander

The examples I have spelled out suggest that, because of the right-handed technology and design of the world, the left-hander is probably at greater risk of accidents than is the right-hander. Surprisingly, although this prediction seems obvious given the design of the environment, when we searched the literature we found virtually no research on this issue. Part of the reason seemed to be that standard accident reporting forms, which go to Worker's Compensation Boards, Health and Labor Departments or Ministries, or insurance companies, do not ask for the handedness of the injured worker, and the data are not readily available.

I decided to determine in a controlled scientific manner whether left-handed university students were at greater risk of accidents. This is a reasonable population to test as younger individuals are generally more accident prone (supplying more accident material to work with). In addition, university students, as part of their studies, leisure activities, or part-time and summer jobs, often work with a broad spectrum of power and hand tools. They are also reasonably active in sports, drive vehicles quite a bit, and also engage in typical home and domestic activities. They were also a population of individuals that I could obtain quickly and inexpensively, considerations not be lightly dismissed!

In the final version of this study, I tested 1,896 university students.[4] First I gave them a handedness questionnaire to determine whether each individual was right- or left-handed. Next I asked each individual to report whether he or she had had any accidents in the past two years. I divided the possible types of accidents up into five different categories, as follows:

1. Accidents of any sort when at work or in the workplace.
2. Accidents while engaged in any activity at home.
3. Accidents while participating in a sports activity.
4. Accidents while using any kind of tool or implement.
5. Accidents while driving a vehicle.

The accidents I was interested in were not the everyday blunders and mishaps, but accidents in which a person suffered an injury. I didn't score things like paper cuts and little nicks with a knife; rather I counted only those accidents that required medical attention. I was interested only in the major accident-related injuries to these people that occurred over a two-year period.

I had expected that left-handers would be more susceptible to accidents than right-handers for all the reasons I have outlined. Pressed to guess the size of the difference, I would have guessed that left-handers would be 5 to 10 percent more accident prone, a modest difference, but one with real implications for the relative safety of left-handers. Finding the expected higher accident rate among left-handers, I was completely unprepared for the true size of the difference.

Across all five accident categories, we found that a left-hander is 89 percent more likely to have an accident-related injury requiring medical attention than is a right-hander. Left-handers have nearly two accidents for every one suffered by right-hander. Further, if we look at the chance that a left-hander will have an accident in more than one category of activity, we find that they are 78 percent more likely to have such a double mishap. Left-handers not only have more accidents but tend to have them in a variety of situations and activities.

Suppose we consider each category of accident-related injury separately. As you can see from figure 14.1, left-handers had a higher risk of an accident-related injury for every single category of activity measured.

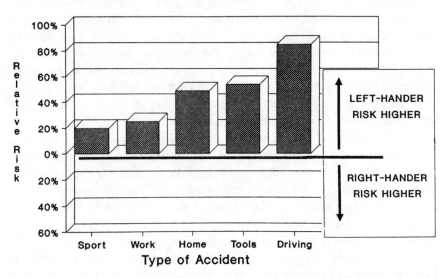

FIGURE 14.1: The relative risk of accidents is always higher for left-handers in every category of accident related injury studied.

They were 20 percent more likely to have an accidental injury when engaged in sports, 25 percent more likely to have such an injury when at work, 49 percent more likely to have an accidental injury when at home, and 51 percent more likely to have accident-related injury when using a tool, machine, or other implement. There was not one accident category in which right-handers were at higher risk.

One of the greatest surprises came in the area of driving. Left-handers seem to have more trouble in traffic than do right-handers. Overall, left-handers were 85 percent more likely to have an accident-related injury when driving a vehicle than were right-handers. The accident risk seems to be greatest for left-handed male drivers.

At first glance this higher traffic-related accident rate in left-handers may seem to be a bit puzzling. Although for most of the world the gear shift is on the right side, gearing up or down is not a major factor in most traffic accidents. The usual driver-related factors that contribute to traffic accidents have to do with speed and the direction in which the car is steered. Yet the steering wheel on cars and trucks is round, and right-handers don't seem to have any immediately apparent advantage in its use, while the brake and accelerator are controlled by the foot, so that handedness shouldn't be a factor in their use.

Careful examination, however, shows that in most of the world traffic patterns are set up with a right-hand bias, at least in those nations where cars are driven on the right side of the road. One might be tempted to think that, with traffic on the right, the most common turn off or onto controlled streets or highways is to the right, the natural turning tendency of the right-hander. However, I do not think that this is the major reason for increased driving-accident risk among left-handers. I believe that part of the reason has to do with a simple reflex response that differs depending upon a person's handedness.

Suppose that you are sitting quietly and suddenly an unexpected or possibly threatening event occurs—a loud noise, a bright flash, or a startling action such as someone taking a poke at your nose or any of a variety of other possibilities. In the presence of such an unanticipated or striking event, people tend to show a *reflex response*, which is an automatic, unlearned pattern of behavior. The pattern shown under conditions of a sudden unexpected happening is called the *startle response*. As part of the startle response, people tend to gasp for breath, their hearts race, they begin to sweat and, most important for us here, they often throw their hands slightly out to the front and sides of their body. Bringing up the hands is a reflex protective pattern that probably evolved as the beginning of a set of movements to protect the individual from frontal attack. Figure 14.2 shows a typical startle reflex. Notice that the hands are out to the side in this example, although sometimes the hands may come up directly in front of the body. Furthermore, notice that the left hand is held somewhat higher than the right hand. This is the startle response pattern typical of the right-hander.

Left-handers tend to have the reverse startle response from the one in the figure. They tend to throw their hands out so that the right hand is high and the left hand is low. We informally verified this in one of the silliest-looking experiments that I have had the opportunity to conduct in more than twenty-five years of research. In this experiment I had a group of students wander around campus carrying a light foam-rubber ball about the size of a softball. The students were required to pick an unsuspecting individual who was not holding anything in either hand (we wanted no broken objects or other disasters). When the person was relaxed, the "experimenter" was to suddenly shout "Now!" or some equivalent and to throw the ball directly at the person's nose. This inevitably produced a startle reaction, and the experimenter simply noted which hand was held high and which was held low. Afterwards (after explanations and apologies were made) the experimenters asked each individual four simple questions to determine his or her handed-

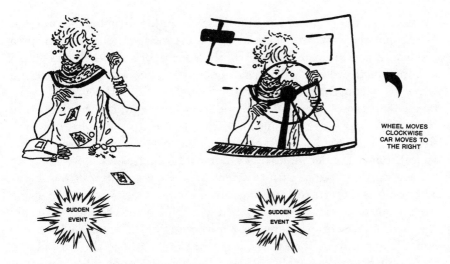

FIGURE 14.2: The startle response of a typical right-hander, with left hand high and right hand low. Notice the effect that this has on the steering of a car. Left-handers reverse this response with the right-hand high and the left-hand low.

ness. After data from 302 people had been collected we stopped the study for safety reasons. The incident that prompted termination of the study occurred in one of the campus snack bars, when one of the student experimenters was scratched on the face by a startled experimental subject who swung at him with a hand that had long fingernails. Her defensive swing was followed by a loud shriek because she thought that she was being attacked. Several of her friends rushed to her rescue, and the issue was a bit sticky for a few minutes until the experimenter and a colleague explained what was going on. They showed the experiment instruction and data sheet and had one of the "rescuers" call me at my office to verify what they were saying. When we stopped the data collection we had observed 260 right-handers and 42 left-handers. Among the right-handers, 79 percent responded to the unexpected event with a startle reaction in which the left hand was high and the right hand was low. Among the left-handers 76 percent responded in the opposite way, with the right hand held high and the left hand held low.

You might wonder why the difference in the startle response of left- and right-handers is significant. Let's turn back to figure 14.2, where we pictured the startle reflex of a right-hander, and place a steering wheel in her hand. Now, instead of a foam ball and a loud sound to startle her, imagine that there is an unexpected traffic situation. It could be a car swerving out of its lane, a child or a cat suddenly appearing in front of the vehicle, a skid or a slide from a grease spot on the road, or a sudden thump from an unseen pothole or debris on the road. If an unanticipated event startles her, notice what happens to the steering wheel as a consequence of her startle reflex. With the typical right-handed pattern of left hand high and right hand low, the steering wheel rotates in a clockwise manner. The car swerves to the right, onto the shoulder of the road and out of traffic. The left-hander, however, is not so fortunate. The left-hander is three and a half times more likely to make a startle response with the right hand high and the left hand low. The result is to turn the steering wheel counterclockwise and to swing the car out to the left. This direction will bring it into contact with cars in other lanes, perhaps even with cars moving in the opposite direction; hence, the possibility of a traffic accident is increased in the left-hander.

One might argue that this relationship between handedness and traffic accidents should probably not hold in countries, such as the United Kingdom, Australia, or South Africa, where drivers drive on the left side of the road. In this case, the reflex of the right-hander is most dangerous (into oncoming traffic) and the left-hander should be somewhat safer (off to the shoulder of the road and out of traffic). This safety for the minority of the population who are left-handers comes at a cost. The cost is increased risk of traffic accidents for the more numerous right-handers. As the right-handers form the majority, this suggests that the overall accident rate should be higher in these "left-handed traffic" countries. To look at this possibility, we obtained statistics published annually by the European Conference of Minsters of Transport.[5] Looking at an eleven-year period, we compared the traffic accident rate of the United Kingdom and Ireland (with left-side driving) to that of the combined statistics of fourteen other European countries who drive on the right side of the road. The data were based on the number of accidents, corrected by the total number of kilometers of highway travelled in that year. We computed these "accidents per kilometer driven" statistics for each year from 1975 to 1986. In every one of the eleven years surveyed, the traffic accident rate was higher in the left-side-driving nations than in the right-side-driving nations, exactly what would be expected if handedness plays a part in road safety. If you bias driving patterns against the reflexes of the right-handed majority, the overall traffic accident rate should go up, as it does in the United Kingdom and Ireland.

Should left-handers still have a higher accident rate in such left-side-driving countries? I would guess that their accident rate would be lower than in right-side driving countries. However, their unexpected (by right-handers) tendency to turn to the left rather than to the right might raise their risk level some, as any form of unexpected or erratic driving might.

More Bad News from California

We have seen that the world is badly set up for the left-hander and that the consequences of this bad design are an increased number of accidents and accident-related injuries. In chapter 12, discussing the shortened life span of left-handers, we concentrated on the medical factors we knew affected the left-hander. Certainly, neurological damage from birth-stress injuries, combined with reduced immune system effectiveness, could be expected to shorten the life span of left-handers, as we found in the baseball-player and the California studies. Could accidents also be a factor in reducing the life span of left-handers?

The research we have just considered has shown that left-handers are 89 percent more likely to have an accident-related injury. It is easy to imagine how that risk might lead to a reduced life span. Certainly, any accident that results in severe injuries might terminate the individual's life immediately. Each accident lays the person's life on the line, and the left-hander is twice as likely to have such accidents.

When accidents result in injuries that are not life threatening, they can still have major consequences. For example, an accident that opens a small, apparently insignificant wound might still expose the individual to infection. In some percentage of cases, such as infection might lead to severe problems and perhaps death. Certainly, the attending physician will not note that a small break in the skin, which resulted from the slip of a knife designed for a right-hander, is the cause of death. Rather the physician would cite the infection contracted later as the problem, or perhaps the secondary effects of such an infection, such as pneumonia or heart failure, as the cause of death.

Even when an accident-related injury does not cause immediate death or death through secondary complications, long-term effects are still possible. Each accidental injury causes damage and requires repair. It is possible that drawing continually upon the body's healing powers may reduce its ability to meet successive new challenges and threats. In addition, the damage associated with each accident-related injury will tend to add up over time. The cumulative effect of many small injuries may eventually add up to a reduction in the person's survival ability by reducing the overall effectiveness of vital organs or systems in the body.

The possibility that accident-related injuries might also be contributing to the reduced life span of left-handers was one of the issues explored in the California study that Diane Halpern and I conducted.[6] When we began the California project, we already knew the results of my other research, indicating that left-handers were more accident prone. It therefore seemed sensible to collect some information on accidental and non-accident-related causes of death. Although we took what information was available on the death records, we knew that accidents are often not reported on death certificates. For this reason, we also asked the next of kin for information about the cause of death and asked whether any accident-related injuries were involved.

Our expectation, of course, was that left-handers were more likely to die of accident-related injuries than were right-handers because they have more accidents than right-handers. Our predictions were confirmed to a degree that startled us. In the California study we found that left-handers were six times more likely to die from causes initiated by accident-related injuries. Though our data were not so finely tuned as to allow us to determine the specific types of activities that caused the accidents, we did single out one group of accidents that seemed to show the largest differences between left- and right-handers. We separated accidents in general from accidents that occurred when the individual was driving a vehicle. Here we found that left-handers were approximately four times more likely to die in accidents while operating a car or truck than was a right-hander.

Considering our original question, namely, "Why do we have so few older left-handers?" this research suggests an answer. Given the fact that the left-hander is six times more likely to die of an accident, the gradual disappearance of left-handers in older groups may be the result of a progressive whittling away at the southpaw population through accident-related deaths. To demonstrate this, at one point I used a procedure called *mathematical modeling*, a way of simulating mathematically what may be expected to happen if a given theory is true. I used mathematical modeling in this instance as a way of estimating what effects the handedness-related difference in accident rate would have on the population of left-handers.[7] All that had to be programmed into the model was that the rate of accidents was 89 percent higher for left-handers (as the data show). This simple assumption led to a decrease in the number of left-handers from 13 percent at age 20 to only 2.5 percent at age 80. This drop in the percentage of left-handers is very similar to the one that we find in real life. The absence of older left-handers could be due to the fact that the right-handed world is, in effect, "devouring" left-handers by arranging the world to make south-paws more accident prone and therefore placing them at higher risk of an early death.

Can anything be done to help the plight of the endangered southpaw? Fortunately there are ways to help, as you will see shortly.

15

Help for the Left-Hander

C an anything be done to make it more likely that the average left-hander will live as long and as happy a life as the average right-hander? Fortunately, the answer is "Yes." Unfortunately, one solution that first springs into many minds—to change the left-hander into a right-hander—is not the correct one.

Many parents and teachers consider left-handedness a problem and feel that training the child to be right-handed makes it disappear. They presume that left-handedness is simply an annoying habit that can be corrected by instruction, cajoling, or punishment. They reason that once the child is performing some common activities, such as writing or eating with the right hand, he or she has been converted to right-handedness. Such parents are simply following the majority opinion. I cannot count the number of times that people have suggested that we should systematically train or, if necessary, force, all left-handers to become right-handers with the idea being that in so doing we would eliminate all of the problems associated with left-handedness.

Forcing right-handed behaviors on everyone is the solution that many industries seem to favor. Recently a former United States Postal Service employee described her experiences working there. She was happily and efficiently sorting mail with her left hand when she was approached by a supervisor. "Excuse me, I'm going to have to get you to case that mail right-handed," the supervisor said. "There's a saying here: 'The post office has no left-handed employees.'"[1]

Pressure from several levels of management was applied to force her to work with her right hand. She tried to accommodate by sorting mail with her right hand but, predictably, she rapidly became fatigued and less accurate. When she returned to her natural left-handed behaviors she was lectured to and chastised. When she complained that it was painful and tiring to work with her right hand she was told that perhaps she needed to exercise her right hand more. When her union eventually came to her support, it was too late, as the Post Office had already terminated her employment. Many other postal employees apparently submit to this pressure, suffering discomfort and reduced efficiency to keep their jobs.

Even if we ignore the ethical issues, such as freedom of choice and freedom of action, changing handedness from left to right is an effort doomed to failure. Left-handedness is not a simple movement preference that has developed into a habit. It probably reflects differences in the pattern of neural circuitry in the brain.

Sadly, even when the effort to change handedness appears to be successful it is only partially so. Those trying to switch a person's handedness tend to focus on one particular skill at a time. Training may improve the ability of the right hand to use a fork or a pen, but this effect will not carry over to other behaviors. Training only creates a mixed-hander or a "modified left-handed." Most importantly, this mixed-hander still has the reflexes of a left-handed, and he or she is just as accident prone as any other left-hander. The modified left-hander will still have the left-turning and counterclockwise-rotation tendencies of most left-handers, will still have the protective reflex in which the right hand goes high and the left goes low, and in times of stress or when rapid action is necessary, will still revert to use of the left hand. In the interactions with the environment that affect safety, this person is still effectively a left-hander.[2]

Forcing use of the right hand will not solve any other problems related to left-handedness. Certainly, to the extent that the brain functions of right-and left-handers differ, forcing a child to eat with the right hand will not change that neural circuitry. It should be equally clear that switching handedness will not repair any malfunctioning of the immune system that may be associated with left-handedness.

The Invisible Left-Hander

The major problem for left-handers seems to be invisibility. The right-handed majority does not worry about "solutions" for the discomfort or risks to which left-handers are subjected. Indeed, most right-handers never bother to think about left-handedness at all. It is a behavior pattern that simply goes unnoticed and its consequences are ignored.

It may be hard to imagine that a set of muscular responses that affects virtually every manipulation of the environment, as well as numerous other body movements, could go unnoticed. Yet it does. Recently I sat down for a cup of coffee with several colleagues, all members of our psychology department faculty. One, the head of the department, had been in that post for about eight years and had been a member of the department for at least twenty years.

I turned to the department head and said, "Richard, I thought that as a left-hander you might interested in something I just learned about southpaws." I was interrupted by one of my colleagues: "Are you really left-handed, Richard? I never noticed that."

"Neither did I," came the voice of a second colleague.

Both of those who expressed surprise at learning that their department head was a left-hander were psychologists who had been with the department for more than 10 years, and both had had extensive interactions with him. Doubtless, over his eight years as head, they had seen him writing, whether signing documents such as grant applications and university forms or taking notes at meetings. Despite seeing him write with his left hand, eat with his left hand, and use a pointer with his left hand, that he was left-handed had not registered in their consciousness.

When I named two other department members who were also left-handed, my colleagues were equally surprised. I asked one of them whether he had noticed that a particular graduate student who had just completed a master's thesis under his supervision was left-handed.

"No way," he emphatically protested. "I would have noticed."

A few days later, he intercepted me in the hallway and apologized for his disbelief. His student was, as I had indicated, definitely left-handed, though he had failed to realize it through three years of close daily association.

Just how commonly left-handedness is overlooked was demonstrated in a study conducted by Clare Porac and me.[3] We tested a group of 159 high school students who ranged in age from fifteen to nineteen. We first determined the handedness of each student using a standard questionnaire. We next asked them about the handedness of their mother and their father. They could answer that each parent was "left-handed" or "right-handed" or admit that they didn't know. Afterwards, we mailed out questionnaires to their parents, asking them to indicate their own handedness directly to us.

The results showed just how invisible left-handers are. Based upon the parent's questionnaires, we determined that 9 percent of the mothers and fathers were left-handed in this particular group. Based upon the reports of their high school aged sons and daughters, however, only 4 percent were left-handed. In other words, 56 percent of the left-handed parents went unnoticed by their young-adult children who had lived with their parents for an average of seventeen years! In every single case in which a parent's handedness was reported wrongly by their child, a left-handed parent was reported to be right-handed. In not one instance was a right-handed parent reported to be left-handed.

Young children tend to watch their parents' every activity with great care. It is through such observation that we learn most of our basic living skills, how to manipulate utensils and perform everyday tasks. Yet, even though these students had watched their parents write with the left hand, use kitchen utensils with the left hand, or wield cleaning implements with the left hand for many years, the fact that a parent was left-handed went unnoticed in more than half the cases. If children are left-handed themselves, they are usually aware of their parents' handedness. However, most right-handed offspring assume that since they and most of the world are right-handed, their parents must be so, too.

If left-handers are invisible to their own children, to their close colleagues, and to their workmates, is it any surprise that they are also invisible to the right-handed people who design our environment and the implements that we use in it? In the university library I looked up fourteen ergonomic and human engineering handbooks, reference works, and texts. (Ergonomists and human engineers are the specialists who design tools and machines to fit the behavior patterns of people.) Only two books mentioned handedness in their indexes. Checking these references, I found that neither contained information on the special needs of the left-hander. Rather, both involved cautionary notes to designers. The first book warned the instrument designer not to overload the right-handed operator by placing all the controls on the right. The possibility of a left-handed operator was not considered, and no thought given to designing the instrument panel for both left- and right-handed use.[4] The second book, in a chapter entitled "People with Disabilities,"[5] asked, "Has a suitable compromise been reached between the requirements of the 90% of people who are right-handed and the 10% who are left-handed?" In the remaining 275 pages of the book, the only mention of handedness was a reminder that 10 percent of the population is left-handed. No specific advice and no suggestions for changing designs to make them more ambidextrous or more usable by the left-hander were given. Furthermore, every diagram of tool or control use depicted a right hand.

Right-handedness is assumed in virtually all ergonomic and design discussions. Several books discuss the importance of proper tool grips, with anatomical drawings and photos of the hand indicating the location of blood vessels and nerves of, of course, only the right hand. They warn that poorly designed hand grips can lead to loss of strength, numbness, and diminished control. The authors then go on to give precise information on the shape of tool handles, citing the importance of indentations for fingers and thumb, with specific suggestions about depth and shape. Of course, all the tool specifications assume right-handed use of the tool, and every illustration shows a right hand using it.

Elaborate charts and tables indicating reaching patterns for male and female operators define the "work-space envelope". Seemingly, only the right hand is expected to reach for things, as only right-handed charts are given.

When safety-switch design is discussed by ergonomists, the engineer is reminded that the most common switching and touching errors involve a movement from right to left, the expected action for a right-hander bringing his arm from the side around to the front and brushing a switch. Thus switches to the right are more likely to be inadvertently triggered. The design recommendation is to place switches that should not be actuated accidentally on the left side of the control panel and to make sure they are activated by a movement from left to right. Of course, these touching errors are errors of the right-handed operator. The left-hander makes touching errors to the left, and inadvertent movements are more likely in the left to right direction. The human engineers are suggesting to make the instrument panel safer for the right-hander with design policy that would make it *more* likely that the left-hander would make errors.[6]

In a similar fashion, one of the ergonomic books that I looked at also discusses the design of an aircraft cockpit control with the similar presumption that every operator is right-handed. This book notes, "Control placement is also dictated by limb assignment and by positioning to achieve maximum efficiency. In general, rapid, precise settings are assigned to the right hand and large, continuous forces to the feet."[7] No mention, consideration or even pity is offered to the poor left-handed aviator. After reading this passage, I found these design recommendations flashing through my mind as boarded a commercial airplane flight.

This immediately made me want to reassure myself that the pilot was right-handed. Of course, I knew that asking the stewardess wouldn't help, because, even if he were left-handed the likelihood that she would notice this is so low. So I suppressed the impulse to make inquiries and contented myself with reading the safety brochure describing emergency evacuation and crash procedures, more closely.

At a recent scientific meeting I asked a human engineering specialist, "When you design instruments and controls, do you make any concessions for the left-handed operator?"

He looked at me and then answered using what I call a "lecture voice". "You have to understand that when we design instruments or tools we are designing them for many users with many different needs. Suppose, for instance, that we are called on to design the cockpit of a plane, or the driver's area of a car. We know that people differ in terms of their size, for instance, so we adopt the principle that we are designing for the 'average' user."

I felt as if either I had missed the point of this "mini-lecture" or the "lecturer" had missed the point of my question, so I pressed him a bit. "Well, it seems to me that that principle doesn't work for handedness. After all, when you average a left-hander and a right-hander what do you get? So what do you do in terms of design and engineering about handedness?"

He looked at me as if I had suddenly lost 50 or 60 IQ points and then said, "If a person is too tall or too short for the cockpit or the car we have engineered, then they simply have to adapt. It may be uncomfortable for them, but they have to make do with the existing equipment. When it comes to handedness the 'average' person is right-handed. Left-handers will have to accommodate the same way that anybody who is very different from the average must. I mean you wouldn't expect us to make every vehicle usable by both giants and dwarfs. When such abnormal people want to use the equipment they simply have to adapt to the design or use some other instrument. The same requirements hold for left-handers, either adapt or don't use the equipment. Besides," he now offered with a little condescending smile, "there really aren't enough left-handers to make much of a difference. If there were a lot of left-handers who were inconvenienced I'm sure that we would have heard about it by now and made appropriate changes."

While about 1 percent of the population suffers from giantism or dwarfism, 13 percent of the population is left-handed. Why hasn't the engineer and designer heard about them and their ongoing inconvenience? Because the left-hander is invisible!

Engineering and Design Solutions for Left-Handers

If left-handers were a visible, recognized minority with specific needs, could any changes be made in the environment and the design of equipment without too much difficulty or expense? Clearly, the answer is "Yes."

Given that 13 percent of the world's population is left-handed, it is probably economically feasible for certain mass-produced items to be specifically designed to make an alternate version available for both left- and right-handers. Candidates for such special designs include kitchen utensils, common drawing instruments, and hand tools. But although this "special equipment" concept may sound attractive to the left-hander, it may not be the optimal solution.

Catering specifically to left-handed needs has been occasionally considered. Already a number of stores and manufacturers appear to have awakened sufficiently to this need to manufacture items specifically designed or marketed for the left-hander. In many major cities, including New York, Chicago, and Los Angeles in the United States, Toronto and Vancouver in Canada, or London in England, one finds shops stocking items for the left-hander, where one can find left-handed cork screws, can openers, scissors, rulers, and spiral notebooks. You can even get a left-handed Swiss Army Knife, with a reversed corkscrew spiral and thumb identations on the left sides of the blades to allow safe opening by left-handers.

This apparent advance is less of a forward movement than one would like. First, the range of items available in such stores is usually quite limited. Major appliances or power tools, properly bevelled knives, a broad range of cooking utensils, and most workshop tools are usually not available. Frequently the merchandise is not of a very high quality and is produced more for its novelty value than for its functional utility. Often the best-selling items in such stores are bumper stickers, coffee mugs, and T-shirts with slogans such as "Lefthanders do it right," "Everyone is lefthanded 'til he commits his first sin," "Lefties are better lovers," "Southpaws—In your heart you know they're right," "Everyone is born righthanded but the greatest overcome it" or simply "Southpaw" printed next to a big animal paw print. Perhaps the most useful items in such stores are instructional booklets, including booklets on needlepoint for the left-hander, left-handed guitar playing, and left-handed calligraphy, in which the diagrams are reversed from the usual right-handed format. This means that the left-hander can actually follow along, matching hand positions and so forth to the printed material, instead of trying to reverse everything mentally to fit instructions to left-handedness.

Most small tools and utensils could be designed for left-handed or ambidextrous use with some thought and ergonomic consideration. However, the engineering and design of some ostensibly left-handed items often does not meet reasonable standards of safety and usability. Some manufacturers produce scissors supposedly for use by both left- and right-handers that turn out merely to be scissors with wider grips and extra sharp edges on both cutting blades. The added sharpness makes them more hazardous because of the added possibility of cuts resulting from slips while one is using them or when one is groping through drawers or sewing bags to find them. Other scissors manufacturers merely leave the blades as they normally are but reverse the handles so that a left-hander can comfortably hold them. This is not a sound design. Normally, scissors devised for right-handed use are biased so that the blades press together during the cutting operation. Using scissors with a right-handed blade bias, even with left-handed handles, forces the blades apart slightly. The result is that the material slips between the blades and the scissors do not cut effectively. Left-handed scissors should include a reversal of the usual bias of the blades to solve this problem. Although some companies produce scissors that meet these requirements, it is often not apparent to the casual observer whether any particular pair is functionally left-handed or only cosmetically so.

A philosophical difficulty is associated with designing items for exclusive left-handed use. If the items are specifically used by one person, such as grooming items, a pocket knife and so on, this strategy makes sense. For example, it would be sensible for parents who know that their child is left-handed to provide him with a pair of left-handed scissors, a left-handed ruler and left-handed notebooks with the spiral on the other side. These are personal items which tend to be used by only one child, rather than shared. For items which may involve community use problems arise. If a left-handed mother outfits her kitchen specifically for herself, what happens to the safety of her right-handed husband and children? One might suggest, of course, that there might be two versions of each tool, one for the left-hander and one for the right-hander. This is both and expensive and an unworkable solution. The expense aspect is obvious, as the cost of every item is now doubled. The unworkable nature of this solution comes from the fact that in many instances careful inspection of the tool or utensil would be needed to determine whether it is left- or right-handed. People would continually be picking up the wrong implement or having to pause in the middle of a task to inspect the bevelling of a knife or the gearing of a can opener. The optimal solution seems to be to strive for instruments that can be used by both hands equally well or be quickly modified to accommodate the handedness of the user.

Some items are easily engineered so as to be ambidextrous. It does not take much effort to notch two pouring lips into a soup ladle or a saucepan, one on either side. It adds little to the cost of a cake knife or a grapefruit sectioning knife to put serrations on both sides of the blade. It does not involve any engineering difficulties, nor add much additional cost to the price of silverware to cast salad or pastry forks so that the outside tine on both sides is thicker to allow either hand to be used to cut a leaf of lettuce or a pie crust. Outside of the kitchen, the common coin-operated coffee machine, with its door that swings open to the left to inconvenience the left-hander is easily modified by making the door lift upwards, giving access regardless of handedness. What is required is, first of all, a sensitivity to the existence of left-handers as a substantial minority whose needs ought to be taken into account and, second, a willingness to alter designs of instruments to meet the needs of both left- and right-handers.

In the workplace similar design considerations can be employed. For example, there is no reason why all tool grips must be designed for the right hand only. It is easy to design grips with finger grooves that can be used by either hand. It is true that the grooves from the right-hand indentations will cross those for the left hand and perhaps not look as aesthetic and sleek. Yet, such a simple design change should render the tool usable by either hand. This design alteration might also assist the right-hander in those rare situations where it becomes necessary to hold the tool in a nondominant left hand, as in situations where the space is limited and access from the right side is difficult.

When it comes to larger equipment and more complex instruments, more thought must be exerted. First, the ergonomists and human engineers must be made aware that left-handers have some different design requirements. The goal, of course, is to make the technology and the environment safer and more comfortable for the left-hander. At the same time, we should not be overly zealous in recommending design changes that might push the pendulum too far to the other side. We certainly don't want to advocate making all machinery safer for the left-handed minority at the expense of increasing the jeopardy and risk of the right-hander majority. That sort of a change would increase the overall rate of accidents and discomfort. What we should strive to do is to increase the safety of the left-hander while not reducing the safety of the right-hander.

In many instances, just taking the left-handers' existence into account can lead to some fairly simple solutions to increase their safety and comfort but not alter the right-handers' risk level or ease of use. Some of these solutions cost little or nothing to bring about. For instance, if you look around a typical machine shop you will find that most of the power tools and large equipment are pushed against the outer walls so that the center of the working area is as open as possible. Unfortunately, when such tools are place against the wall they are often placed in an orientation where the machine is open on the right side and partially blocked on the left side. The virtue in such an arrangement is that it gives the right arm of the normally left-handed operator the most freedom. The negative aspect of this arrangement is that it tends to block free movement of the left arm and thus increases the difficulty that the left-hander will have in using the tool. Simply moving machines out a foot or so from a wall or corner, or orienting them so that one side is not blocked will often increase the safety of the left-hander without affecting the right-hander at all.

In some production lines the problem of handedness is simply solved either by having the left-handed individual sit on the other side of the line or by having the person work facing the direction opposite that faced by the other workers. For example, in the case of the postal employee who was pressured to use her right hand for all sorting activities,[1] her supervisors argued that the mail-sorting cases were set up for right-handers. With the slots to the front and the right, the supervisor felt that it was inefficient for the left-handed employee to have to cross over her body with her arm. One possible resolution offered by the employee was quite simple. She could turn her body 90 degrees clockwise, so that the slots would be in front and to her left. This former postal worker reports, "This logic did not impress my supervisor. Apparently they wanted all their soldiers moving in the same direction, regardless." It might not look as neat and orderly to have every tenth employee facing in a different direction or seated on the opposite side of the work line; however, it would be more efficient and in some cases safer to employ this easy solution. It would certainly improve the working conditions of the left-hander.

For smaller power tools, such as hand drills and certain saws, some simple design changes might be useful. For example, the safety or run switch, engineered to be triggered by the right thumb when the machine is held in the right hand, can be placed on both sides of the pistol grip to be activated by either thumb. If two switches seem too costly, one safety switch could be placed below the trigger to be activated by the middle finger of either hand or placed at the back of the pistol grip, much like the safety on a standard .45 caliber automatic pistol, to be activated by the palm when the hand squeezes down on the handle.

For some tools, an added grip or lever might be all that is needed to assist the southpaw. The drill press pictured in figure 13.9 could be made safer and more comfortable for the left-hander by simply adding a second handle on the left so that either hand could lower the rotating drill bit.

Other modifications to major machines should not be very complicated, although some may increase the cost of a tool slightly. The band saw shown in figure 13.10 requires only a modification of the blade to be made safer for the left-hander. If the blade had teeth on both sides, then the left-hander could simply walk around to the other side of the machine to cut material. He would then have the opportunity to hold the work to be cut in his dominant left hand, as can be seen in figure 15.1. In effect, this change means that the saw is set up for right-handers when approached from one side and for left-handers when approached from the other.

Many tools and machines could be made safer by centering the controls in front of the body to be easily reached by either hand. On the obviously left-handed video cameras discussed in chapter 13, the eyepiece of the viewer could be placed in the center rather than off to the left.

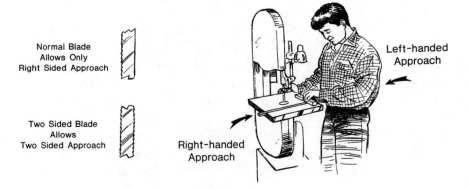

FIGURE 15.1: Left-handed operators of a band saw with teeth in both side of the blade can approach from the opposite side effectively making the saw "left-handed" without affecting the right-handers usual use of the tool in any way.

In some instances, it is probably worth the additional cost to duplicate the controls and safety switches to be accessible to either the left or the right hand. On some cranes and heavy earth-moving equipment, duplication has already been tried and seems to work out well.

For many machines it should be possible to convert the operation to either left- or right-handed use by providing means to temporarily adapt the apparatus to fit the handedness of the operator. Often all that is necessary is a removable set of handles that can be switched around and screwed into place. Sometimes it means that a swing arm is removed and reattached to the other side. This solution has been used in some convertible dental stations. Often the needed changes take only a minute or so to effect, and they can be made at the beginning of each shift to make the machine more useful to the left- or right-handed operator.

In some realms, of course, major redesign will be needed. It is here that the ergonomists and human engineers should begin to exercise their special skills to make the environment equally safe for both varieties of handedness. For instance design and engineering textbooks should acknowledge the different needs of left- and right-handers and try to recommend how both might be accommodated.

A first step in the process of redesign of apparatus and the environment for the use of both hands should involve gathering information about the places and situations in which left-handers have the most accidents when using tools and machines. Suppose that the accident-reporting forms used by most governments, unions, worker's compensation boards, and insurance companies included information on the handedness of the individual who had the accident as well as a description of the tool, machine, or activity involved. In a few years we would have a picture of the left-handers' "accident hot spots." Designers and engineers could isolate these and begin to apply individual redesign and modification to correct the problems involving specifically dangerous machines and situations.

Non-engineered Solutions for Left-Handers

The technological aspects of the construction and layout of our machines and environment can be addressed by changes in design. In some instances, however, other, more behavioral, solutions are needed.

One place where we can't immediately find a technological solution has to do with the higher traffic accident rate of left-handers. We know that the right-hand-driving rule of the road is biased in favor of the right-hander; about the only place where left-handers seem to have an advantage is in paying tolls at a tollbooth. It is certainly not a solution to shift driving to the left side of the road. Left-side-driving means a higher overall accident rate because it increases the risks for the right-handed majority.

If we can't change the traffic environment, is there something that we can do to change the left-hander's risk, given current driving practices? Remember that the left-hander's problem lies in the reflexes. In some instances, reflex tendencies can be overcome by specific training. Where snow and ice are a problem in winter, driving instructors explain the procedures for safe driving on ice-slicked streets. One specific instruction given to novice drivers has to do with skidding. When a car goes into a skid, the natural and most common reflex is to turn the steering wheel so that the wheels are pointing in the direction opposite the direction that the car is skidding. Unfortunately, this action actually reduces the driver's control. Driving instructors therefore drill students so that when a skid occurs they know that they should turn the car in the direction of the skid. This information now "sits on top" of the usual reflex. If you watch a driver who has been so trained encounter a skid, the original instinct is still to steer away from the skid and the steering wheel momentarily flicks in that direction. Once the correct information is remembered, however, the driver quickly adjusts to the situation by turning into the skid.

The same type of procedure could be used to instruct left-handers if they were visible to driving instructors. The instructor who recognized that he or she was dealing with a left-hander would add additional defensive driving instruction to their usual training. The left-hander would be instructed to steer to the right whenever a traffic situation develops. This *Turn Right on Trouble Rule* would be applied to every traffic situation, making the left-hander more likely to swerve out of the way of oncoming traffic and more likely to respond in the way that the other (mostly right-handed) drivers on the road expect. Of course, the right-hand-high, left-hand-low defensive reflex would still be there, but it would cause only a brief twitch on the steering wheel, which would be quickly compensated for by the learned defensive turning response. The untrained left-hander does not know that he has a left-side-turning tendency and hence does not know that he needs to correct it. The trained left-handed driver can compensate. The major requirement is that left-handers be visible to driving instructors, who must know that left-handers have different requirements.

The invisibility of the left-hander also damages his or her ability to get a decent education. How many primary school teachers know how to teach a child how to write with the left hand? I once asked several professors of primary education at my university how they trained elementary school teachers to teach printing and handwriting to left-handers. Their responses provided more proof that the needs of the left-hander are not visible. Not one of the three that I spoke with indicated that they provided any special instruction on how to teach the left-hander to write. One said that she did caution her students to watch the handedness of the children:

"I tell my student teachers that if a child picks up a pencil in the left hand they might suggest that the child try to use the other hand instead. I point out to them that they may have to repeat the suggestion several times, and sometimes reinforce it by physically moving the pencil to the right hand and showing the child the correct hand grip. I also tell them that if the child persists in using the left hand they should not force the child to write right-handed."

"Yes, but do you specifically show teachers how to change the sequence of strokes so that the left-hander can write more comfortably if you have a persistent left-hander who will not switch to right-handedness?" I asked.

"As I just said, if the child stubbornly continues to use their left-hand for writing we certainly allow them to do so. The child is given the same instruction that all of the other children are given, with the only difference being that they are holding their pencil in their left-hand."

In other words, the standard sequence of instruction taught to primary school teachers is first to try to change left-handedness to right-handedness for the purpose of writing and then, if that fails, to ignore the fact that the child is left-handed. Conscientious teachers will probably give individual attention to each child to correct problems in pencil grip and the pattern of strokes used to make individual letters, but no special instruction will be given to the left-hander. The teacher might stop to try to demonstrate proper writing movements. However, it is likely that he or she will demonstrate only the basic right-handed set of hand movements, emphasizing clockwise movements on the upward segment of the motion and counterclockwise on the lower stroke, while the left-hander needs to be taught a different set of movements emphasizing the opposite pen strokes. Most teachers, even if well-intentioned, give left-handed children inappropriate writing instruction or benignly ignore them. One left-hander complained to me that in grade school, "Right-handed kids are taught to write while we left-handers are supposed to teach ourselves."

Here again the problem is invisibility. It should not be difficult for teachers to learn how to instruct left-handed children to write properly. Teachers are given instruction on how to deal with many special-needs children and left-handers are a very large group with special needs of their own. In an average class of thirty children, the teacher will have three to five left-handers, who should be entitled to the same instructional opportunity as the other members of the class.

One realm in which it is difficult to assist the left-hander is medicine. Although we can not repair the neurological damage that may have caused left-handedness, certain things might medically assist the left-handers if they were visible. For example, if left-handers' special physiological conditions were better known to medical doctors, certain treatment programs might be expedited or tried more quickly. In some instances, left-handedness might serve as a marker to indicate some problems that might be more likely to occur in left-handers.

For example, when a patient show up with what doctors call "diffuse nonspecific complaints" such as headache, fatigue, depression, and nonspecific muscle aches, practitioners often have difficulty knowing where to begin their diagnostic search. If the patient is left-handed, this might suggest some possibilities to check out early in the examination. The physician should be alerted to the possibility of allergies, as left-handers suffer from these more commonly. Also, certain autoimmune conditions should immediately be considered. The possibility of thyroid and thymus problems might also be considered. Thus, left-handedness may provide a clue as to a starting place for the search for the individual's present medical problem.

If left-handers were more visible, then physicians might also be aware of the fact that left-handers have reduced immune system efficiency. This means that left-handers may be more susceptible to infections.[8] During the course of treatment such knowledge might also be useful. It might suggest that when prescribing antibiotics to left-handers, the dosage level should be a bit higher, or the course of treatment should be a bit longer, on the assumption that the immune response system of the left-hander will be less capable of defending itself.

As in the cases of technological solutions to the left-hander's problems, more information is needed. Death records and hospital records could routinely list handedness information. In this way it could be learned which diseases and which types of infection the left-hander is most susceptible to. Such information could be used by medical practitioners to gather the data that would allow them to better serve their left-handed patients. Of course, such information will only be collected if left-handers are visible to the people who keep such records.

16

An Action Plan
for Left-Handers

It should be clear, by now, that our man-made technological and physical environment is unsafe for left-handers. It also should be clear that there are many ways in which left-handers differ physically and psychologically from right-handers. Unfortunately, simple knowledge is not enough to improve the lot of left-hander. As the English biologist Thomas Henry Huxley pointed out, "The great end of life is not knowledge but action".

If left-handers want to better the quality of their lives, to make their world more comfortable and safer, they must take certain actions. These actions must be oriented toward changing the attitudes of society toward left-handers.

The first step toward solving many of the left-hander's problems and discomforts is for society to become aware that they exist. Left-handers are a very large minority. The largest single racial minority in the United States, blacks, comprise only 12 percent of the American population. The left-handed minority comprises 13 percent. Combining the United States and Canada, more than 33 million North Americans are left handed.

In the United States, struggles to make the lives of minorities, particularly visible minorities such as Afro-Americans, more comfortable have resulted in decisions that have the force of law behind them. One cannot, discriminate against an individual because he or she is of a particular race, age, or sex. One can not restrict the educational opportunities of minorities. Strong social sanctions prevent people from making slurs against racial minorities and discourage the use of language that makes minorities uncomfortable or demeans them. There still is some controversy about the degree to which society should assist minorities in their attempts to live safe and healthy lives. Yet, it is certainly true that if there was evidence of systematic lack of attention to a minority group's safety, or if segments of society were acting in a manner which threatened the health of some minority, attempts would be made to stop the relevant practices. Most North Americans are uncomfortable about overt discrimination, and such a situation would not be tolerated. Numerous and vocal forces can be rallied in support of almost any persecuted minority, even to the point of forcing protective legislation.

Yet for our largest minority, this group of 33 million left-handers, there is no formal protection. Left-handers are the butt of humiliating jokes and biased language. They can be subtly denied employment by making it impossible for them to perform in workplaces specifically designed for right-handers. I wonder, for instance, how many left-handers fail in courses designed to lead to a pilot's license, or a license to drive heavy equipment, because their performance appears imprecise, although the problem lies in the right-handed design of the equipment. Even after left-handers are hired in many industries, their very lives can be put in jeopardy by environmental and technological design that make the workplace unsafe for them.

When women protested that many jobs were being denied them because of physical requirements incompatible with their body build or equipment ill-suited for the female hand size and capabilities, feminist organizations and women's groups backed them. Human rights commissions supported their claims, and legislative and economic pressure was brought to bear. Various industries then modified their equipment and job requirements so that women could operate in their work environments. Now ergonomic textbooks commonly include cautions such as "Separate tools with different size grips are needed for large people (most men and large women) versus small people (most women and small men)."[1]

What happens when left-handers complain about similar problems, such as tools that do not conform to their body's normal use patterns and restrict their ability to perform adequately? Are they offered a customized set of tools, as women were? Are their job requirements changed to accommodate their needs and abilities? Certainly not. Instead, they are laughed at. They are told to become right-handed. They are told to adapt to the situation or to get out. Such a response to a woman or a member of an ethnic minority group would be grounds for legal action.

When it comes to education, the left-handed minority is again discriminated against. Teachers are trained to deal with the handicapped student, to communicate with the student for whom English is not the first language, to integrate the retarded child into the classroom, to enrich the experience of the culturally deprived child, and to accept the cultural and religious differences of various special groups of children in their care. For left-handers, however, there is no additional educational attention. They are told to adjust their behavior to match that of the right-handed majority, and when they fail they are ignored and left to struggle along on their own. They are given lower grades because their handwriting is messy when they have not been give the individualized instruction that would allow them to learn to write correctly and neatly. In arts and crafts they get lower grades because they are forced to use rulers, scissors, and other tools designed for the right-hander. Such a history of lower grades and lack of support and understanding in the early years in the educational system is very likely to have serious psychological effects on the left-hander. His or her attitude toward education is apt to sour, and the likelihood that he or she will have the motivation or ability to continue on to university is lowered. Nonetheless, left-handers have no protection and no legal recourse. Why?

The issue is visibility. Ethnic minorities have an advantage over left-handers in that their minority status is readily visible. Left-handers are not easily labelled unless one asks about their handedness or monitors their behaviors carefully.

Left-handers also seem to want to remain invisible. On call-in talk shows, a very common complaint that I hear from left-handers is that I shouldn't be talking about them as somehow different. Left-handers object to my references to their higher accident rate or their immunity problems because of the possible negative impact of this information on their lives. They envision higher personal insurance rates, or they worry that they will not be hired for particular jobs because the fact that they are more accident prone might cause the employer's insurance rates to go up. Most fundamentally, they are understandably concerned about being singled out as "odd" or "tainted" in some way.

During the early stages of the union, civil rights and feminist movements in the United States, similar fears were expressed by union supporters, blacks, and feminists. One should not "make noise" because the nonunion, white, or male forces would somehow make things worse. Each of these groups learned, however, that it was through publicizing their cause rather than by hiding and remaining quiet that they became visible. Society as a whole can ignore invisible groups, but once a group is seen and acknowledged it becomes a force of its own, a force that must be dealt with. The invisible left-hander has to become visible.

The evidence that left-handers suffer from more accidents has been amply documented in this book. Nonetheless, the attempts of my research group to get Departments or Ministries of Labor and Health to assist us in gathering data about impact of handedness in the workplace has met with little cooperation. Often, a right-handed administrator will simply laugh at our proposals. One looked at me in disbelief and said, "Let's be serious now, what are you really interested in? Left-handedness is not a problem. If it were a problem then we would have currently have a policy dealing with it. Even if it is a problem, it must be minor. A few people out of a hundred just don't make enough of a difference to affect anything or to require policy decisions to be made. Look, I'm told that 8 percent of the population thinks that Elvis Presley is still alive. Do we have to change our policies to take them into account too?"

Left-handers have never really made an effort to become visible. They have a few organizations, such as *Lefthanders International*, but for the most part these groups are not activist or political. Left-hander groups tend to be associations of people who band together in an attempt to glorify or celebrate their left-hander identity and their differences from the majority. Celebration is fine if you are an accepted and visible minority. For example, in the United States and Canada there are many Scottish groups of various sorts. They promote Scottish dancing and Scottish games. They play the bagpipes, celebrate Robert Burns day, organize Scotch whisky tasting parties, and have a good time. They often sponsor or publish newsletters and magazines filled with articles about what it is like to be Scottish, how people respond to you when they learn that you are Scottish, the origin of the various clans, stories of famous and successful Scottish-Americans, advertisements for Scottish regalia and trinkets, and so forth. They even pick a Scottish-American Man of the Year. They never engage in politics because they do not need to. Nobody discriminates against someone simply because he is Scottish.

To date most organizations of left-handers have behaved similarly, as though handedness were not a problem but rather a simple difference to be revelled in, like being Scottish. Their newsletters and magazines describe what it is like to left-handed, the history of left-handedness, how people become left-handed, and stories about famous left-handers and also pick a Left-Hander of the Year. Oh yes, and they also include a section that advertises a few useful household items and lots of left-hander regalia and trinkets, such as coffee mugs that read "Lefty on the move." Their failing is that they never engage in the politics or political activism needed to make left-handers visible.

Left-handers need a group, or perhaps several groups, devoted to the advocacy of the rights of left-handers, rights that are being limited by a right-handed society. What is needed is an activist group that will serve as the spokesman for left-handers. It has to be vocal. It has the fight *handism* in a very noisy and radical manner if left-handers are ever to become visible. It has to lobby people in power and get them to help collect the information that is needed if left-handers are to be kept alive, healthy, and comfortable. It must approach the newspapers, magazines, television, and radio stations. To make left-handers visible, the group may even have to be outrageous at times, simply to catch the attention of the society at large.

A left-hander advocacy group should be willing to use legal options when necessary. The same laws that protect individuals from the effects of discrimination on the basis of religious, racial, or national background, as well sex, physical disability, or sexual orientation, could probably be extended to help insure the rights and privileges of left-handers.

In the case of accidents, left-handers should bring forward more legal actions. There are a number of relevant legal precedents bearing on design flaws. For example, in the case of Campo vs. Scofield (1950) the court dealt with a plaintiff who was injured by a hazardous part of a machine. In their ruling the court established the principle that a "concealed danger" or a "latent defect" is grounds for establishing liability. In the preceding chapters I noted many examples of machinery and other apparatus with a fairly subtle and concealed right-handed bias that would not be obvious to the average user, especially in the absence of safeguards and warnings. Left-handers should cite such legal precedents. They will not win every case, but they will win some and will establish new precedents; they will also enhance the credibility of left-handers' rights and needs. Even those cases that are lost or settled out of court will be important. The publicity and the awareness of potential legal liability will begin to sensitize designers and engineers to the needs of the left-hander. Visibility will insure that the left-hander's concerns will be taken into account.

If left-handers fail to stand up for themselves, we have seen that they will continue to be ignored by the right-handed majority, including the teachers, engineers, designers, and others that should serve them. They will continue to suffer risk and discomfort and to live nine fewer years than right-handers. Edmund Burke's warning that "Dangers by being despised grow great"[12] applies here.

There are 30 million left-handers in the United States alone. They represent a sizable voting bloc with considerable economic clout. They deserve some recognition and a better quality of life. The key is visibility.

There once was a gentle spokesman for the left-hander. He was Benjamin Franklin, the early American statesman, scientist, philosopher, inventor, author, and left-hander. He was moved to write a note to society about his concerns:

A Petition to Those Who Have the Superintendency of Education
I address myself to all the friends of youth, and conjure them to direct their compassionate regard to my unhappy fate, in order to remove the prejudices of which I am the victim. There are twin sisters of us; and the eyes of man do not more resemble, nor are capable of being on better terms with each other than my sister and myself, were it not for the partiality of our parents, who made the most injurious distinction between us.

From my infancy I have been led to consider my sister as a being of more educated rank. I was suffered to grow up without the least instruction, while nothing was spared in her education. She had masters to teach her writing, drawing, music and other accomplishments, but if by chance I touched a pencil, a pen, or a needle I was bitterly rebuked; and more than once I have been beaten for being awkward, and wanting a graceful manner. It is true that my sister associated with me upon some occasions; but she always made a point of taking the lead, calling upon me only from necessity, or to figure by her side.

But conceive not, sirs, that my complaints are instigated merely by vanity. No; my uneasiness is occasioned by an object much more serious. It is the practice of our family, that the whole business of providing for its subsistence falls upon my sister and myself. If any indisposition should attach my sister—and I mention it in confidence, upon this occasion, that she is subject to the gout, the rheumatism, and cramp, without making mention of other accidents— what would be the fate of our poor family? Must not the regret of our parents be excessive, at having placed so great a difference between sisters who are so perfectly equal? Alas! we must perish from distress; for it would not be in my power to even scrawl a suppliant petition for relief, having been obliged to employ the hand of another in transcribing the request which I have now the honor to prefer to you.

Condescend, sir, to make my parents sensible of the injustice of an exclusive tenderness, and of the necessity of distributing their care and affection among their children equally.

I am, with profound respect Sirs,

Your obedient servant
THE LEFT HAND[3]

Right-handers and left-handers can coexist in the same environment, but their mutual rights to dignity, opportunity, and safety must be respected. Both have needs, which can be jointly met if we set our minds to it. As the late president John Fitzgerald Kennedy said in 1963, "If we cannot now end our differences, at least we can help make the world safe for diversity."[4]

Notes

Chapter 1   Beliefs and Stereotypes About Handedness

1. *Oxford English dictionary* (2nd ed.). Oxford: Clarendon Press, 1989.
2. Joness, EE, Farina A, Hastorf AH, Markus H, Miller DT & Scott RA. *Social stigma: The psychology of marked relationships.* New York: Freeman, 1984.
3. Sherif M, Harvey LJ, White BJ, Hood WR & Sherif CW. *The Robbers Cave experiment: Intergroup conflict and cooperation.* Middletown, CT: Wesleyan University Press, 1988.
4. Byrne D, Clore GL & Smeaton G. *J Pers Soc Psychol.* 1986;51:1167–1170; Hill JP, Rubin Z & Peplau LA. *J Soc Issues.* 1976;32:147–168.
5. Rosenbaum ME. *J Pers Soc Psychol.* 1986;51:1156–1166.
6. Zajonc RB. *J Pers Soc Psychol Monogr Supl.* 1968;9:1–27.
7. Mita TH, Dermer M & Knight J. *J Pers Soc Psychol.* 1977;35:597–601.
8. Domhoff GW. *Psychoanalytic Rev.* 1969;56:586–596.
9. Cholmeley RJ. *The Idylls of Theocritus.* 1919 (3rd Idyllium).
10. Stoddart A. *Treatise on moles.* New York: A. Stoddart, 1805.
11. Brand J. *Popular Antiquities* (vol. 3). London: Charles Knight, 1842.
12. Hertz R. *Rev Philos de la France et de l'etranger.* 1909;68:553–580.
13. Westermarck EA. *Ritual and belief in Morocco.* London: Macmillan, 1926.
14. Burdel C. *Tarot classic cards.* Muller & Cie: Switzerland, 1751.
15. Boguet H. *Discours des Sorciers.* 1608.
16. Murray MA. *The Witch-cult in Western Europe.* Oxford, 1921.
17. Leviticus 21:17–21.
18. Jewish Publication Society. *The holy scriptures: According to the Masoretic*

text. Philadelphia: Jewish Publication Soc Amer, 1955. Preuss J. *Biblical and Talmudic medicine*, trans. F. Rosner. New York: Sanhedrin Press, 1978.

19. Scholem G. *Major trends in Jewish mysticism*. London, 1955.
20. Leviticus, VIII: 23, 24.
21. Psalms 118:15–16.
22. Jonah IV:11.
23. Matthew XXV:31–46.
24. Hécan H & de Ajuriaguerra J. *Left-handedness: Manual superiority and cerebral dominance*. New York: Gruen & Stratton, 1964.
25. Hughes TP. *Dictionary of Islam*. New York: Scribner, Welford, 1885.

Chapter 2   The Lopsided Animal

1. Darwin C. *The descent of man and selection in relation to sex* (2d ed.). London: John Murray, 1874, p. 193.
2. Lovejoy OC. *Science*. 1981;221:341–350; Miyamoto M, Slighton JL & Goodman. *Science*. 1987;238:369–373.
3. Gould SJ. *Hen's teeth and horse's toes*. Harmonsworth, England: Penguin Books, p. 240.
4. Gardner RA & Gardner BT. *Ann NY Acad Sci*. 1978;309:37–76.
5. Premack D. *Amer Scientist*. 1976;64:674–683.
6. Goodall J. In Lehrman DS, Hinde RA & Shaw E (eds.). *Advances in the study of behavior* (vol. 3). New York: Academic Press, pp. 195–249.
7. Griffin DR. *Behav Brain Res*. 1983;10:399–403.
8. See Annett M. *Left, Right, hand and brain: The right shift theory*. London: Erlbaum, 1985, for a review.
9. MacNeilage PF, Studdert-Kennedy MG & Lindblom B. *Behav Brain Sci*. 1987;10:247–303, includes a source article and 25 commentaries.
10. Porac C, Rees L & Buller T. In Coren S (ed.). *Left-handedness: Behavioral implications and anomalies*. Amsterdam: North-Holland, Elsevier, 1990.
11. Yakovlev PI. In *Proceedings of the 18th Annual convention of the Society of Biological Psychiatry*, June, 1973.
12. Porac & Coren S. *Lateral preferences and human behavior*. New York: Springer-Verlag, 1981.
13. Porac C & Coren S. *Psychol Bulletin*. 1976;83:880–897.
14. Coren S. *Developmental Psychol*. 1974;10:304.
15. Coren S & Porac C. *Bull Psychonomic Soc*. 1977;9:269–271.
16. Coren S & Porac C. *Am J Optom Physiol Optics*. 1982;59:987–990.
17. Porac C & Coren S. *Canad J Psychol*. 1984;38:610–624.
18. Porac C & Coren S. *Vision Research*. 1986;26:1709–1713.
19. Balfour, E. *The cyclopedia of India*. London, 1885.
20. De Lee JB. *The principles and practice of obstetrics*. Philadelphia: WB Saunders, 1913, p. 13.

Chapter 3   Measuring Sidedness

1. Crovitz HF & Zener K. *Am J Psychol.* 1962;75:271–276.
2. Satz P, Achenback K & Fennel E. *Neuropsychologia.* 1967;5:295–310.
3. Raczkowski D, Kalat JW & Nebes R. *Neuropsychologia.* 1974;12:43–47.
4. Coren S & Porac C. *Brit J Psychol.* 1978;69:207–211.
5. Peters M. In Coren S (ed.). *Left-handedness: Behavioral implications and anomalies.* Amsterdam: North-Holland, Elsevier, 1990.
6. For example, Steenhuis RE & Bryden MP. *Cortex.* 1989;25:289–304.
7. Results that are generally similar have also been reported by Healey JM, Liederman J & Geschwind N. *Cortex.* 1986;22:33–53, although these researchers think that specific muscle and movement patterns may be important as well.
8. Provins KA & Cunliffe P. *Percept & Motor Skills.* 1972;35:143–150.
9. Porac C & Coren S. *Lateral preferences and human behavior.* New York: Springer-Verlag, 1981.
10. Kimura D & Vanderwolf CH. *Brain.* 1970;93:769–774: Parlow S. *Cortex.* 1978;14:608–611.
11. Coren S, Porac C & Duncan P. *J Clin Neuropsychol.* 1979;1:55–64.
12. deKay JT. *Left-handed kids.* New York: M Evans, 1989.
13. Reichler JL. *The baseball encyclopedia.* New York: Macmillam, 1979.

Chapter 4   Does Society Make Right-Handers?

1. Porac C & Coren S. *Lateral preferences and human behavior.* New York: Springer-Verlag, 1981.
2. Ellis SJ, Ellis PJ & Marshall E. *Cortex.* 1988;24:157–163; Lansky LM, Feinstein H & Peterson J. *Neuropsychologia.* 1988;26:465–477; Tambs K, Magnus P & Berg K. *Percept & Motor Skills.* 1987;64:155–170; Tan LE. *Percept & Motor Skills.* 1983;56:867–874.
3. Godfrey J. *A treatise upon the useful science of defence, connecting the small and back-sword, and shewing the affinity between them.* London: T Gardner, 1747 (cited in 6).
4. Hall GS & Hartwell EM. *Mind.* 1884;9:93–109.
5. Burt C. *The backward child.* New York: Appleton-Century, 1937.
6. An excellent, more technical treatment of this material can be found in the chapter by Lauren J. Harris in Coren S (ed.). *Left-handedness: Behavioral implications and anomalies.* Amsterdam: North-Holland, Elsevier, 1990.
7. Plato. Laws 7. 795.
8. Watson JB. *Behaviorism.* New York: Peoples Institute Publishing Co., 1924, p. 101, emphasis is as in the original text.
9. Clement F. *The petie schole with an English orthographie.* Facimilie of the 1587 edition with an introduction by RD Pepper. Gainesville, Florida: Scholars' Facsimiles & Reprints, 1966, p. 55 (cited in 6).

10. Quoted in Parson BS. *Left-handedness: A new interpretation.* New York: Macmillan, 1924, p. 102.

11. Selzer CA. *Lateral dominance and visual fusion.* Harvard Monographs in Education, No. 12: Studies in educational psychology and educational measurement. Cambridge, Mass. Harvard Univ Press, 1933.

12. Hildreth G. *J Genetic Psychol.* 1950;76:101–144. Quotes from p. 104.

13. Hertz R. *Rev Philos de la France et de l'etranger.* 1909;68:553–580.

14. Shaw J. *Lancet.* 1902;2:1486 (cited in 6).

15. Blau A. *The master hand.* New York: American Orthopsychiatric Assoc., 1946.

16. Ibid., p. 91.

17. Lindsay B. *Northumberland & Durham Med J.* 1904;12:129–136.

18. The dates that I give for Reade's letters are for publication in *Harper's Weekly.*

19. Jackson J. *Ambidexterity.* London: Kegan Paul, 1905.

20. Crighton-Browne J. *Proceedings of the Royal Institution of Great Britain.* 1907;18:623–652 (cited in 6).

21. Baldwin JM. *Science.* 1890;16:247–248 and *Popular Science Monthly.* 1894;44:606–615.

22. Woolley HT, *Psych Rev.* 1910;17:37–41.

23. Clark MM. *Left Handedness: Laterality characteristics and their education implications.* London: Univ London Press, 1957.

24. Broun H. *Collier's Magazine.* 1920;65:22–62 (cited in 6).

25. Laponce JA. *Left and right: The topography of political perceptions.* Toronto: Univ Toronto Press, 1981.

26. Hardyck C, Goldman R & Petrinovich L. *Hum Biol.* 1975;47:369.

27. Porac C, Coren S & Searleman A. *Behav Genet.* 1986;16:251–261.

28. Porac C, Rees L & Buller T. In Coren S (ed.). *Left-handedness: Behavioral implications and anomalies.* Amsterdam: North-Holland, Elsevier, 1990. This publication reports two separate studies; however, only the first one, which used normal adults and a technique similar to that used in the previous study are analyzed here, and we select only the left-to-right shifts.

29. Teng EL, Lee P-H & Chang PC. *Science.* 1976;193:1148–1150; Teng El, Lee P-H, Yang K-S & Chang PC. *Neuropsychologia.* 1979;17:41–48.

30. Annett M. *Brit J Psychol.* 1970;61:303–321.

Chapter 5   Is Handedness Inherited?

1. *Journal of the Royal College of General Practitioners.* 1974;24:437–439.

2. Bryden P. *Laterality: Functional asymmetry in the intact brain.* New York: Academic Press, 1982.

3. Coren S & Porac C. *Science.* 1977;198:631–632.

4. Semenov SA. *Prehistoric technology.* London: Cory, McAdams & MacKay, 1964.

5. Keeley LH. *Scientific American.* 1977 (November);237:108–127 (p. 126).
6. Toth N. *J Human Evolution.* 1985;14:607–614.
7. Porac C & Coren S. *Neuropsychologia.* 1979;17:543–548.
8. Coren S & Porac C. *Behavior Genetics.* 1980;10:333–348.
9. Rameley F. *American Naturalist.* 1913;47:730–738; Chamberlain HD. *J Heredity.* 1928;19:557–559; Rife DC. *Genetics.* 1940;25:178–186; Merrell DJ. *Human Biology.* 1957;29:314–328; Falek A. *Am J Human Genetics.* 1959;11:52–62; Annett M. *Ann Human Genetics,* 1973;37:93–105; Bryden MP. 1979, reported in Bryden MP. 1982, op. cit.; Porac C & Coren S. 1979, op. cit.; Coren S & Porac C. 1980, op. cit.; Carter-Saltzman L. *Science.* 1980;209:163–165; McGee MG & Cozad T. *Behavior Genetics.* 1980;10:263–276.
10. Corballis MC. *Human laterality.* New York: Academic Press, 1983.
11. Carter-Saltzmann L, Scarr-Salapatek S, Barker WB & Katz S. *Behavior Genetics.* 1976;6:189–203; Loehlin JC & Nichols RC. *Heredity environment and personality: A study of 850 sets of twins.* Austin: University of Texas Press, 1976; McManus IC *Psychological medicine.* Monograph Supplement No 8, 1985 (cites NCDS data); Newman HH, Freeman FN & Holzinger DH. *Twins: A study of heredity and environment.* Chicago: University of Chicago Press, 1937; Rife DC. *Genetics.* 1937;25:178–186; Rife DC. *Human Biology.* 1950;22:136–145; Springer SP & Searleman A. In Herron J (ed.). *Neuropsychology of left-handedness.* New York: Academic Press, 1980, pp. 139–158.; Stocks PA. *Annals of Eugenics.* 1933;5:1–55; Wilson PT & Jones HE. *Genetics.* 1932;17:560–572; Zazzo R. *Les jumeaux: Lè couple et la personne.* Paris: Presses Universitaires de France, 1960 (includes citations of Bouterwek 1938; Thyss 1946; Dechaume 1957).
12. Corballis MC. In J Herron (ed.). *Neuropsychology of left-handedness.* New York: Academic Press, 1980, pp. 159–176, quote from p. 166.

Chapter 6   The Two Brains

1. Broca P, cited in Harris LJ. In Herron J (ed.). *Neuropsychology of left-handedness.* New York: Academic Press, 1980, pp. 3–78.
2. Broca P, cited in Dimond S. *The Double Brain.* London: Churchill-Livingstone, 1972.
3. Jackson JH. In Taylor J (ed.). *selected writings of John Hughlings Jackson.* New York: Basic Books, 1958.
4. Wada JA & Rasmussen T. *J Neurosurgery.* 1960;17:266–282; Milner B. In Purpura DP, Penry JK & Walters RD (eds.). *Advances in neurology* (vol. 8). New York: Raven, 1975.
5. Pratt RTC & Warrington EK. *Brit J Psychiatry.* 1972;21:327–328; Warrington EK & Pratt RTC. *Neuropsychologia.* 1973;11:423–428.
6. Weisenberg T & McBride KE. *Aphasia: A clinical and psychological study.* New York: Commonwealth Fund, 1935.

7. Alajouanine T. *Brain.* 1948;71:229–241.

8. Heilman KM, Scholes R & Watson RT. *J Neurology, Neurosurgery & Psychiatry.* 1975;38:69–72.

9. Gazzaniga MS. *Scientific American.* 1967 (August).

10. Mavlov L. *Cortex.* 1980;16:331–338.

Chapter 7   Psycho-Neuro-Astrology

1. Doyle AC. *Scandal in Bohemia.* 1891.

2. Goleman D. *Psychology Today.* 1977;11:88–90.

3. Sagan C. *Broca's Brain.* New York: Balantine Books, 1979.

4. Regelski TA. *Music Educators Journal.* 1977;63:30–38 (cited in 9).

5. Hunter M. *Today's Education.* 1976;65:45–48 (cited in 9).

6. Meyers JT. *J Creative Behav.* 1982;16:197–211 (cited in 9).

7. Edwards B. *Drawing on the right side of the brain.* Los Angeles: Jeremy P Tarcher, 1989.

8. Beckman L. *Gifted Child Quarterly.* 1977;21:113–116 (cited in 9).

9. Many of the quotes and advertisements in this section have been taken from a marvelous, scholarly chapter by Lauren J. Harris, who is probably my favorite historian on issues of laterality. Those noted are from Harris L J. In Best CT (ed.). *Hemispheric function and collaboration in the child.* Orlando. Academic Press, 1985, pp. 231–275.

10. Rubenzer RL. *ERIC Clearinghouse on Handicapped and Gifted Children.* Report #ISBN-0-86586-141-2 (cited in 9).

11. Fincher J. *Sinister People.* New York: GP Putnam's Sons, 1977.

12. Allport GW & Postman LJ. *The psychology of rumor.* New York: Holt, Rinehart and Winston, 1947.

13. This discussion is based, in part, upon Coren S. Is left-sidedness pathological? Invited address delivered at Western Psychological Association meetings held in Seattle, Washington, 1986, May.

14. Although I no longer remember the exact details of the paper presentation (my own form of leveling has taken place), the study was published in a standard journal form as Kimura D. *Quart J Exp Psychol.* 1974;16:355–358.

15. Gazzaniga M. *The bisected brain.* New York: Appleton-Century-Crofts, 1970.

16. Ornstein RE. *The psychology of consciousness.* San Francisco: WH Freeman, 1972.

17. Gazzaniga MS & LeDoux JE. *The integrated mind.* New York: Plenum Press, 1978.

18. Corballis MC. *American Psychologist.* 1980;35:284–295.

19. Hardyck C & Haapanen R. *J School Psychology.* 1979;17:219–230 (cited in 9).

20. Arndt S & Berger DE. *Cortex.* 1978;14:78–86; Ornstein RE & Galin D. In Lec P, Ornstein RE, Galin DK, Deichman A & Tart C. (eds.). *Symposium on consciousness.* New York: Viking Press, 1976.

21. Coren S & Porac C. *Perceptual & Motor Skills.* 1982;54:787–792.

22. Mebert CJ & Michel GF. In Herron J (ed.). *Neuropsychology of left-handedness.* New York: Academic Press, 1980.

23. Peterson JM & Lansky LM. *Perceptual & Motor Skills.* 1974;38:547–550 and 1977;45:1216–1218.

24. Cranberg L & Albert M. In Obler L & Fein D (eds.). *The exceptional brain.* New York: Guilford, 1988; Mankin A & Benbow CP. Reported in O'Boyle MW & Benbow CP. In Coren S (ed.). *Left-handedness: Behavioral implications and anomalies.* Amsterdam: North-Holland, Elsevier, 1990.

25. Byrne B. *Brit J Psychol.* 1974;65:279–281; Deutsch D. In Herron J (ed.). *Neuropsychology of left-handedness.* New York: Academic Press, 1980.

26. Some of the data reported in this section is based upon unpublished results (hot off the press, so to speak) that are currently being prepared for submission to the regular scientific journals. These data have been collected over the past four years at the University of British Columbia.

Chapter 8   Is Left-Handedness Pathological?

1. Wile IS. *Handedness: Right and left.* Boston: Lathrop, Lee & Shepard, 1934.

2. Brewster ET. *McClure's Magazine.* 1913:168–183.

3. Burt C. *The backward child.* London: London Univ Press, 1937.

4. Jordan HE. *Good Health.* 1922;57:378–383.

5. See, for instance, Satz P, Orsini DL, Saslow E & Henry R. *Brain & cognition.* 1985;4:27–46 or Orsini DL & Satz P. *Arch Neurol.* 1986;43:333–337.

6. Gordon H. *Brain.* 1921;43:313–368.

7. Green MF, Satz P, Smith C, Nelson L. *J Abnormal Psychol.* 1989;98:57–61; Gur RE. *Arch Gen Psychiatry.* 1977;34:33–37; Katsanis J, Iacono WG. *Amer J Psychiatry.* 1989;146:1056–1058; Manoach DS, Maher BA, Manschreck TC. *J Abnormal Psychol.* 1988;97:97–99.

8. An excellent review may be found in Harris LJ & Carlson DF. In Molfese DL & Segalowitz SJ (eds.). *Brain lateralization in children.* New York: Guilford Press, 1988.

9. Paoluzzi C & Bravaccio F, 1967, reported in Subirana A. In Vinken PJ & Bruyn GW. *Handbook of clinical neurology* (vol. 4). Amsterdam: North-Holland, 1969.

10. Corballis M. *Human laterality.* New York: Academic Press, 1983; Corballis MC & Morgan MJ. *Behav & Brain Sciences.* 1978;2:261–336; Morgan MJ & Corballis MC. *Behav & Brain Sciences.* 1978;2:270–277.

11. Gerschwind N & Galaburda AM. *Cerebral lateralization: Biological mechanisms, associations and pathology.* Cambridge, Mass: MIT Press, 1987.

12. Blondel, James (1729), cited in Oakley KA, Macfarlane A, Chalmers I. In AR Rees and HJ Purcell (eds.). *Disease and the environment.* Chichester: Wiley and Sons, 1982.

13. An excellent summary of the history and current research in this area, as

it pertains to handedness, may be found in Bakan P. In Coren S (ed.). *Left-handedness: Behavioral implications and anomalies.* Amsterdam: North-Holland, Elsevier, 1990.

14. Bakan P, Dibb G, Reed P. *Neuropsychologia.* 1973;11:363–366.

15. Coren S, Searleman A, Porac C. *Canadian J Psychol.* 1982;36:478–487. Some earlier work from our lab on the same issue is Coren S & Porac C. *Behavior Genetics.* 1980;10:123–138.

16. O'Callaghan MJ, Tudehope DI, Dugdale AE, Mohay H, Burns Y & Cook F. *Lancet.* 1987;May 16:1155.

17. Ross G, Lipper EG & Auld PAM. *Developmental Medicine and Child Neurology.* 1987;29:615–622.

18. Strien JW van, Bouma A & Bakker DJ. *J Clinical & Experimental Neuropsychology.* 1987;9:775–780.

19. Schwartz M. *Neuropsychologia.* 1988;15:341–344.

20. Coren S. *New England J of Medicine.* 1990;322:1673.

21. Bakan, P. *Canadian Psychology.* 1987;28:2a, abstract 18.

22. Searleman A, Porac C, & Coren S. *Psychological Bulletin.* 1989;105:397–408.

Chapter 9   The Sign of the Left

1. A much fuller list can be compiled by consulting Coren S (ed.). *Left-handedness: Behavioral implications and anomalies.* Amsterdam: North-Holland, Elsevier, 1990; and Porac C & Coren S. *Lateral preferences and human behavior.* New York: Springer-Verlag, 1981.

2. A full discussion of this issue may be found in Bell RQ & Waldrop MF. In porter R & Collins GM (eds.). *Temperamental differences in infants and young children.* London: Pitman, 1982; Campbell M, Geller B, Small AM, Petti TA & Ferris SH. *Amer J Psychiatry.* 1978;135:573–575; Krouse JP & Kauffman JM. *J Abnormal Child Psychology.* 1982;10:247–264.

3. Coren S & Searleman A. In Coren S (ed.). *Left-handedness: Behavioral implications and anomalies* Amsterdam: North-Holland, Elsevier, 1990.

4. Satz P. *Neuropsychologia.* 1973;11:115–117; Satz P. *Cortex.* 1972;8:121–135.

5. Fuller technical discussions of handedness control may be found in Brodal A. *Neurological anatomy in relation to clinical medicine* (3rd ed.). New York: Oxford Univ Press, 1981; Harris LJ & Carlson DF. In Molfese DL & Segalowitz SJ (eds.). *Brain lateralization in children: Developmental implications.* New York: Guilford Press, 1988; Kupyers HGJM. In Swash M & Kennard C (eds.). *Scientific basis of clinical neurology.* Edinburgh: Churchill-Livingstone, 1985.

6. Pipe M-E, In Coren S (ed.). *Left-handedness: Behavioral implications and anomalies* Amsterdam: North-Holland, Elsevier, 1990. You might also look at Porac C, Coren S & Duncan P. *J Clin Neuropsychology.* 1980;35:173–187, to see a typical set of experimental results on this issue.

7. Flor-Henry P. In Coren S (ed.). *Left-handedness: Behavioral implications and anomalies* Amsterdam: North-Holland, Elsevier, 1990.

Chapter 10   Left-Hander Difference and Deficiencies

1. Some descriptions of this slow growth of lateral preferences and its implications and associations with other factors, such as retardation and cognitive difficulties, can be found in: Berman A. *Cortex.* 1971;7:372–386; Delecato CH. *Neurological organization and reading.* Springfield IL: CC Thomas, 1966; Lenneberg EH. In Carterette EC (ed.). *Brain function, Vol. 3: Speech, language, and communication.* UCLA Forum in Medical Sciences, No. 4. Los Angeles: Univ of Calif Press.
2. Coren S, Searleman A & Porac C. *Developmental Neuropsychology.* 1986;2:17–23.
3. Reichler JL (ed.). *The baseball encyclopedia.* New York: Macmillan, 1979.
4. Coren S. *Journal of the American Medical Association.* 1989;262:2682–2683.
5. Gaddes WH. *Learning disabilities and brain function: A neurophysiological approach.* New York: Springer-Verlag, 1980.
6. For example, the same argument is made in Porac C, Coren S & Duncan P. *J Clin Neuropsychol.* 1980;2:173–187.
7. Geschwind N & Behan P. *Proc National Acad Sci USA.* 1982; and in Geschwind N & Galaburda AM (eds.). *Cerebral dominance: The biological foundations.* Cambridge, Mass.: Harvard Univ Press, 1984; also see the review of this topic in Porac C & Coren S. *Lateral preferences and human behavior.* New York: Springer-Verlag, 1981.
8. Porac C & Coren S. *Lateral preferences and human behavior.* New York: Springer-Verlag, 1981.
9. Williams SM. *J Genet Psychol.* 1987;148:469–478.
10. Temple CM. *Neuropsychologia.* 1990;28:303–308.
11. Cranberg L & Albert M. In Obler L & Fein D (eds.). *The exceptional brain.* New York: Guilford.
12. Peterson JM & Lansky LM. *Percept Mot Skills.* 1974;38:547–550; and 1977;45:1216–1218; Mebert CJ & Michel GF, In Herron J (ed.). *Neuropsychology of left-handedness.* New York: Academic Press, 1980.
13. Benbow CP. *Neuropsychologia.* 1986;24:719–725; Benbow CP & Benbow RM. In DeVries G, Debruin J, Uylings H & Corner M (eds.). *Sex differences in the brain: The relation between structure and function. Progress in Brain Research,* 61 Amsterdam: Elsevier, 1984; O'Boyle MW & Benbow CP. In Coren S (Ed.). *Left-handedness: Behavioral implications and anomalies.* Amsterdam: North-Holland, 1990.
14. Lombroso C. *Nor Am Rev.* 1903;177:440–444 (quote p. 444).
15. The first such study was Smith LG. *Pedagogical Seminary.* 1917;24:19–35.
16. Grace WC. *J Clin Psychol.* 1987;43:151–155.

17. Burt C. *The backward child*. London: Univ London Press, 1937 (quote p. 317).
18. Gabrielli WF & Mednick SA. *J Abnorm Psych*. 1980;89:654–661.
19. Lanyon RI. *J Consulting & Clinical Psych*. 1970;35 (No. 1, part 2):1–24.
20. Blau A. *The master hand*. New York: Amer Orthopsychiatric Assoc (quotes pp. 112 & 113 and 96).
21. Hicks RA & Pellegrini RJ. *Cortex*. 1978;14:119–121.
22. Schuenenman AL, Pickleman J & Freeark RJ. *Surgery*. 1985;98:506–514.
23. Dillon KM. *Psych Reports*. 1989;65:496–498.
24. Orme JE. *Brit J Soc Clin Psychol*. 1970;9:87–88.
25. Schachter SC, Bernard BJ & Geschwind N. *Neuropsychologia*. 1987;25:269–276.
26. Chayatte C, Chayatte C & Altoff D. *S African Med J*. 1979;56:505–506.
27. Hannay EJ, Ciaccia PJ, Kerr JW & Barrett D. *Percept Mot Skills*. 1990;70:451–457.
28. Fry CJ. *Percept Mot Skills*. 1988;67:168–170.
29. James WH. *J Theor Biol*. 1989;122:243–245.

Chapter 11   Health and the Left-Hander

1. Mortimer J. *Observer*, 20 Aug 1978.
2. Bernal JF. *Dev Med Child Neurol*. 1973;15:760–769; Bhatia VP et al. *Arch Dis Child*. 1980;55:134–138; Moore T & Ucko LE. *Arch Dis Child*. 1957;32:333–342.
3. Coren S & Searleman A. *Sleep*. 1985;8:222–226.
4. Coren S & Searleman A. *Brain & Cognition*. 1987;6:184–192.
5. Lessell S. *Arch Ophthamol*. 1986;104:1492–1494.
6. Bonvillian JD, Orlansky MD & Garland JB. *Brain & Cognition*. 1982;1:141–157.
7. Geschwind N & Galaburda AM. *Cerebral lateralization: Biological mechanisms, associations, and pathology*. Cambridge, Mass: MIT Press, 1987; Habib M, Touze F & Galaburda AM. In Coren S (ed.). *Left-handedness: Behavioral implications and anomalies*. Amsterdam: North-Holland, Elsevier, 1990.
8. Geschwind N & Behan P. *Proc National Acad Sci USA*, 1982; and in Geschwind N & Galaburda AM (Eds.). *Cerebral dominance: The biological foundations*. Cambridge, Mass: Harvard Univ Press, 1984; Geschwind N & Galaburda AM. *Arch Neurol*. 1985;42:428–459, 521–552, 634–654.
9. Smith, J. *Neuropsychologia*. 1987;25:665–674.
10. Weinstein RE & Pieper DR. *Brain Behav & Immunity*. 1988;2:235–241.
11. Kilty T, Charney N & Leviton A. *Percept Mot Skills*. 1987;65:159–163.
12. See references in note 7, this chapter, and Searleman A & Fugagli AK, *Neuropsychologia*. 1987;25:367–374.
13. For a review see London WP. In Coren S (ed.). *Left-handedness: Behavioral implications and anomalies* Amsterdam: North-Holland, Elsevier, 1990.

14. Smith V & Chayatte C. *J Studies on Alcohol.* 1983;44:553–555.
15. London WP. *Alcohol: Clin Exper Res.* 1985;9:503–504.
16. Harburg E. *Percept Mot Skills.* 1981;52:279–282; Harburg E, Feldstein A & Papsdorf J. *Percept Mot Skills.* 1978;47:1171–1174.
17. Irwin P. *Neuropsychologia.* 1985;23:61–67.
18. McCulloch MJ & Waddington JL. *Brit J Psychiat.* 1981;139:341–345.
19. Meyer-Bahlburg HFL. *Arch Sexual Behav.* 1977;6:297–325.
20. Lindesay J. *Neuropsychologia.* 1987;25:965–969.
21. McCormick CM, Witelson SF, Kinstone E. *Soc Neurosci Abstr.* 1987;13:851.
22. McCormick CM, Witelson SF & Kingstone E. *Psychoneuroendocrinology.* 1990;1:69–76.
23. Salk L, Lipsitt L, Sturner WQ, Reilly BM & Levat RH. *Lancet.* 1985; 1:624–627; Jacobson B, Eklund G, Hamberger L, Linnarsson KD, Sedvall G & Valverius M. *Acta Psychiat Scand.* 1987;76:364–371.
24. For example, Bruder GE, Quitkin FM, Stewart JW, Marein C, Voglmaier MM & Harrison WM. *J Abnorm Psych.* 1989;98:177–186; Hicks RA & Pellegrini RJ. *Cortex.* 1978;14:119–121.
25. Sackeim HA & Decina P. In Flor-Henry P & Gruzelier (eds.). *Laterality and Psychopathology.* Amsterdam: North-Holland, Elsevier, 1983.
26. Lishman WA & McMeekan ERL. *Brit J Psychiat.* 1976;129:158–166; Flor-Henry P & Yeudall LT. In Gruzelier J & Flor-Henry P (eds.). *Hemisphere asymmetries of function in psychopathology.* Amsterdam: North-Holland, Elsevier, 1979.
27. Bruce LC. *Brain.* 1895;18:54–65.
28. Chayatte C & Smith V. *Military Medicine.* 1981;146:277–278.

Chapter 12   Do Left-Handers Die Younger?

1. For instance, the same decrease in left-handers for older groups was found by Ellis SJ, Ellis PJ & Marshall E. *Cortex.* 1988;24:157–163; Fleminger JJ, Dalton R & Standage KF. *Neuropsychologia.* 1977;15:471–473; Lansky LM, Feinstein H & Peterson J. *Neuropsychologia.* 1988;26:465–477; Tambs K, Magnus P & Berg K. *Percept Mot Skills.* 1987;64:155–170; Tan LE. *Percept Mot Skills.* 1983;56:867–874.
2. From an article published by Hertz R. *Revue philosphique* trans. R Needham. 1909;68:553–590. In R. Needham (ed.). *Right and left.* Chicago: Univ Chicago Press, 1973.
3. Holden, C. *Science.* 1987;238:158–160.
4. Reichler JL. (ed.). *The baseball encyclopedia.* New York: Macmillan, 1979.
5. Small differences in death rate do have large effects on any group of people. This was demonstrated more formally in Coren. S. *Amer J Public Health.* 1990;80:353.
6. Halpern D F & Coren S. *Nature.* 1988;333:213.
7. Wood, E.K. *Nature.* 1988;335:212.

8. Heitz LH. *Lefthander Magazine.* 1990 (Mar/Ap);15:6–7.
9. Anderson, M.G. *Nature.* 1989;341:112.
10. Coren S & Halpern DF. *Psychological Bulletin.* 1991;109:90–106. Halpern DF & Coren S. *New England J Medicine.* 1991;324:998.

Chapter 13 A World for Right-Handers

1. Barsley M. *The left-handed book.* London: Souvenir Press, 1966 (p. 204).

Chapter 14 The Hazardous Life of the Southpaw

1. Burt C. *The backward child.* London: London Univ Press, 1937, p. 287.
2. Bradshaw JL & Bradshaw JA *Int J Neuroscience.* 1988;39:229–232.
3. See, for instance, Bell J. *San Francisco Examiner and Chronicle,* 20 October 1974.
4. Coren S. *Am J Public Health.* 1989;79:1040–1041.
5. European Conference of Ministers of Transport. *Annual Reports including the Statistical Report on Road Accidents.* Paris: OECD Publications Service (the latest available to us was the 1987, 37th Annual Report, published 1988).
6. Various aspects and phases of the California study are described in chapter 14 of this book and in Halpern DF & Coren S. In Coren S (ed.). *Left-handedness: Behavioral implications and anomalies.* Amsterdam: North-Holland, Elsevier, 1990; Coren S & Halpern DF. *Psychological Bulletin.* 1991;109:90–106; Halpern DF & Coren S. *New Eng J Med.* 1991;324:998.
7. Coren S. *Amer J Public Health.* 1990;80:353.

Chapter 15 Help for the Left-Hander

1. Harris L. *Lefthander Magazine.* 1990(Nov-Dec);15:16–17.
2. A full discussion of the implications of trying to shift handedness can be found in chapter 6.
3. Porac C & Coren S. *Percept Motor Skills.* 1979;49:227–231.
4. Salvendy G (ed.). *Handbook of human factors.* New York: Wiley, 1987.
5. Pheasant S. *Bodyspace: Anthropometry, ergonomics and design.* London: Taylor & Francis, 1986.
6. See, for instance Bradley JV. *Human Factors.* 1969;11:227–238 for touching errors and McCormick EJ. *Human factors in engineering and design* (4th ed.). New York: McGraw Hill, 1976, as an example of design recommendations.
7. Huchingson RD. *New horizons for human factors in design.* New York: McGraw Hill, 1981 (quote p. 151).
8. Geschwind N & Galaburda AM. *Cerebral lateralization: Biological mechanisms, associations, and pathology.* Cambridge, Mass: MIT Press, 1987, discuss

the relationship between handedness and susceptibility to infections as well as the overall reduced immune system response.

Chapter 16 An Action Plan for Left-Handers

1. Kantowitz BH & Sorkin RD. *Human factors: understanding people-system relationships.* New York: Wiley, 1983 (quote p. 332).
2. Burke E. Speech, British House of Commons, 11 May 1792.
3. Wile IS. *Handedness: Right and left.* Boston: Lothrop, Lee & Shepard, 1934 (pp. 356–357).
4. Kennedy JF. Speech, American University (Washington DC), 10 June 1963.

Name Index

Subject Index